Color Atlas of the

Brain and Spinal Cord

Commissioning Editor: Inta Ozols
Project Development Manager: Siân Jarman
Project Manager: Jess Thompson
Design Direction: George Ajayi
Illustration Manager: Bruce Hogarth
Illustrator: PCA Creative
Marketing Manager(s) (UK/USA): John Gore and Valerie Maciejczyk

Color Atlas of the
Brain and
Spinal Cord SECOND EDITION

An Introduction to Normal Neuroanatomy

Marjorie A. England

Formerly Senior Lecturer in Anatomy, Medical Sciences, University of Leicester and
Lately, Honorary Senior Research Fellow, Royal College of Surgeons of England and
Lately, The Helen Waddell Visiting Professor, School of Biomedical Science, The Queen's University of Belfast, U.K. and
Visiting Professor to the School of Medicine, University of Split, Croatia

Jennifer Wakely

Formerly Lecturer in Anatomy, Medical Sciences University of Leicester,
Lecturer, School of Archaeology and Ancient History, University of Leicester and Visiting Lecturer,
School of Health and Life Sciences, De Montfort University, Leicester

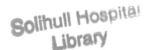
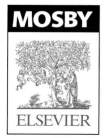
MOSBY
ELSEVIER

MOSBY
ELSEVIER

An imprint of Elsevier Limited.

© 2006, Elsevier Limited. All rights reserved.

First edition 1991, Wolfe Publishing Ltd
Second edition 2006

EAN 9780323036672
ISBN 0323036678

British Library Cataloguing in Publication Data
A catalogue record for this book is available from the British Library

Library of Congress Cataloging in Publication Data
A catalog record for this book is available from the Library of Congress

Notice
Medical knowledge is constantly changing. Standard safety precautions must be followed, but as
new research and clinical experience broaden our knowledge, changes in treatment and drug
therapy may become necessary or appropriate. Readers are advised to check the most current
product information provided by the manufacturer of each drug to be administered to verify the
recommended dose, the method and duration of administration, and contraindications. It is the
responsibility of the practitioner, relying on experience and knowledge of the patient, to
determine dosages and the best treatment for each individual patient. Neither the Publisher nor
the authors assume any liability for any injury and/or damage to persons or property arising from
this publication.

The Publisher

Printed in China

Last digit is the print number: 9 8 7 6 5 4 3 2 1

Contents

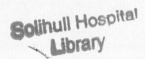

CONTENTS

To the memories of
Dr. John M. England
Haematologist
and
Mr. Richard H. Wakely
Photographer

Acknowledgments to the First Edition

Many of the illustrations in this book show our own preparations. In addition, the authors are deeply grateful to many people who generously contributed to this book with their advice and time, and who often provided access to their personal collections of materials or those prepared for their institutions. Their enthusiasm for this subject was both a delight and an encouragement to us.

In particular we are grateful to Professor T. W. A. Glenister, CBE, Charing Cross and Westminster Hospital Medical School, London (CXWMS) and to the Anatomy Department for allowing us to photograph some of the specimens in their collection.

Professor B. A. Wood. Middlesex Hospital Medical School, London (MHMS), also allowed us to photograph materials from the departmental collection.

Professor R. E. Coupland, University of Nottingham Medical School (UN), generously allowed us to photograph specimens from his departmental collection.

We are also indebted to Professor N. Gluhbegovic, University of Utrecht, The Netherlands, who advised us on many occasions on the preparation of frozen dissected brains. He also allowed us to use one of his preparations.

Professor V. Chan-Palay, Neurology Institute, University Hospital of Zurich, generously supplied two photomicrographs of neuropeptide Y neurons from her research studies. Professor Dr. Eva Braak, Klinikum der Johann Wolfgang Goethe-Universitat, Frankfurt, West Germany, kindly supplied micrographs of somatostatin–immunoreactive neurons.

Dr. N. A. Lassen, Department of Clinical Physiology, Bispebjerg Hospital, Copenhagen, Denmark, provided Xenon-133 intracarotid technique photographs of the auditory cortex.

Dr. E. Motti, Instituto Di Neurochirurgia, Milano, Italy, provided scanning electron micrographs of the blood vessels of the choroid plexus.

Professor H. M. Duvernoy, Université de Franche-Comte, Besançon, Cedex, France, generously allowed us to use a preparation from his book, *Hianan Brainstem Vessels*.

Professor F. Walker and Professor I. Lauder, Department of Pathology, University of Leicester, provided some materials for this book.

Professor John Marshall, Institute of Ophthalmology, London, provided two histological sections of the retina.

Dr. G. H. Wright, University of Cambridge, advised one of us about the materials available in the Anatomy Department collection.

Miss E. Allen, Qvist Curator, The Hunterian Museum, The Royal College of Surgeons of England (RCS), kindly allowed us to photograph specimens in the museum. She was ably assisted by Miss A. Serrant.

Dr. V. Navaratnam and Dr. E. Ford, Department of Anatomy, University of Cambridge (CAM), very kindly provided materials from the departmental collection. Mr. B. Logan generously advised and assisted us with some preparations for which we are very grateful.

Dr. M. R. Matthews, Department of Human Anatomy, University of Oxford (OXF), generously allowed us to photograph materials in the department.

Dr. G. Batcup, Consultant Pathologist, University of Leeds, provided and prepared fetal materials and we are very grateful for her generosity and to Dr. M. O. Mohamdee, her Senior Registrar, for her help.

Dr. E. C. Blenkinsopp, Consultant Pathologist, and Dr. W. K. Blenkinsopp, Consultant Pathologist, Watford General Hospital, both very generously provided specimens.

Dr. J. Lowe, Department of Pathology, University of Nottingham, prepared electron micrographs of a synapse, nerve fibers and immunocytochemical preparations for us.

Dr. M. Ingle Wright, University of Manchester, kindly provided her own special preparations of the ear.

Dr. J. Southgate, Leicester Royal Infirmary, generously provided three histological sections of the eye.

Dr. B. Bracegirdle, Wellcome Museum of the History of Medicine, kindly allowed one of us to examine and photograph histological sections of the nervous system prepared in the 19th century. These included preparations by Martin Cole from the 1890s; Dr. Needham's collection amassed in the 1870s; specimens prepared in the 1860s for Smith, Beck and Beck Co., and Martin Cole in 1884.

Dr. D. C. Bouch, Consultant Histopathologist, Leicester Royal Infirmary, generously provided facilities for sectioning half-brains. We are very grateful for this privilege and to his staff for their advice.

Dr. N. Messios, Consultant Radiologist, Leicester Royal Infirmary, assisted greatly with photographs from the CT scanner.

Dr. A. Fletcher, Consultant Pathologist, Leicester Royal Infirmary, kindly provided immunocytochemical preparations of nervous tissue.

Dr. D. James, Consultant Radiologist, Leicester Royal Infirmary, kindly assisted us on several films.

Professor A. R. Fielder, Birmingham University, and Mr. H. Harris, Leicester Royal Infirmary, generously donated images of the retina.

Nuclear magnetic resonance figures were provided by Dr. G. Bydder, Senior Lecturer, Royal Postgraduate Medical School, London.

The color-enhanced magnetic resonance image (MRI) was provided through the courtesy of Dr. M. W. Vannier, Associate Professor of Radiology, Mallinckrodt Institute of Radiology at Washington University Medical Center, St. Louis, Missouri, USA.

Elscint Ltd., Watford, provided CT scans and NMR images.

Dr. I. Talbot, Reader in Pathology, Dr. M. Levene, Reader in Child Health, Dr. A. Fletcher, Consultant Histopathologist, and Mrs. L. Palmer and Mr. R. Stewart, Mr. R. Cullen and Mrs. G. Hayward, Leicester Royal Infirmary, also advised us on materials. Dr. Fletcher additionally gave us immunocytochemical and silver-stained preparations.

Mr. G. A. Bell, Principal, Schools of Radiography, Leicester Royal Infirmary, assisted us with a special brain preparation, as did Dr. M. A. Goodwin, University of Leicester.

We are also grateful to Mr. P. A. Runnicles, Chief Technician, and to Mr. C. Syms, The Middlesex Hospital School of Medicine, who assisted greatly. Mr. R. Watts, Chief Technician, and Mr. P. A. Ryan, Charing Cross Hospital Medical School; Mr. E. T. Williams, University of Cambridge; and Mr. R. White, University of Oxford; Mr. B. Logan, Prosector, Department of Anatomy, The University of Cambridge, and Miss M. Hudson, Charing Cross and Westminster Hospital School of Medicine all advised and generously assisted us.

Assistance and advice were also received from Mr. J. E. Cartledge, Leicester General Hospital; Mr. F. Young, Chief Technician, Nottingham University Medical School; and from Mr. G. Bottomley, Chief Technician; Mr. G. L. C. McTurk, Chief Technician; Mr. C. R. d'Lacey, Mrs. A. Lea, Mrs. C. Libetta, Mrs. B. Hayward, Miss S. Uppal, Mr. I. Indans, Mr. S. Byrne, Mr. L. Paterson, Mr. C. Brooks, and Mr. H. Kowalski, University of Leicester.

Mr. D. Adams, University of Leicester, generously advised us on the preparation of materials and prepared some of the histological specimens.

Professor A. R. Lieberman. Dean, University College, London, generously assumed the task of reading the final manuscript and we are deeply indebted to him for all his work and for his suggestions on Golgi staining.

We are also grateful to Mr. G. Tresidder, Consultant Surgeon and Anatomist, to Dr. L. Howard, University of Leicester and Dr. A. Lawson, University of Ghana, who very generously read the manuscript and commented upon the book. Miss S. Pattani, a medical student, assisted us in some photographs. We are deeply grateful for all their constructive suggestions and interest.

The authors are very grateful to Dr. J. M. England, Consultant Haematologist, Watford General Hospital, and to Mr. R. H. Wakely, Photographer, who kindly assisted us and encouraged us throughout the preparation, writing and production of this book.

We are also grateful to J. B. Lippincott Company for permission to reproduce one figure from *The Human Brain: a photographic guide* by Gluhbegovic and Williams, 1980.

Springer-Verlag Publishers gave permission to use one figure from *Human Brainstem Vessels* by Professor H. M. Duvernoy. Dr. M. B. Carpenter gave permission to reproduce an illustration from his book, *Core Text of Neuroanatomy*. The original photograph was produced by Dr. Harry A. Kaplan. The publishers Williams and Wilkins also gave permission for us to use this picture.

An especial acknowledgment is made to Mr. K. Garfield, Chief Technician, Central Photographic Unit, University of Leicester, who produced many of the photographs in this book. His expertise and interest have contributed greatly.

The authors are deeply grateful for all the work contributed by Mr. Anton Lawrencepulle and Lara Last, Wolfe Publishing, towards the production of this book.

Acknowledgments to the Second Edition

In addition to those individuals who kindly allowed us access to their collections of material for the First Edition, the following people and their institutions have generously helped us to prepare this second edition.

We are particularly grateful to the following people who provided us with various neurological imaging techniques: Dr. R. J. Abbott, Consultant Neurologist, Leicester Royal Infirmary (LRI), Mr. J. Wasserberg, Consultant Neurosurgeon, Queen Elizabeth Hospital (QEH), Birmingham, and Professor F. W. Zonneveld, Department of Radiology, Utrecht University Hospital (UUH), Utrecht, The Netherlands. It is a great pleasure to thank them for allowing us the use of their materials.

We are also very pleased to thank for their anatomical and histological preparations : Professor H. Duvernoy, Laboratoire d'Anatomie, Université de Franche-Comte (UFC), Besançon, France, Dr. A. Fletcher, Consultant, Department of Pathology, Leicester Royal Infirmary, Professor J. S. Lowe, Consultant, Department of Pathology, Queen's Medical Centre, Nottingham (QMC), Dr. M. Rossi, Consultant, Department of Pathology, Walton Centre for Neurology and Neurosurgery (WCNN), Liverpool, Professor R. Rübsamen, Institut für Zoologie (IZ), Leipzig, Germany, Professor N. Scolding, Institute of Clinical Neurosciences, Frenchay Hospital, Bristol(FH), Professor Dr. K. Zilles, Institut für Neuroanatomie, Universtität Düsseldorf (UD), Germany. Their generosity is much appreciated and greatly enhances our book.

Dr. J. S. Morris, Leopold Muller Functional Imaging Laboratory, Institute of Neurology, London (INL), Dr. M. A. Rutherford, Robert Steiner Magnetic Resonance Unit, Imperial College School of Medicine (ICSM), Hammersmith, London, and Dr. S. C. R. Williams, Neuroimaging Research, Institute of Psychiatry (IP), London, all gave generously from their collections of neurological images.

We are also very grateful to Dr. G. Clowry and to Dr. S. Lindsay, Department of Child Health, University of Newcastle (UN), Newcastle-upon-Tyne, and Dr. H. Hilbig, Institut für Anatomie, Universität Leipzig (UL), Germany, for giving us histological and histochemical images of developing and adult nervous tissue. Their contributions are invaluable. Excellent histological preparations were also generously given by I. Bazwinsky Dip. Biol., Institut für Zoologie, University of Leipzig, Germany, Mr. J. Wills, Technician, Department of Pathology, Leicester Royal Infirmary, and from Dr. K. Vilović, Professor M. Saraga-Babić, and Dr. D. Sapunar, Department of Anatomy, Histology and Embryology, School of Medicine, University of Split, Croatia (US).

Valuable advice and constructive comments were also made by Dr. H. Crick, Department of Pre-Clinical Sciences, University of Leicester (LU), Dr. R. Donga, Department of Pre-Clinical Sciences, University of Leicester, and Mr. J. N. James, Emeritus Consultant in Oral Surgery, Leicester Royal Infirmary.

We are grateful to the Wellcome Library, London, for permission to reproduce images from their collection.

The final manuscript was read by Mr. I. V. Fussey, Lecturer, Department of Pre-Clinical Sciences, University of Leicester and former Consultant Surgeon, Lincoln County Hospital and also by Professor Emeritus P. N. Dilly, St. George's Hospital Medical School, London. Their comments and constructive suggestions have been invaluable and we are deeply grateful for their advice and expertise. Any errors and misconceptions are purely our own misinterpretations and mistakes. They should in no way reflect upon any of our contributors.

The authors are deeply grateful for all the work of Siân Jarman and Richard Furn toward the production of this book and to Jess Thompson and Inta Ozols, Elsevier.

An especial acknowledgement is made to Mr. George L. C. McTurk, Chief Technician, Leicester University Scanning Electron Microscope Unit, for his invaluable advice and expert assistance with materials and photographic techniques. His suggestions, expertise and interest have contributed greatly to this edition. We are very indebted for his many contributions.

Preface to the First Edition

This Atlas is intended to illustrate those aspects of the normal human brain and spinal cord which are of importance in the study of neuroanatomy. Neuroanatomy is a very difficult subject for the student of medicine or nursing and is often so even for the postgraduate, not only because of the three-dimensional nature of the material but because of its complexity and associated vocabulary. However, once knowledge of the vocabulary is acquired, then the functional aspects may be better appreciated: we have designed this book to reflect this approach to learning.

The book is divided into two parts. In the first part the morphology of the brain and spinal cord is presented and the second part illustrates their functional relationships. All of the illustrations in this book are from human material and it is our intention to limit the text wherever possible to the central nervous system. The student should be aware, however, that this separation is an artificial one and that the central nervous system is integrated with the peripheral system. It is suggested that the reader consult the textbooks listed in "Suggestions for Further Reading" and use them in conjunction with this Atlas.

The descriptions accompanying the photographs are intended to link them and to indicate the relevant features or orientation. It is not the intention to label every structure present on a specimen. Photographs illustrating more than one feature may be used on more than one occasion. In general, the terminology used is based on the 6th edition of the *Nomina Anatomica*. Several older names have been retained, however, because of their current usage in texts and in the medical profession.

Points of historical, physiological or clinical interest have been presented as footnotes marked by a spot. Important terminology appears on gray-coloured pages.

A guide for a student examination of the brain has been included. The pages should be followed sequentially to illustrate the main morphological features of the brain.

This Atlas has been written both as an introduction to neuroanatomy for medical, nursing and paramedical students and as a review for those familiar with this subject. It is our sincere hope that having completed his or her study the reader will have not only an understanding of a very complex and difficult subject, but also an appreciation of the three-dimensional beauty and mystery of the human brain and spinal cord.

Preface to the Second Edition

Since the first edition of this Atlas was published, new techniques have advanced our knowledge and understanding of the brain beyond what we envisaged at that time. Selection from this vast body of new knowledge was very difficult. Therefore, we have included only those aspects of neuroanatomy relevant to a general textbook. Further detail may be obtained from more specialist texts or research papers.

New imaging methods display structural detail in the living brain. The complex forms and chemical composition of nerve cells, using specific staining methods at the cellular level, can now be revealed with ever increasing precision. In addition to the Guide for Student Examination of the Brain in the first edition, we have added a Student Guide to Imaging. It is our sincere hope that this new edition reflects many of these advances, as well as retaining all that has been gained by the tried and tested methods of traditional anatomical science.

Section 1
STRUCTURAL FEATURES OF THE CENTRAL NERVOUS SYSTEM

1 An Introduction to the Human Nervous System

Central and Peripheral Systems

The brain is an active controller of the body. It receives and processes information from the various sense organs about its external and internal environments. The brain then selects from several possible courses of action, and generates and controls the body's responses. The information received from the sense organs may also be stored as a "memory" to integrate past history and present experience.

The main centers of nervous correlation and integration are the brain and spinal cord. Together they are called the central nervous system (or CNS). Information is transmitted to and from the brain and spinal cord by the peripheral nervous system composed of the cranial and spinal nerves and their associated ganglia. Nerves that carry impulses toward the central nervous system are called afferent (or sensory) and those that carry nerve impulses away from the central nervous system are called efferent (or motor). Afferent or efferent nerves supplying the body wall or extremities are also referred to as *somatic*; those supplying the smooth muscles of internal organs, the blood vessels, and cardiac muscle are called *visceral*; and those supplying glands are called *secretor*.

The brain and spinal cord lie protected in the bony skull and vertebral column. They are bathed and suspended in cerebrospinal fluid which is also found in a series of interconnected cavities inside the brain called the ventricles. The peripheral nervous system, however, usually lies outside the bones and so is not protected by them.

The brain and spinal cord are composed of nerve cells (neurons) supported by specialized cells called neuroglia. Each neuron has a cell body (perikaryon) and several processes.

Neurons have traditionally been classified by their shape, size, and by the number, length, and branching of their processes. These processes are classified as axons or dendrites.

An axon is a long process, usually single, that is clearly demarcated from the cell's body at its point of origin from the cell. It generally, but not exclusively, conducts impulses (action potentials) away from the cell body. Axons greater than 1 μm in diameter in the peripheral nervous system and 0.25 μm diameter in the CNS are myelinated. Axons tend to be of a uniform diameter along their length. A distinctive ultrastructural feature of the axon hillock (site of origin from the cell body) and initial segment of the axon is that the microtubules are grouped into bundles and linked by side-arms. In the initial segment, but not in the axon hillock, and also at nodes of Ranvier, an undercoating of dense material underlies the membrane (axolemma) of the axon. Dendrites merge with the contours of the cell body where they arise from it. They are usually multiple, shorter than axons, and branch extensively. They form the receptor sites of the cells and so tend to conduct information towards the cell body.

A nerve fiber consists of an axon and its supporting cells. A surrounding basal lamina is present in the peripheral nervous system. Neurons are functionally connected by synapses, specialized sites where information is transmitted across a small gap between one neuron and another by chemical messengers, the neurotransmitters.

Neurotransmitters interact with receptors on the cell body or processes and this interaction leads to a change in a cell function. Neurotransmitters are classified into three groups: excitatory, inhibitory, and those that play a modulatory role in neuronal function. The commonest excitatory neurotransmitter in the central nervous system is glutamic acid (glutamate), an amino acid.

The most widespread inhibitory neurotransmitters are gamma-aminobutyric acid (GABA) in the brain and glycine in the spinal cord. Neurotransmitters that play a modulatory role do not directly excite or inhibit neurons but may, for example, alter their response or sensitivity to an excitatory or inhibitory neurotransmitter. Other common neurotransmitters in the CNS are acetylcholine, dopamine, norepinephrine (noradrenaline) and the neuropeptides. A further complicating factor is that a given transmitter substance may have either excitatory or inhibitory effects depending on the nature and response of receptors on the postsynaptic membrane of the cell concerned.

Listed below are the stains and injection media used to prepare specimens illustrated in this Atlas, and the purpose for which they were used.

Stains and injection media used on specimens in this Atlas

1 **Stains for thick brain slices**
   With Mulligan's stain the gray matter is blue and the white matter remains unstained.
2 **Myelin stains, distinguishing gray matter from white matter by selectively staining myelin sheaths of nerve fibers**
   Weigert stain
   Weigert-Pal stain
   Weil's stain
   Luxol fast blue stain
   Solochrome cyanin stain
3 **Stains to show the shape and structure of individual nerve cells or fibers**
   Cresyl violet stain
   Toluidine blue stain
   Thionin stain
   Golgi Cox stain
   Most silver stains including Bodian and Palmgren's stain
   Stains for glial cells, including Holtzer's stain
4 **Stains to show the general structure and organization of tissues**
   Hematoxylin and eosin stain
   Phosphotungstic acid and hematoxylin stain
   Van Gieson's stain
   Light green and orange G stain
   De Castro stain (embryos)
   Masson's trichrome stain
   Carmine stain
5 **Counterstains, used to provide a background contrasting color to the major stain**
   Nuclear fast red stain
   Hematoxylin stain
   Light green stain

Fuchsin stains
Neutral red stain
For example, a section stained with Luxol fast blue might be counterstained with acid fuchsin.
6 **Specific immunocytochemical stains for particular components of tissues**
   A) Stains for cytoskeletal components
      Neurofilament antigen stain
      Glial fibrillary acidic protein (GFAP) stain
      Alpha-B crystallin stain
      SMI (Sternberger Monoclonals Inc) stain for non-phosphorylated neurofilaments
   B) Stains for neurotransmitters and their receptors
      Stains for neuropeptides, e.g. neuropeptide Y and somatostatin
      Autoradiography for receptor localization
   C) Stains for proteins found at synapses, e.g. synaptophysin
   D) Stains for cell surface molecules
      CD68 immunostain
      Ricinus communis agglutinin stain
      Leukocyte common antigen stain
7 **Other stains identifying particular tissue components**
   Elastin stain for elastic tissue
   Osmium tetroxide for lipids
   Block staining with silver nitrate for connective tissue
8 **Injection media used to demonstrate the distribution of blood vessels at tissue level**
   Gelatine and carmine
   Gelatine and India ink
9 **Stains for transmission electron microscopy to make the tissue electron dense**
   Lead citrate stain

● *In some cases the precise identity of the stain in a loaned section was not known because of the age of the specimen. These sections have been indicated as "myelin stain"or "silver stain". The general nature of the stain is apparent from an examination of the structures displayed in the section.*

● *The depth and color of Weigert and Weigert-Pal staining may vary according to the staining and the section-mounting conditions, or may fade with time. It is normally a shade of brown, but may fade to a golden or purplish tone.*

● *Chromatolysis is the disappearance of Nissl substance staining if the cell's axon is cut.*

A textbook of physiology or pharmacology should be consulted for further detailed information.

The brain and spinal cord are organized into two tissues: gray matter and white matter. The gray matter is composed of neuropil, an intermingling of axons and dendrites where they establish synaptic contact. Gray matter also contains neuronal cell bodies and neuroglia. The white matter is composed of nerve fibers and the surrounding neuroglia. Bundles of nerve fibers in the central nervous system with a common origin and destination are called nerve tracts. In the peripheral nervous system, bundles of nerve fibers form peripheral nerves and nerve roots. A pathway is a chain of functionally interconnected neurons.

Additionally, the nerve fibers present in the central and peripheral nervous system may be described as myelinated or unmyelinated fibers. Myelinated nerve fibers are those axons surrounded by an insulating myelin sheath. This myelin sheath is produced by supporting neurological cells called oligodendrocytes in the CNS and by Schwann cells in the peripheral nervous system; the latter facilitate the regeneration of injured fibers.

Autonomic System

This system, a component of both the central and peripheral systems, is responsible, with the endocrine system, for the stability and maintenance of the internal environment. For the most part, the autonomic system functions at the subconscious level, i.e. structures supplied by the autonomic system have an involuntary innervation. The autonomic system contains both afferent (sensory) and efferent (motor or secretor) fibers, myelinated and unmyelinated fibers, and ganglia. Its activities are, however, integrated with those of the endocrine glands. Nerves pass to involuntary (i.e. smooth or cardiac) muscles in organs of the gastrointestinal tract, bladder, heart, etc., and to exocrine glands, e.g. salivary glands, sweat glands, etc.

The autonomic system is further divided into two parts: the sympathetic and parasympathetic parts. The sympathetic part prepares the body for emergencies, i.e. fear, rage, strenuous exercise. The heart rate increases and a relative redistribution of the circulation occurs. Blood vessels are constricted in the skin and intestines, and blood leaves these areas. The blood pressure rises and the increased supply of blood is made available to the brain, heart and skeletal muscles. Intestinal peristalsis is inhibited and the rectal and bladder sphincters closed. The pupils of the eyes dilate and the body is ready for a "fight or flight" response.

The parasympathetic part of the autonomic nervous system is responsible for conserving energy and the routine maintenance of bodily activities. It promotes digestion by stimulating peristalsis and the secretions of the glands of the gastrointestinal tract. Stimulation of the parasympathetic system also constricts the pupil, decreases the heart rate and relaxes the rectal and bladder sphincters.

It is characteristic of the autonomic nervous system that the pathway from the central nervous system to the organ supplied is always interrupted by a ganglion. It, therefore, has two components: preganglionic, between the CNS and the ganglion, and postganglionic, between the ganglion and the organ.

While many viscera have both sympathetic and parasympathetic supplies, by which a functional "balance" is effected, some have only one supply. Equally important is the fact that some viscera are constantly inhibited by one or other of the two components of the autonomic nervous system, e.g. the heart.

The classical concept of autonomic nervous system function includes only two neurotransmitters: acetylcholine and norepinephrine (noradrenaline). Acetylcholine occurs throughout the parasympathetic system and in the synapses between preganglionic sympathetic fibers and postganglionic cells in sympathetic ganglia. Norepinephrine occurs in postganglionic sympathetic innervation.

Recent studies on this system have identified other autonomic neurotransmitters. For example, some cells in the ganglia supplying postganglionic sympathetic fibers to the gut contain peptide transmitters (somatostatin, substance P, enkephalin). Similar non-adrenergic, non-cholinergic nerves are present in the wall of the bladder. Their cell bodies lie in the pelvic ganglia.

Nervous Tissue

All nervous tissue consists of nerve cells (neurons), supporting cells (glial cells or neuroglia) and blood vessels.

A neuron consists of the cell body or perikaryon, which contains the nucleus and other organelles, and one or more cell processes. The cell bodies are concentrated in areas of gray matter. A neuronal process together with its sheathing cells constitutes a nerve fiber. Fibers in the peripheral nervous system have an additional covering of basal lamina. Nerve fibers are concentrated in areas of white matter. Cytoplasmic components and neurotransmitters are synthesized in the cell body and can be transported along the processes by cytoplasmic flow. This mechanism is best understood in axons (axoplasmic flow).

LIST OF COMPONENTS OF NERVOUS TISSUE

Neuronal fibers (axons and dendrites) Myelinated and unmyelinated	**Neuroglia (supporting cells)** Astrocytes, oligodendrocytes
Neurons Unipolar, bipolar, multipolar	**Immune cells** Microglia, perivascular macrophages
	Blood vessels

A

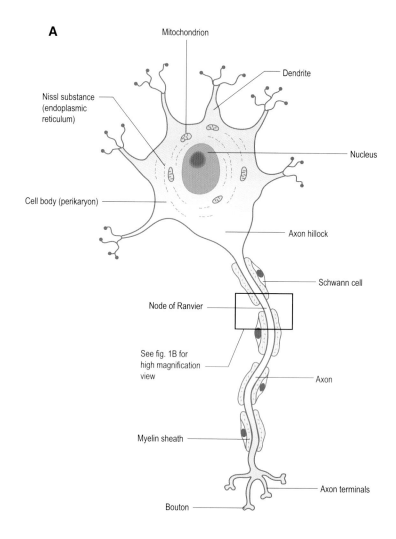

Diagram **A** to illustrate the structure of a neuron.

B

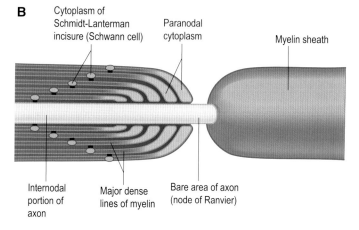

Diagram **B** to show the interruption of the myelin sheath at a node of Ranvier.

Reproduced by permission of Prof. J. S. Lowe QMC

Neurons throughout the central nervous system vary in size and shape. In humans, the largest are the giant Purkinje cells of the cerebellum, with cell body diameters of 50–70 μm. (1 μm [micrometer] = one thousandth of a millimeter.) The granule cells of the cerebellum are on average less than one tenth of that size. Neurons are classified according to their shape. This is determined by the number of processes arising from the cell body. Most are multipolar, with many processes, enabling them to contact other neurons over a wide field. Bipolar cells have two processes, one at each end of the cell. They are found in developing neural tissue and in the retina, and as interneurons providing local connections within the central nervous system (CNS). Unipolar cells, with only one process, are found in the dorsal root ganglia of the spinal cord.

Figures 1.1–1.3 Low power histological preparations to show the distribution of areas of neurons in nervous tissue.

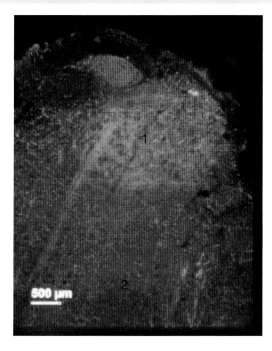

Fig. 1.1
Low power photomicrograph of the brainstem, fluorescently stained to localize neuronal cell bodies and dendrites. Aggregations of neurons are known as nuclei. They stain intensely against a faintly stained background of white matter. This section shows the abducens nucleus. Scale on picture.

1 Abducens nucleus
2 White matter

Prof. R. Rübsamen and I. Bazwinsky Dipl.-Biol. UL

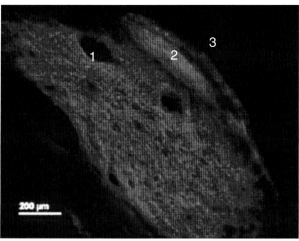

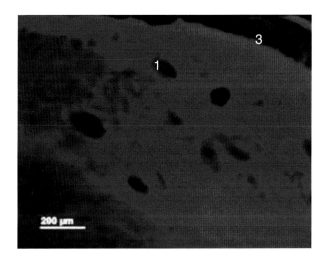

Figs 1.2 and 1.3
Low power photomicrographs of consecutive sections of the dorsal cochlear nucleus of the brainstem stained in Fig. 1.2 for neurons and synapses (synaptophysin stain) and in Fig. 1.3 for neuroglia (GFAP stain). Both stains are fluorescently labeled. While neurons and glia are present in all parts of the section, areas rich in glia are relatively poorer in neurons and vice versa. Scale on picture.

1 Blood vessel
2 Dorsal cochlear nucleus
3 External surface

Prof. R. Rübsamen and I. Bazwinsky Dipl.-Biol UL

TABLE SHOWING THE VARIETY OF NEURONAL SHAPES.

	Unipolar Embryonic only
	Pseudo-unipolar Dorsal root ganglia
	Bipolar Retina
	Multipolar Most numerous throughout the CNS*

* For exception, see Amacrine cells p. 241.

Figures 1.4–1.17 Histological preparations to show neurons and nerve fibers.

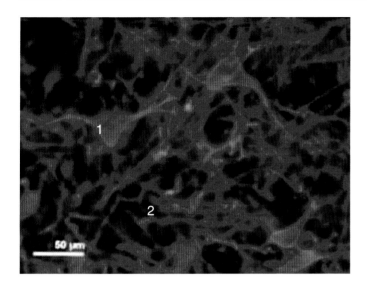

Fig. 1.4
A group of neurons from the abducens nucleus showing cell bodies and processes. SMI neurofilament antigen stain. Scale on picture.

1 Neuronal cell body
2 Neuronal processes

Prof. R. Rübsamen and I. Bazwinsky Dipl-Biol. UL

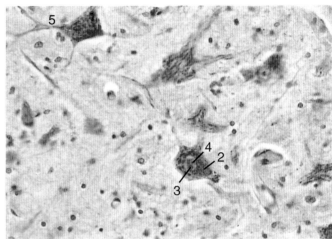

Fig. 1.5
A histological section to show the parts of a neuron. Cresyl violet stain. ×798

1 Cell body
2 Nissl substance
3 Nucleolus
4 Nucleus
5 Process

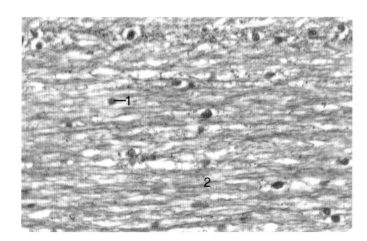

Fig. 1.6
An area of white matter in the cerebrum, to show nerve fibers in longitudinal section. Palmgren's stain. ×780

1 Glial cell nucleus
2 Nerve fibers

Dr. A. Fletcher LRI

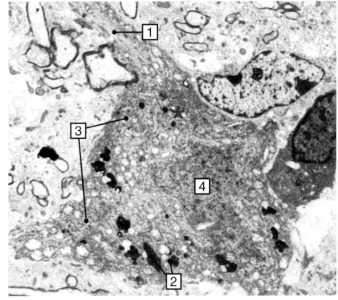

Fig. 1.7
Electron micrograph to show the structure of a neuron.

1 Axon (⋆ = axon hillock)
2 Lysosomes
3 Nissl substance
4 Nucleus

Reproduced by permission of Prof. J. S. Lowe QMC

Neurons are very active cells and this is reflected in their internal structure, e.g. their large numbers of energy-generating mitochondria. They have an extensive cell membrane which requires continual maintenance and repair. Hence, they have large nuclei and contain large volumes of rough endoplasmic reticulum (Nissl substance) for protein synthesis, and many lysosomes for the recycling of membrane components. They also have to maintain an electrical gradient across their cell membranes and synthesize the transmitter substances used to communicate with one another. Their complex shapes are supported by an extensive cytoskeleton of neurofilaments, a type of intermediate filament.

Substances such as neurotransmitters and structural components of the cell are made in the cell body and are continually transported down the axon. Some axons are as much as 1 meter long, such as those connecting the spinal cord to the lower limb. Microtubules form tracks along which this axonal transport operates. Substances such as cytoskeletal proteins travel slowly, 1–5 mm per day. Fast transport mechanisms, 300–400 mm per day, convey neurotransmitters to the nerve ending packaged in membrane vesicles, and return substances to the cell body for recycling.

Most adult neurons are unable to divide, so that cell bodies lost by disease or injury are not normally replaced. However, there is some plasticity in the ability of neurons to form new connections, either during development or during recovery from damage.

Figures 1.4–1.17 Histological preparations to show neurons and nerve fibers.

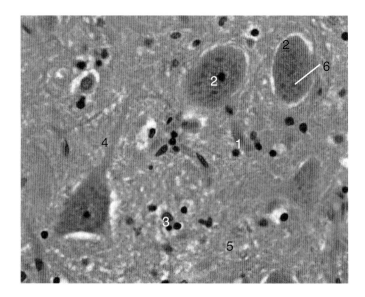

Fig. 1.8
High power photomicrograph of a large motor neuron from the spinal cord to show the nucleus and Nissl substance. The neuron is surrounded by a dense entanglement of processes from other neurons, neuroglia and blood vessels, often referred to as neuropil. Hematoxylin and eosin stain. ×350

1 Capillary
2 Cell body of neuron
3 Neuroglial nuclei
4 Neuronal cell processes
5 Neuropil
6 Nissl substance

Prof. J. S. Lowe QMC

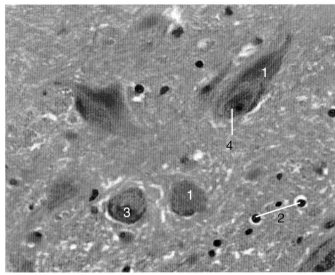

Fig. 1.9
Cells from the substantia nigra stained to show their supporting cytoskeleton of neurofilaments. Neurofilament antigen stain. ×350

1 Cells containing neurofilaments
2 Glial cell nuclei
3 Neuronal cell body
4 Neuronal nucleus

Prof. J. S. Lowe QMC

Figures 1.4–1.17 Histological preparations to show neurons and nerve fibers.

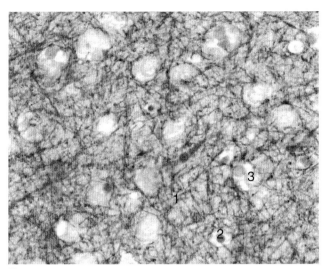

Fig. 1.10

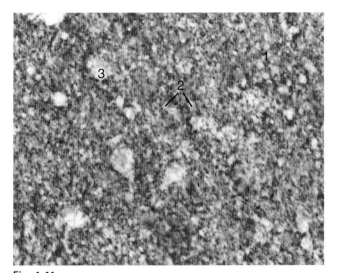

Fig. 1.11

Figs 1.10 and 1.11
Sections of gray matter (1.10) and white matter (1.11) stained immunocytochemically for neurofilament protein. In gray matter, stained nerve fibers are relatively sparse, but in the white matter most of the field is filled by images of sectioned and stained nerve fibers. Neurofilament antigen stain. ×250

1 Nerve fibers containing stained neurofilaments
2 Neuroglial nucleus
3 Neuronal cell body

Prof. J. S. Lowe QMC

Fig. 1.12
An area of cerebellar cortex to show the variation in neuronal size. Hematoxylin and eosin stain. ×280

1 Granule cell
2 Purkinje cell

Prof. J. S. Lowe QMC

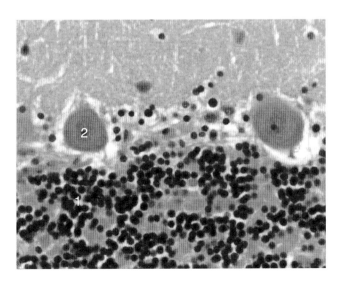

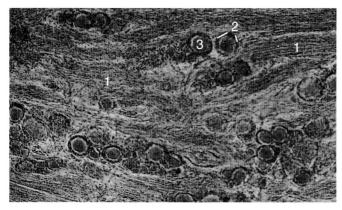

Fig. 1.13
Unipolar neurons appear circular in section, having only one process. They are usually surrounded by glial cells, the satellite cells. A histological section showing a group of unipolar neurons in a dorsal root ganglion. Unknown stain. ×139

1 Nerve fibers
2 Satellite cells
3 Unipolar neuron   Wellcome Museum

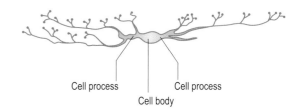

Fig. 1.14
A bipolar cell from the retina, stained with silver to show its cell body and two major cell processes. Redrawn from an original drawing by Santiago Ramón y Cajal published in 1892.

Wellcome Library, London

Figures 1.15 and 1.16 Sections showing variations in the shape of multipolar neurons.

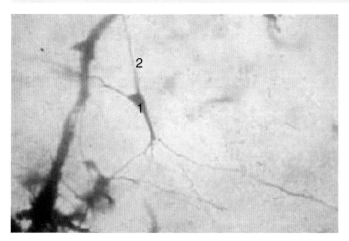

Fig. 1.15
A multipolar neuron from the superior colliculus. Its processes are orientated in the vertical plane. Golgi stain. ×63

1 Neuronal cell body
2 Neuronal cell processes   Dr. H. Hilbig UL

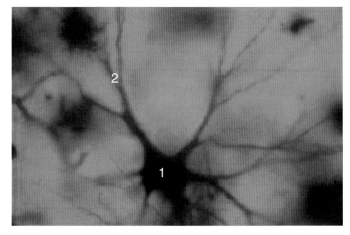

Fig. 1.16
A wide field neuron from the superior colliculus. Golgi stain. ×260
Dr. H. Hilbig UL

Information is transferred from one neuron to another at specialized regions of the cell known as synapses. Synaptic vesicles contain the substances known as neurotransmitters by which means neurons communicate. The transmitters are released into the gap between the two neurons at the synapse. Specific receptors exist at synapses for neurotransmitters. When the transmitter binds to its receptor, the neuron is stimulated and changes occur in the gradient of electrical potential across its cell membrane. These changes are propagated along the membrane as a nerve impulse or action potential. Nerve fiber diameters vary from 0.5 μm to 100 μm. The thicker the nerve fiber, the faster the impulse travels, up to 100 m/sec for the largest diameter axons. Myelin also increases the conduction rate.

● *Brain tissues have no sensations. Pain or pressure on nonnervous tissue (e.g. blood vessels, meninges) produces sensations (e.g. headache).*

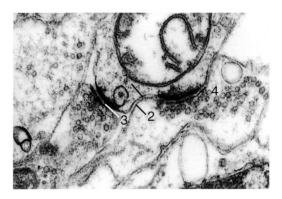

Fig. 1.17
A transmission electron micrograph to show a synapse in the cerebral cortex of a 4-month-old infant. Lead citrate stain. ×42 000

1 Postsynaptic membrane
2 Presynaptic membrane
3 Synaptic cleft
4 Synaptic vesicles

Prof. J. S. Lowe QMC

Glial Cells

The supporting tissues of the central nervous system are called glial cells. There are three basic types of glial cells: astrocytes, which have many processes; oligodendrocytes, which have few processes; and microglia, which are irregular in shape. Astrocytes and oligodendrocytes are often referred to together as macroglia. Although glial cells and neurons have a common ancestry, in the stem cell, glial cells are more numerous than neurons. There are about ten glia to each neuron in the adult brain.

Macroglia: Astrocytes

Astrocytes have many functions. They produce neurotrophic substances which neurons need for their development and long-term survival. They can take up potassium released during neuronal activity. They may also have a role in nutrition of the nervous tissue, since they transport glucose from the blood to the neurons, and store glycogen. Their presence is necessary for the normal development and functioning of synapses. Astrocytes can also phagocytose degenerating synaptic terminals. Functionally, they share some characteristics with neurons. They can retrieve GABA and glutamate after these transmitters have been released at nerve terminals. They do not retrieve catecholamine transmitters such as epinephrine (adrenaline), which are either destroyed by enzymes or taken up into nerve endings. They can also produce neurotransmitters themselves, especially glutamate and adenosine triphosphate (ATP). Astrocytes make contact with each other and with neurons at gap junctions, where small molecules and calcium ions can flow from cell to cell. However, communication between astrocytes is much slower than neuronal transmission.

● *Camillo Golgi (1843–1926) introduced a silver staining method which led to significant advances in the histological study of nervous tissue. In 1906, he was awarded the Nobel Prize jointly with Santiago Ramón y Cajal (1852–1934) for his many contributions to histology. Golgi believed that neural tissue was a syncytium, with all the cells in continuity, but Cajal showed that they were separated at synapses.*

● *In the elderly, accumulations of lipid material can be seen in neuronal cell bodies. These are called lipofuscin granules and are probably residual products of membrane recycling by lysosomes.*

● *In Alzheimer's disease, disorganized neurofilaments accumulate in damaged neurons, forming neurofibrillary tangles and plaques.*

● *In multiple sclerosis, nerve fibers become demyelinated.*

Astrocytes have many long processes. They may be identified by immunocytochemical staining to demonstrate glial fibrillary acidic protein in the cell (GFAP staining). These glial filaments are a class of intermediate filaments, part of the cell's cytoskeleton.

Astrocytes frequently contact blood vessels. They control the permeability of the vessels by determining that the endothelial cells of the vessels develop tight junctions. They themselves form a barrier outside the capillary wall, part of the blood–brain barrier (see p. 90). On the outer surface of the brain, astrocyte processes interweave to form a limiting layer. Together with the basal lamina, these astrocytic processes form a surface layer, the glia limitans.

Figure 1.18 Astrocytes and their processes.

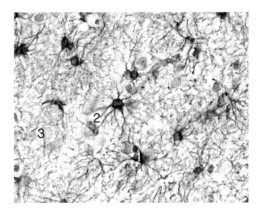

Fig. 1.18
A group of astrocytes in gray matter. GFAP stain. ×375

1 Astrocyte
2 Astrocyte processes
3 Neuronal nucleus

Prof. J. S. Lowe QMC

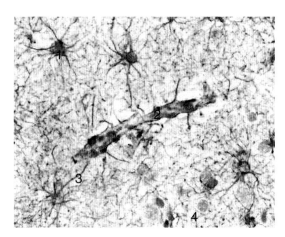

Fig. 1.19
A section to show astrocyte foot processes on a
capillary. GFAP stain. ×320

1 Astrocyte   3 Foot process
2 Capillary   4 Neuronal nucleus

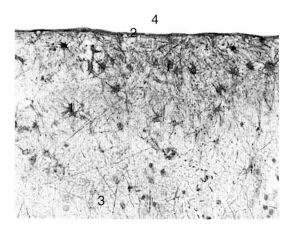

Fig. 1.20
The glia limitans on the outside of the cerebral cortex.
GFAP stain. ×130

1 Astrocyte   3 Neural tissue
2 Glia limitans   4 Subarachnoid space

- *Monoamine oxidase is the enzyme which breaks down
  catecholamine transmitters such as serotonin and adrenaline when
  their function is completed. Some antidepressant drugs inhibit this
  process.*

Macroglia: Oligodendrocytes

Oligodendrocytes make the myelin sheaths of myelinated
nerve fibres in the central nervous system. Myelin is formed
when the oligodendrocyte extends a flap of cell membrane
around one or more axons and wraps the membrane many
times around the axon, creating a many-layered arrangement
of fused cell membranes. The ability to form new myelin

reduces as the cell ages. Because of their association with
nerve fibres, oligodendrocytes are more prevalent in white
matter than in grey matter. Their nuclei are commonly seen
in rows between the nerve fibres.

Each oligodendrocyte forms a short segment of myelin.
the gaps between consecutive segments are known as 'nodes
of Ranvier'. As a nerve impulse passes along a myelinated
nerve fibre, it jumps from one node to the next. This is
called saltatory.

Figures 1.21–1.27 Histological preparations to show the structure of oligodendrocytes.

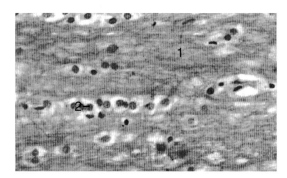

Fig. 1.21
Oligodendrocyte nuclei and nerve fibres in the white matter of the
pons. Haematoxylin and eosin stain. ×570

1 Nerve fibres
2 Oligodendrocyte nuclei

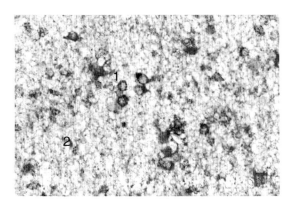

Fig. 1.22
Oligodendrocytes in white matter. Alpha B crystalin stain. ×660

1 Oligodendrocyte
2 White matter

1.19–1.22 Prof. J. S. Lowe QMC

Figures 1.23 and 1.24 Oligodendrocytes stained with monoclonal antibody, fluorescein (FITC) labeled ×850.

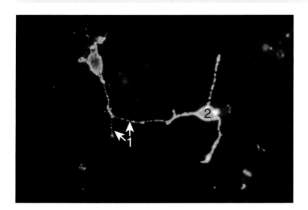

Fig. 1.23
Human oligodendrocyte progenitor cells *in vitro*.

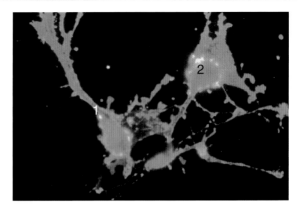

Fig. 1.24
Mature human oligodendrocytes *in vitro*.

1 Cytoplasmic processes
2 Nucleus
Prof. N. Scolding FH

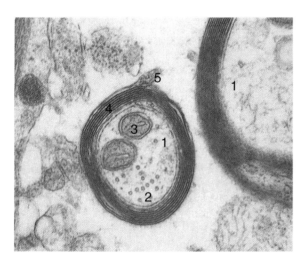

Fig. 1.25
A myelinated nerve fiber from the cerebral cortex to show
the relationship between the oligodendrocyte, the myelin
sheath and the axon as seen by transmission electron
microscopy. Lead citrate stain. ×36 000

1 Axon   **4** Myelin
2 Microtubules **5** Oligodendrocyte cytoplasm
3 Mitochondrion

Prof. J. S. Lowe QMC

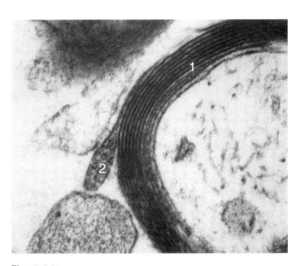

Fig. 1.26
Detail of the myelin sheath as seen by transmission electron
microscopy. Lead citrate stain. ×65 000

1 Myelin lamellae   **2** Oligodendrocyte cytoplasm
Prof. J. S. Lowe QMC

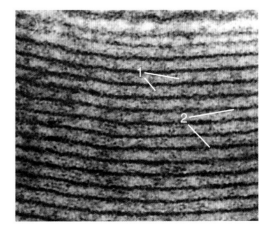

Fig. 1.27
High magnification transmission electron micrograph to show details of the layered
structure of myelin. Alternating major dense lines (dark) and intraperiod lines (light)
show where the cell membranes have fused. ×175 000

1 Intraperiod line   **2** Major dense line
Prof. J. S. Lowe QMC

Microglia

Microglia are the specialized macrophages of nervous tissue. They become activated during inflammatory reactions and participate in immunological defense mechanisms.

Throughout the body, monocytes of the blood can transform into macrophages. This cell type also exists in the brain. Lymphocytes, the main immune cell type outside the CNS, are extremely rare in nervous tissue.

Figures 1.28–1.30 Microglia and other immune cells can be identified by histochemical staining for specific components of their surface.

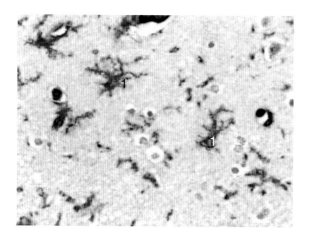

Fig. 1.28
Ricinus communis agglutinin specifically labels microglial cells in nervous tissue. ×225

1 Microglial cell

Prof. J. S. Lowe QMC

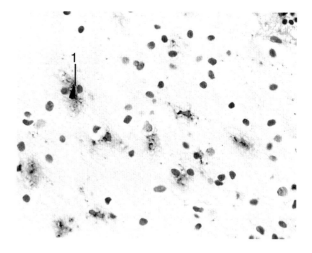

Fig. 1.29
CD68 immunostain specifically stains microglial cells. In this section of white matter, the unstained cells are astrocytes or oligodendrocytes. ×190

1 Microglial cell

Prof. J. S. Lowe QMC

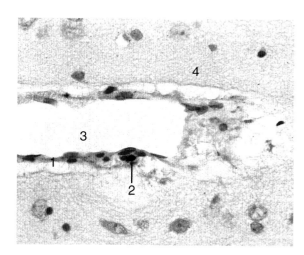

Fig. 1.30
A monocyte-derived macrophage in the perivascular space. Leukocyte common antigen stain. ×275

1 Endothelium
2 Macrophage
3 Vessel lumen
4 White matter

Prof. J. S. Lowe QMC

- *Astrocytes retain their ability to divide throughout life.*

- *In multiple sclerosis, a loss of myelin occurs and, in consequence, a slowing of impulse conduction. This condition may be an autoimmune reaction directed against oligodendrocytes.*

- *Gliosis is the formation of a scar in damaged neural tissue by the astrocytes.*

- *The commonest origin of cerebral tumors is from the glial cells. They are oligodendroglioma, astrocytoma, neuroblastoma and glioblastoma. Specific staining methods are used to identify the cell type giving rise to the tumor.*

- *Generally, tumors arising in the CNS do not metastasize to other parts of the body, but metastases from other regions often lodge in the brain.*

Summary

1. Nervous tissue is composed of neurons and neuroglial cells.
2. Neurons and glial cells can be distinguished histologically by specific staining techniques that identify their characteristic intracellular and cell surface components.
3. Neurons consist of a cell body and cell processes (axons and dendrites).
4. Axons and dendrites are known collectively as nerve fibers.
5. Neurons can be classified according to their shape. Unipolar neurons have one process, bipolar two and multipolar many processes.
6. Areas of nervous tissue in the CNS containing mainly cell bodies are known as gray matter. Collections of cell bodies outside the CNS are called ganglia.
7. Areas of nervous tissue containing mainly nerve fibers are known as white matter.
8. There are three types of neuroglial cells: astrocytes, oligodendrocytes and microglia.
9. Astrocytes provide structural support for neurons and transport nutrients and other substances between blood and nervous tissue.
10. Oligodendrocytes form myelin sheaths around some nerve fibers.
11. Microglia are phagocytic.
12. Astrocytes and oligodendrocytes can give rise to malignant tumors of the brain or spinal cord.
13. Mature neurons are normally unable to divide, so damaged cell bodies usually cannot be replaced.
14. A physiological barrier exists between cerebral blood vessels and the nervous tissue.

2 Terminology

In topographical anatomy, the directional terms used are based on the standing human body and are described as **superior** (towards the head), **inferior** (towards the feet), **anterior** (ventral or abdominal surface of the body) and **posterior** (dorsal or back of the body). In neuroanatomy this terminology remains applicable to the spinal cord, but not to the brain.

The brain is bent across the vertical axis and is too convoluted to employ usefully the same terminology as that for the upright body. Imagine the human body as a straight cylinder, like an earthworm's body, and the central nervous system inside it is stretched out straight. The parts of the central nervous system then lie behind one another in a straight line. This line is the neuraxis. The following terminology can be applied: **rostral** (towards the nose) and **caudal** (towards the tail), and these terms are still used when the neuraxis is bent as in the developing and adult human brain.

An alternative terminology is used in relation to the brain inside the head. **Anterior** is towards the face, **posterior** towards the occipital region, **superior** towards the top of the head, and **inferior** towards the base of the skull.

Another set of terms is used in relation to the spinal cord. Imagine a dog: the spinal cord will have a **dorsal** surface running along its back and a **ventral** surface towards the belly. If the dog stands on its hind legs to imitate the human upright posture, these surfaces become **posterior** and **anterior**, respectively. These two pairs of terms may be used interchangeably in relation to the spinal cord.

If the brain is sectioned along the neuraxis in the median plane, the section is termed **sagittal** or **median**. Those sections parallel to the sagittal (median) plane are called **paramedian**. Brain sections at right angles to the neuraxis of the forebrain are termed **coronal** while those cut parallel with its superior and inferior margins are **horizontal**. Sections at right angles to the axis of the brainstem are **transverse**; those parallel with its long axis are **longitudinal**.

In association with these spatial terms are the words used to describe the direction of nerve fibers, i.e. **ascending** (running in a rostral direction) and **descending** (running in a caudal direction). If a fiber remains on the same side of the body, it is **ipsilateral** to the parent cell body, and if it crosses the midline it is said to **decussate** and then it becomes **contralateral** (on the opposite side to the parent cell body).

External structures can be seen on the surface of the brain or spinal cord without cutting it. **Internal** features do not appear on the surface and so can be seen only in sections.

Terminology

Terminology used to indicate directions of the brain.

Fig. 2.1
An external and lateral view of the brain (left side). ×0.71

1 Anterior
2 Inferior
3 Lateral
4 Medial (curved arrows at top)
5 Posterior
6 Superior

- *Because the brain bends during development, the orientation is described in relation to two axes.*

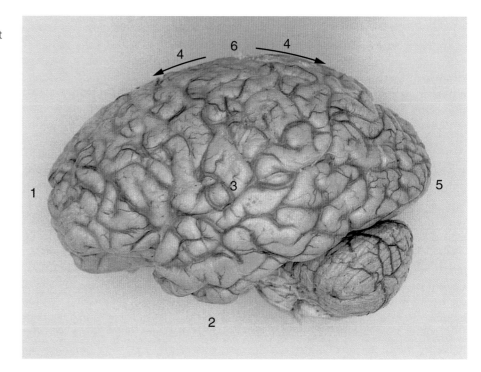

Fig. 2.2
Orientation in a medial view of the cerebral hemispheres. ×0.71

1 Anterior (ventral)
2 Caudal
3 Inferior
4 Neuraxis (dashed line)
5 Posterior (dorsal)
6 Rostral
7 Superior

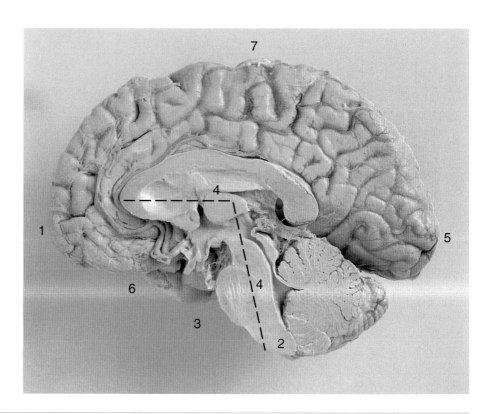

Planes of Section

A brain is usually sectioned in the following planes.

Fig. 2.3
A sagittal or median section through the brain. ×0.5

1 Caudal
2 Lateral
3 Medial
4 Posterior
5 Rostral (anterior)

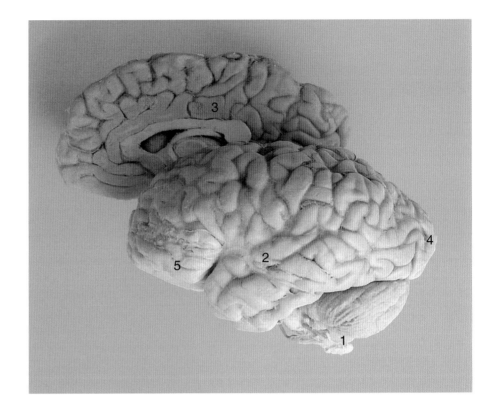

Fig. 2.4
A sagittal section parallel to the median plane of the brain (paramedian section). ×0.64

1 Anterior (rostral)
2 Dorsal or superior
3 Lateral
4 Medial
5 Posterior
6 Ventral or inferior

● *The term "parasagittal" is becoming redundant and "sagittal" refers to all sections parallel to the median plane. Many authors, however, still use "paramedian" to refer to these sections.*

      O'Rahilly, R. Acta Anat.,
      ***131**, 1-2: 1988*

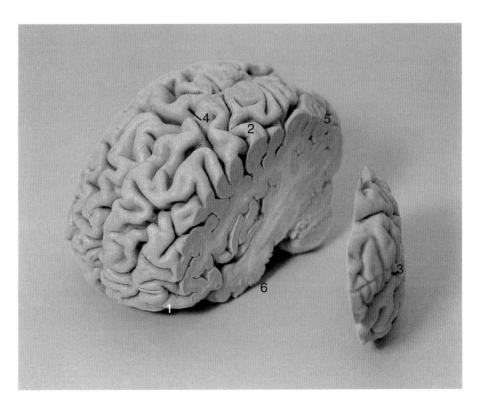

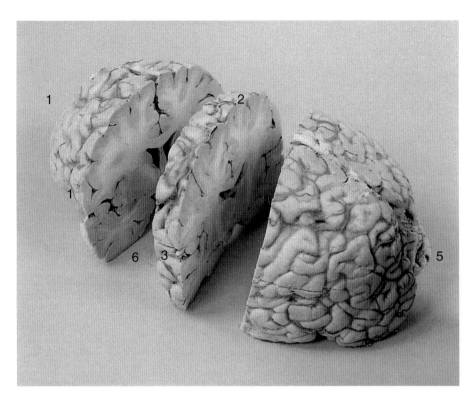

Fig. 2.5
Coronal sections (the cerebellum has been removed). ×0.5

1 Anterior (rostral)
2 Dorsal or superior
3 Lateral
4 Medial
5 Posterior
6 Ventral or inferior

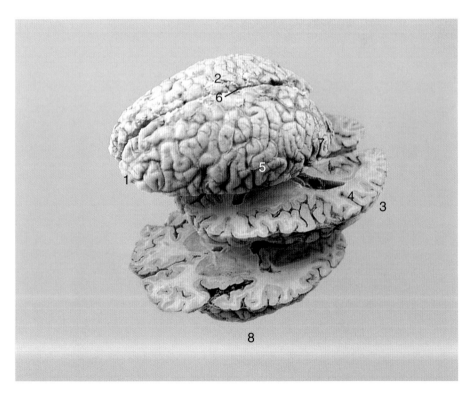

Fig. 2.6
Horizontal sections. ×0.42

1 Anterior (rostral)
2 Dorsal or superior
3 External
4 Internal
5 Lateral
6 Longitudinal fissure
7 Posterior
8 Ventral or inferior

3 Embryology

Early Development

The central nervous system develops from a midline ectoderm neural plate (Stage 8, Week 2). Neural folds form, rise and fuse to form a neural tube. Initially, fusion is in the caudal hindbrain and proceeds cranially and caudally until only the two ends of the tube remain open (neuropores). The rostral and caudal neuropores eventually close. When the rostral neuropore closes, this region is known as the lamina terminalis.

The cranial end of the neural tube expands and the main divisions of the central nervous system are established (Week 4); these are the forebrain (prosencephalon), midbrain (mesencephalon), hindbrain (rhombencephalon) and spinal cord. The optic cup is an outgrowth of the forebrain. The midbrain and part of the hindbrain become the brainstem. The cerebellum is also a hindbrain derivative.

In Week 5 the three areas of the brain subdivide to form five regions.

A series of diagrams to show the formation of the neural tube (neurulation).

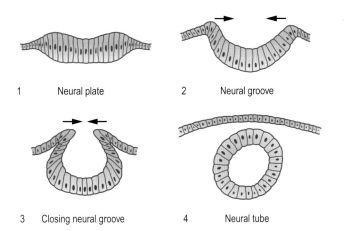

1   Neural plate   2   Neural groove

3   Closing neural groove   4   Neural tube

● *Many homeobox genes have been identified with neurulation.*

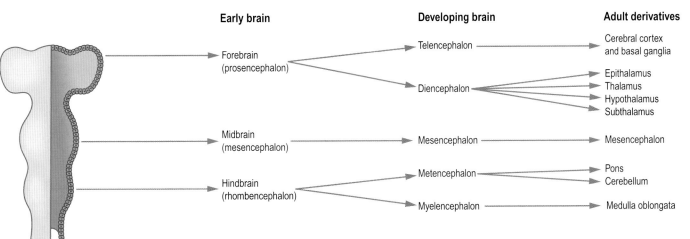

Diagram showing the regions of the developing brain and their adult derivatives.

● *Some alternative definitions of brainstem also include the diencephalon.*

● *The nervous system is largely symmetrical but there are anatomical and functional asymmetrical areas. Some structures are different in females and males.*

Flexures of the Brain

The brain flexures appear early in development. The first, the midbrain flexure, arises in Week 3 between the forebrain and midbrain. At this flexure the forebrain bends in a ventral direction. During Week 4 the second flexure, the cervical or neck flexure, forms between the hindbrain and spinal cord.

This flexure disappears after the head extends during Week 8. The third flexure, the pontine flexure, is seen during Week 5 in the region of the pons. The appearance of this flexure causes the roof of the rhombencephalon to splay and form a diamond shape.

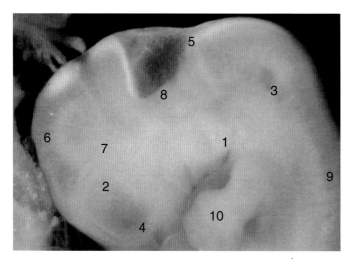

Fig. 3.1
The early brain flexures of a 12-mm CR (Stage 16) embryo viewed from the side. ×14.8

 1 Branchial arches
 2 Cerebral hemisphere
 3 Cervical flexure
 4 Forebrain
 5 Hindbrain
 6 Midbrain
 7 Midbrain flexure
 8 Pontine flexure
 9 Spinal cord
10 Upper limb and handplate

Fig. 3.2
The primary brain flexures illustrated on a 27-mm CR embryo. Hematoxylin and eosin stain. ×5.4

1 Cephalic (midbrain) flexure
2 Cerebral hemispheres
3 Cervical flexure
4 Forebrain
5 Hindbrain
6 Midbrain
7 Pontine flexure
8 Spinal cord

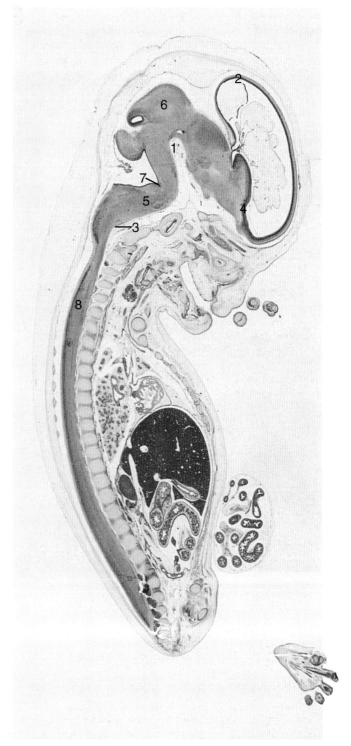

MHMS

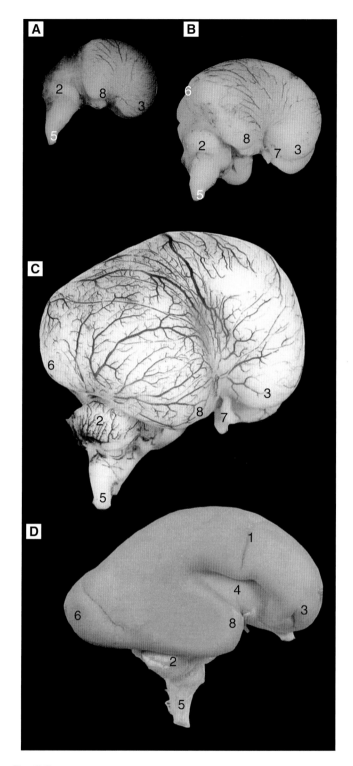

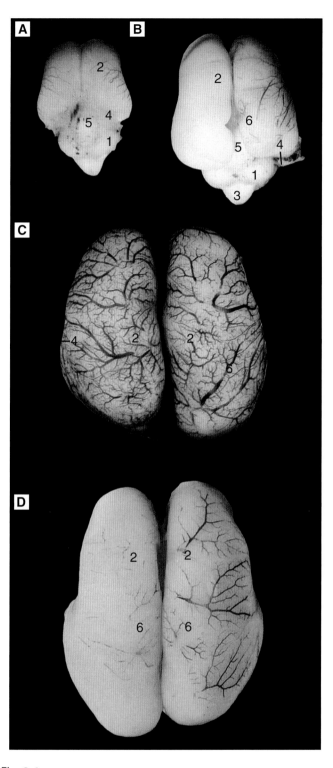

Fig. 3.3
Sequential development of the brain (lateral view).

A Weeks 11–12 ×1.54   **C** Weeks 17–18 ×2.5
B Weeks 13–14 ×1.54   **D** Months 6–7 ×1.1

1 Central sulcus   **5** Medulla oblongata
2 Cerebellum   **6** Occipital lobe
3 Frontal lobe   **7** Olfactory bulb
4 Insula   **8** Temporal lobe

A–C Dr. G. Batcup; **D** RCS

Fig. 3.4
Sequential expansion of the cerebral hemispheres in relation to the midbrain viewed from above. The meninges have been removed on one side in **B** and **D**.

A Weeks 11–12 ×1.54   **C** Week 15 ×1.54
B Weeks 13–14 ×1.54   **D** Weeks 17–18 ×1.54

1 Cerebellum   **4** Meninges
2 Cerebral hemispheres **5** Midbrain
3 Medulla oblongata   **6** Parietal lobe   A–C Dr. G. Batcup

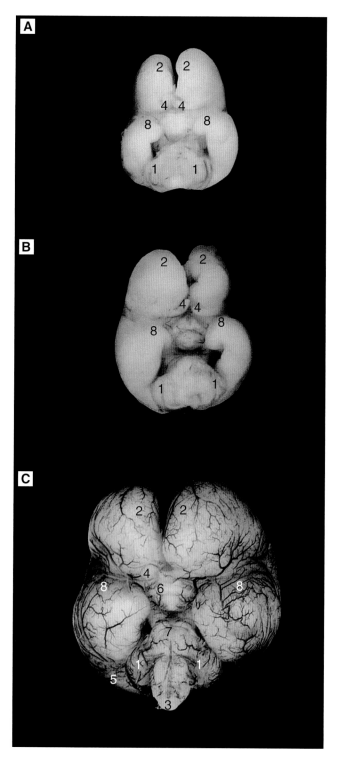

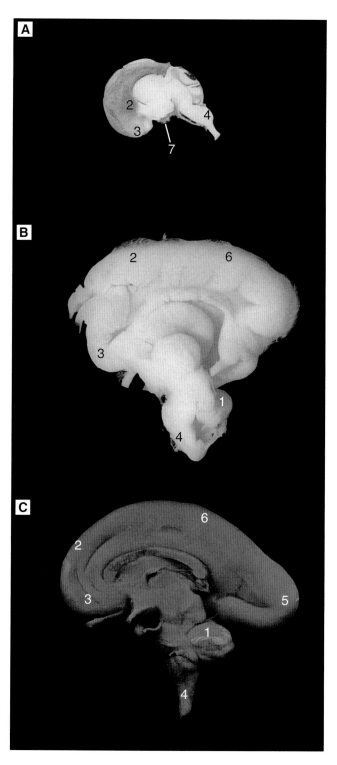

Fig. 3.5
Sequential series of development of the brain viewed from below.

A Weeks 13–14 ×1.8   **C** Weeks 17–18 ×1.4
B Week 15 ×1.8

1 Cerebellum   5 Occipital lobe
2 Frontal lobe   6 Optic nerve
3 Medulla oblongata   7 Pons
4 Olfactory bulb   8 Temporal lobe

A–C Dr. G. Batcup

Fig. 3.6
Sagittal sections of fetal brain to illustrate sequential development.

A Week 8 ×1.54   **C** Months 6–7 ×1.1
B Weeks 13–14 ×1.3

1 Cerebellum   5 Occipital lobe
2 Cerebral hemispheres   6 Parietal lobe (medial extent of)
3 Frontal lobe   7 Temporal lobe
4 Medulla oblongata

A Dr. G. Batcup; C RCS

Cavities of the Brain

The lumen of the early neural tube is retained in the adult brain and spinal cord.

Two balloon-like cerebral vesicles grow out at the rostral end of the forebrain (telencephalon). The hollow space inside each hemisphere is called the lateral ventricle and is continuous through the interventricular foramen with the original space in the forebrain (diencephalon), which becomes the third ventricle. The third ventricle is continuous with the lumen of the midbrain (cerebral aqueduct) which, in turn, is continuous with the lumen of the hindbrain (fourth ventricle). At the boundary between the midbrain and hindbrain is a distinct constriction, or isthmus. The diamond-shaped hindbrain's fourth ventricle and the central canal of the spinal cord merge without a distinct boundary. The floor of the fourth ventricle is diamond shaped.

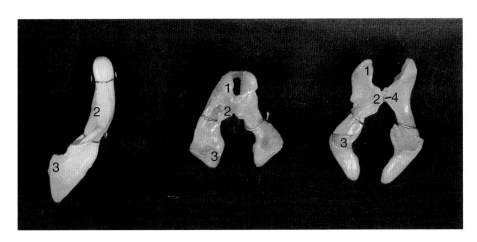

Fig. 3.7
Plastic casts of the developing ventricles in weeks 12–24. ×1.01

1 Anterior horn of the lateral ventricle
2 Body of lateral ventricle
3 Inferior horn of the lateral ventricle
4 Third ventricle

RCS

Fig. 3.8
Ventricular cast superimposed on the base of the brain (130 mm CR fetus) to show its position in relation to the external features of the brain. ×2.1

  1 Anterior horn of the lateral ventricle
  2 Body of lateral ventricle
  3 Cerebellum
  4 Frontal lobe
  5 Inferior horn of the lateral ventricle
  6 Occipital lobe
  7 Spinal cord
  8 Temporal lobe

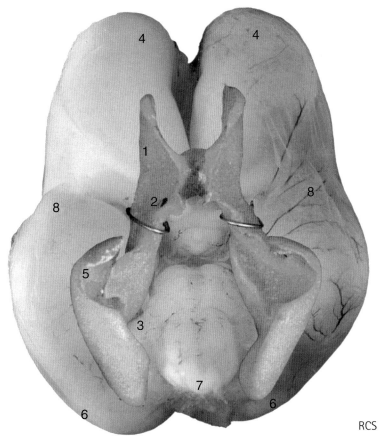

RCS

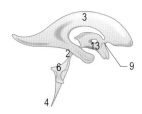

Diagram of a lateral view of the ventricles.

Choroid Plexus

The choroid plexus forms when blood vessels and pia mater invaginate the thin, ependymal medial wall of the cerebral hemispheres (choroidal fissure), and the thin, ependymal roofs of the diencephalon and hindbrain. These plexuses form the choroid plexuses of the lateral, third and fourth ventricles.

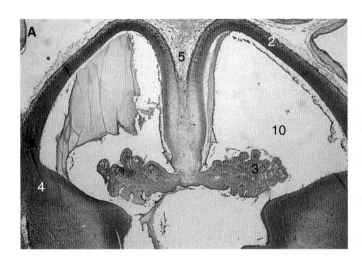

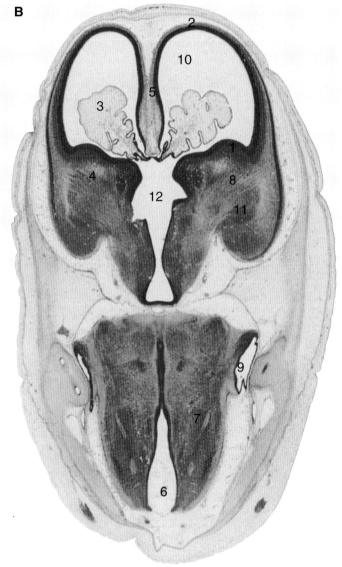

Fig. 3.9
The developing choroid plexus. **A**, A coronal paraffin wax section through the lateral ventricles of a 22-mm CR embryo. De Castro stain. ×23.5. **B**, A Week 10 (57 mm CR) fetus sectioned through the midbrain. Hematoxylin and eosin stain. ×10.7

1 Caudate nucleus
2 Cerebral hemisphere
3 Choroid plexus
4 Corpus striatum
5 Forebrain
6 Fourth ventricle
7 Hindbrain
8 Internal capsule
9 Lateral recess
10 Lateral ventricle
11 Lentiform nucleus
12 Third ventricle

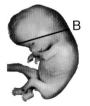

MHMS

● *Stem cells which give rise to new olfactory system neurons line the walls of the lateral ventricle.*

Corpus Striatum

As the two cerebral hemispheres (telencephalon) expand they develop a C-shape, with the formation of the temporal lobe. The lateral ventricle inside each hemisphere similarly becomes C-shaped.

A swelling, the corpus striatum, develops in the floor of each lateral ventricle. As the ventricle becomes C-shaped, the caudal end of the corpus striatum becomes drawn out with it, forming the tail of the caudate nucleus and the amygdaloid nucleus on its distal end. Thus, the caudate nucleus assumes the C-shaped conformation seen in the adult brain.

Expansion of the cerebral hemisphere brings the medial aspect of the hemisphere into contact with the lateral side of the diencephalon in the region of the future thalamus. The surfaces adhere and tissue continuity is established, with the thalamus and corpus striatum adjacent to each other.

Projection fibers begin to form to link the cerebral hemisphere with the diencephalon and brainstem. These split the corpus striatum into two parts, the caudate nucleus medially and the lentiform nucleus laterally. They grow through the region between the corpus striatum and the thalamus, forming the internal capsule.

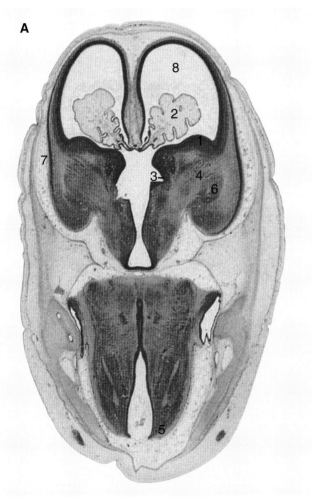

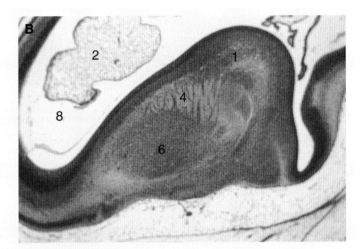

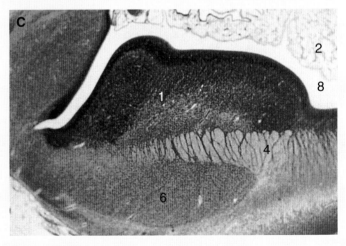

Fig. 3.10
The development of the corpus striatum, internal capsule, caudate and lentiform nuclei. Hematoxylin and eosin stain. **A**, A week 10 (57-mm CR) fetus sectioned through the basal ganglia. Hematoxylin and eosin stain. ×8.8. **B**, A paraffin wax section through the basal ganglia of a 35-mm CR fetus. Hematoxylin and eosin stain. ×24.5. **C**, A paraffin wax section through the basal ganglia of a 3-month fetus. Hematoxylin and eosin stain. ×24.5

1 Caudate nucleus
2 Choroid plexus

3 Hypothalamic sulcus
4 Internal capsule
5 Hindbrain

6 Lentiform nucleus
7 Meninx
8 Ventricle (lateral)   MHMS

● *The embryonic meninx (see p. 33) contributes to the development of the three adult meninges: pia mater, arachnoid mater and dura mater.*

Histological Development of the Cerebral Cortex

Four fundamental layers are formed in the embryonic central nervous system (CNS). From them, all the adult components develop. Initially, there is one pseudostratified layer of neuroepithelial cells, the ventricular zone. A second zone is formed when the nuclei of these cells congregate around the lumen of the neural tube, leaving an outer layer made up mainly of cell processes, the marginal zone. Cells then migrate out of the ventricular zone to create a third layer between the ventricular and marginal zones; this is the intermediate zone. The fourth layer is the subventricular zone, lying between the ventricular and the intermediate zones (Boulder Committee terminology. *Anat. Rec.,* **166**: 257-262, 1970). In the developing cerebral cortex, cells migrate out from the intermediate zone to form an extra layer, the cortical plate between the intermediate and marginal zones. Cell rearrangement within the cortical plate creates the layers of mature neocortex. Nerve fibers, the corticopetal fibers, entering the developing cortex from other parts of the brain are a trigger for neuronal maturation.

Most of the adult cortex is called neocortex and has six layers, numbered I to VI. Layer I forms first in the marginal layer. Layers II to VI form in the cortical plate from the inside outwards. Successive waves of cells migrate into the cortical plate across the intermediate zone.

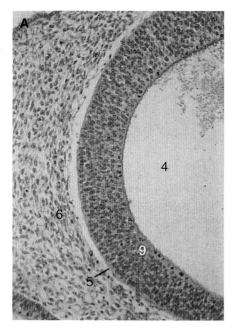

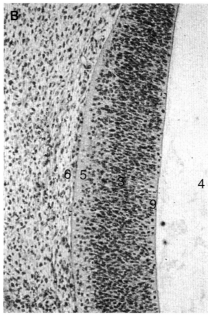

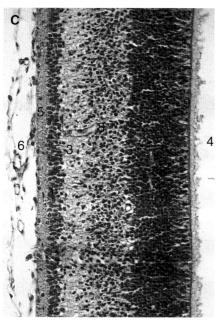

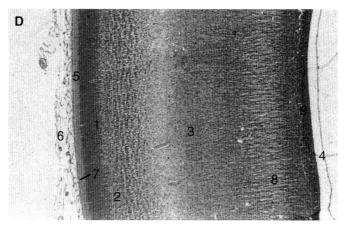

Fig. 3.11
The histological development of the cortex. Transverse paraffin wax sections of the cerebral cortex. Hematoxylin and eosin stain.

A 3-mm CR embryo. ×190
B 10-mm CR embryo. ×194
C 35-mm CR fetus. ×42
D 150-mm CR fetus. ×33.3

1 Cortical plate
2 Inner zone of cortical plate; loosely packed cells
3 Intermediate (mantle) zone
4 Lumen
5 Marginal zone
6 Meninx
7 Outer zone of cortical plate; closely packed cells
8 Subventricular zone
9 Ventricular (ependymal) zone

A, B, D CXWMS; **C** MHMS

Cerebellum

The cerebellum develops from the metencephalon of the hindbrain. Two areas on its dorsal aspect, known as the alar lamina and the rhombic lip, enlarge and grow backwards.

They overlap first the rostral end of the fourth ventricle, then the pons and medulla. The formation of the cerebellum begins at around 10 weeks of gestation.

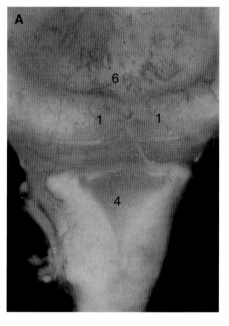

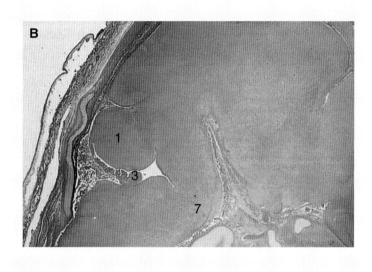

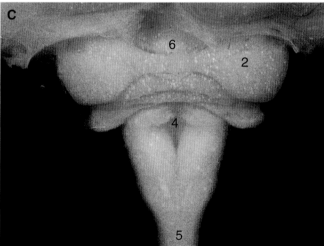

Fig. 3.12
Development of the cerebellum.

A Week 10, 57-mm CR fetus. ×15.6
B Week 10, 57-mm CR fetus, De Castro stain. ×8.3
C Week 15, 123-mm CR fetus. ×4

1 Cerebellum
2 Cerebellar hemisphere
3 Choroid plexus in fourth ventricle
4 Fourth ventricle with roof removed
5 Medulla oblongata
6 Mesencephalon
7 Pontine flexure

B CXWMS

● *The cerebellar cortex forms by cell migration in a different manner to the cerebral cortex. Stellate and granular cells are formed from a superficial secondary germinal layer, the outer granular layer from which cells migrate inwards to populate the cortex. The Purkinje cells are formed from the ventricular zone.*

Cranial Nerves

The olfactory nerves (I) are processes of bipolar neurons in the olfactory epithelium. The optic nerve (II) is a brain pathway. The remaining cranial nerves (III–XII) can be divided into those without ganglia (III, IV, VI, XI, XII) and those that possess ganglia (V, VII, VIII, IX, X). Those with ganglia contain sensory or autonomic components, or both. The ganglia are formed by a combination of neural crest cells and cells derived from a thickening (placode) of the ectoderm. In this they differ from dorsal root (sensory) ganglia of the spinal cord and the autonomic ganglia of the sympathetic chain, which do not have a placodal component.

A

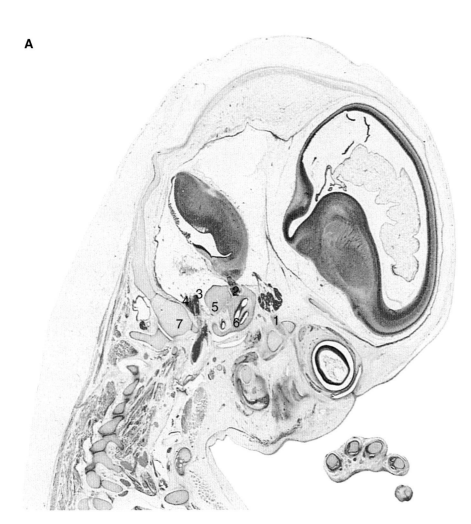

- *Cranial nerves can also be classified by their function, into four groups.*
  Nerves I, II and VIII are purely sensory.
  Nerves III, IV, VI, XI and XII are purely motor.
  Nerves V, VII, IX and X are mixed, with sensory and motor components.
  Nerves III, VII, IX and X contain autonomic fibers.
  The accessory nerve (XI) may contain some proprioceptive fibers (see p. 185).

Fig. 3.13
The development of the cranial nerves. **A,** A longitudinal paraffin wax section of a 35-mm CR fetus. Hematoxylin and eosin stain. ×6.9. **B,** A close-up of the brainstem showing the emergence of nerves V, VIII, IX and X and their associated ganglia. Hematoxylin and eosin stain. ×8.6

1 V nerve and ganglion
2 VIII nerve
3 IX nerve and ganglia
4 X nerve and ganglia
5 Petrous temporal cartilage
6 Semicircular canals
7 Skull base

MHMS

Meninges

The meninges form from mesoderm condensing around the neural tube to form the primitive meninx. The outer part of the meninx forms dura mater, and the inner forms pia–arachnoid. The neural crest contributes to the latter layer. The subarachnoid space forms as fluid accumulates in the pia–arachnoid layer. A layer of cells on the outside of the arachnoid acts as a barrier to the fluid. This fluid is the cerebrospinal fluid and is produced by the choroid plexus (see p. 93).

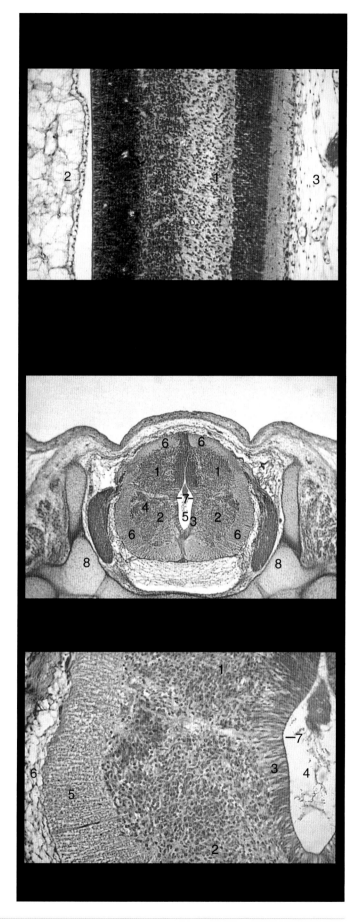

Fig. 3.14
Medial side of the cerebral hemisphere with meninx of a 3-month fetus. Hematoxylin and eosin stain. ×47.4

1 Brain		**3** Meninx
2 Choroid plexus		MHMS

Alar and Basal Plates

Cell bodies of developing neurons collect around the lumen of the neural tube forming the intermediate zone, while their processes (nerve fibers) form the marginal layer on the outside. The cross-sectional profile of the lumen becomes diamond-shaped. The sulcus limitans in the side wall of the lumen divides the mantle layer into alar plate above and basal plate below. Structures that are derived from the alar plate will have sensory functions and those from the basal plate will be motor.

Fig. 3.15
A transverse paraffin wax section through the thoracic level of the spinal cord in a 22-mm CR embryo. The alar and basal plates are shown. De Castro stain. ×24

1 Alar plate	**4** Intermediate zone	**7** Sulcus limitans
2 Basal plate	**5** Lumen	**8** Vertebra
3 Ependyma	**6** Marginal layer	MHMS

Fig. 3.16
A higher magnification of Fig. 3.15 showing the alar and basal plates. The alar plate becomes the dorsal (posterior) horn and the basal plate becomes the ventral (anterior) horn and the lateral horn. The marginal layer becomes the white matter. De Castro stain. ×97

1 Alar plate	**4** Lumen	**6** Meninx
2 Basal plate	**5** Marginal layer	**7** Sulcus limitans
3 Ependyma		
		MHMS

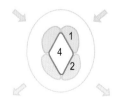

Diagram showing the alar and basal plates in a transverse section of neural tube, and the direction of afferent and efferent nerves. Alar plate and afferent – green; basal plate and efferent – blue. Other labels as Fig. 3.16.

Figures 3.17–3.19 Sequential stages in the development of the brainstem showing the fate of the alar and basal plates.

Fig. 3.17
A paraffin wax section through the head of a 22-mm CR embryo passing through the hindbrain (myelencephalon) and forebrain (diencephalon and telencephalon), to show the formation of the lateral, third and fourth ventricles and the alar and basal plates. De Castro stain. ×7.5

MHMS

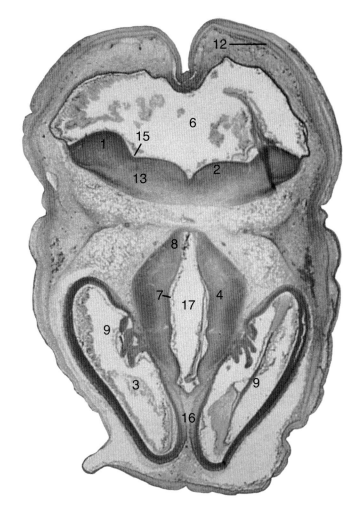

● *The diencephalon has no basal plate; the alar plate forms both thalamus and hypothalamus.*

Fig. 3.18
Transverse histological section through the basal plate of the myelencephalon showing the formation of cell columns which will become motor cranial nerve nuclei. Cell columns in the alar plate become sensory nuclei. De Castro stain. ×26

1 Alar plate
2 Basal plate
3 Choroid plexus
4 Diencephalon
5 Ependyma
6 Fourth ventricle
7 Hypothalamic sulcus
8 Hypothalamus
9 Lateral ventricle
10 Mantle (intermediate) layer
11 Marginal layer
12 Meninx
13 Myelencephalon
14 Somatic motor cell column
15 Sulcus limitans
16 Telencephalon
17 Third ventricle
18 Visceral motor cell column

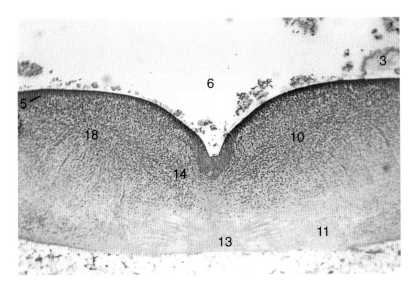

MHMS

Fig. 3.19
A coronal paraffin section through the head and neck of a 3-month fetus to show the formation of nuclei in the midbrain and medulla. Hematoxylin and eosin stain. × 3.3. Structures for orientation have been italicized in the list.

1 Alar plate
2 Basal plate
3 *Base of skull*
4 Cerebral aqueduct
5 *Cerebral hemispheres*
6 Cerebral peduncle
7 Choroid plexus
8 Dorsal root ganglion
9 Epiphysis
10 External ear
11 First cervical nerve root
12 Humerus
13 Hypoglossal nerve
14 Hypoglossal nucleus
15 Inferior olivary nucleus
16 *Inner ear*
17 Internal jugular vein
18 Jugular foramen
19 Lateral ventricle
20 Medulla oblongata
21 Meninx
22 Mesencephalic trigeminal nucleus
23 Midbrain
24 Nuclei of vestibulocochlear nerve
25 Oculomotor nucleus
26 Pyramid of medulla oblongata
27 Red nucleus
28 *Shoulder*
29 Solitary nucleus
30 Spinal cord
31 Spinal trigeminal nucleus
32 Substantia nigra
33 Sulcus limitans
34 Tectum
35 Vertebral artery
36 *Vertebral column*
37 Vestibulocochlear nerve

MHMS

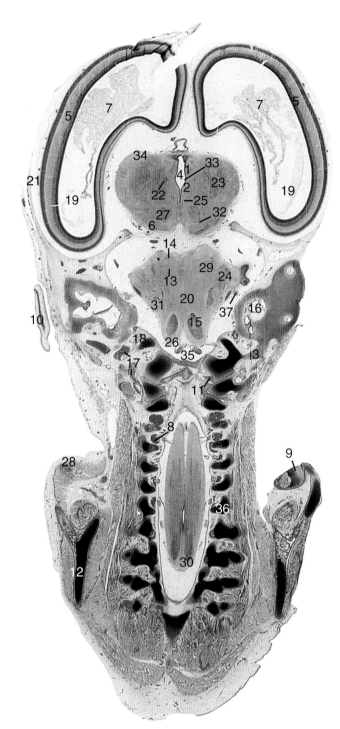

● *The presence of cervical, pontine and midbrain flexures between the divisions of the developing central nervous system explains why forebrain, midbrain, hindbrain and spinal cord are all cut in the same coronal section.*

Spinal Cord

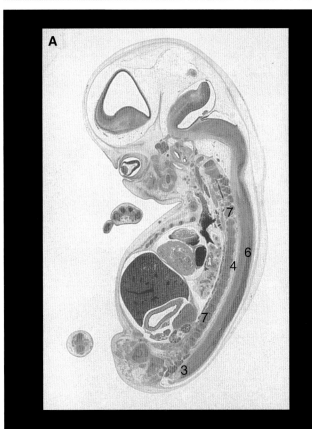

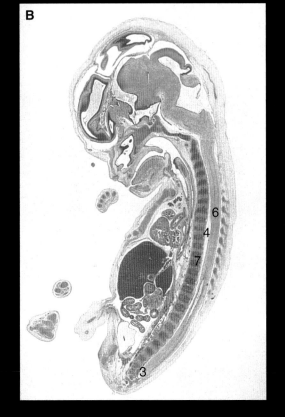

Fig. 3.20

The sequential changes in spinal cord development, showing its change in relative length compared with the vertebral column. **A**, The spinal cord occupies the length of the spinal column, 25-mm CR embryo. Hematoxylin and eosin stain. ×3.5. **B**, The spinal cord in a 40-mm CR fetus in a longitudinal histological section. Hematoxylin and eosin stain. ×.2.2. **C**, A dissection of the spinal cord in a fetus ×1.1.

1 Cervical expansion	**5** Spinal nerves
2 Lumbar expansion	**6** Thoracic cord
3 Sacral cord	**7** Vertebral column
4 Spinal canal	

A,B CXWMS; **C** RCS

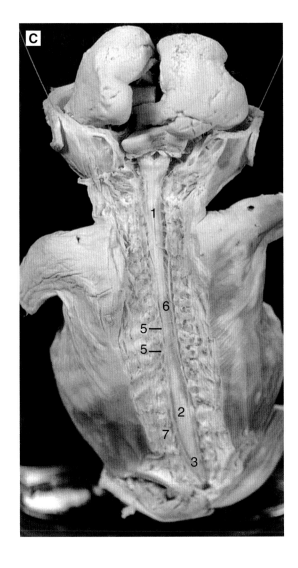

Cellular Differentiation in the Nervous System

Specific staining for neural development in the brain and spinal cord

By using immunocytochemical techniques, it is possible to show changing patterns of expression of various proteins during development.

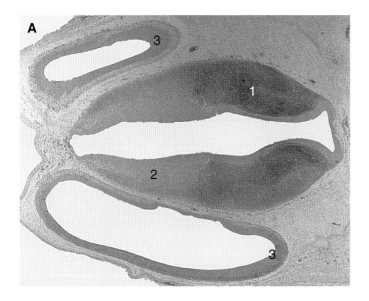

Fig. 3.21A
Forebrain of a 7–8-week embryo stained with MAP-2/counterstained toluidine blue to show developing dendrites and neurons. ×18

1 Developing dendrites and neurons
2 Diencephalon
3 Telencephalon

Dr. G. Clowry and Dr. S. Lindsay UN

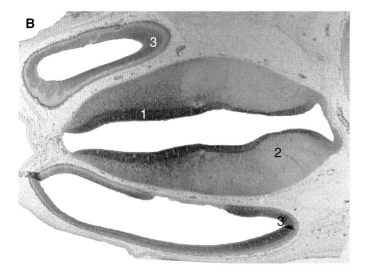

Fig. 3.21B
Forebrain of a 7–8-week embryo stained with nestin/counterstained toluidine blue to show developing radial glia, neuroblasts and glioblasts. ×18

1 Developing glioblasts, radial glia and neuroblasts
2 Diencephalon
3 Telencephalon

Dr. G. Clowry and Dr. S. Lindsay UN

Fig. 3.22A
Spinal cord of a 7–8-week embryo stained for growth associated protein (GAP 43) to show developing nerve fibers. Counterstain toluidine blue. The green/brown of GAP 43 is concentrated in future areas of white matter, peripheral nerves and dorsal root zone. ×50

1 Dorsal root entry zone
2 Dorsal root ganglion
3 Peripheral nerve fiber tracts
4 Spinal cord
5 Ventral funiculus
6 Vertebral body

Dr. G. Clowry and Dr. S. Lindsay UN

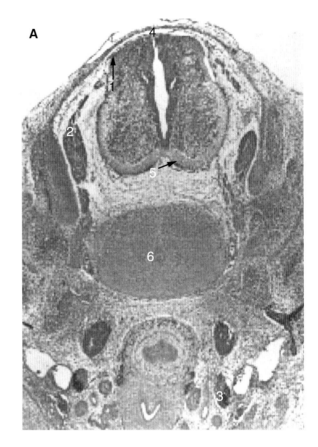

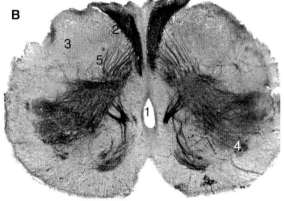

Fig. 3.22B
Cervical spinal cord (C5/6) of an 11 week fetus stained for parvalbumin (PV) to show those neurons that are highly electrically active due to the arrival or maturation of afferent inputs. ×40

1 Central canal
2 Dorsal funiculus
3 Dorsal horn
4 Motor neuron pools
5 Proprioreceptive axons

Dr. G. Clowry UN

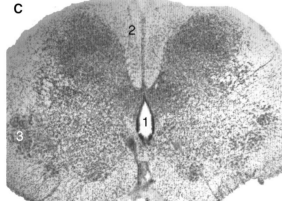

Fig. 3.22C
Cervical spinal cord (C5/6) of an 11 week fetus stained for cresyl violet. Larger cells are clearly present in the motor columns. ×44

1 Central canal
2 Dorsal columns
3 Motor columns

Dr. G. Clowry UN

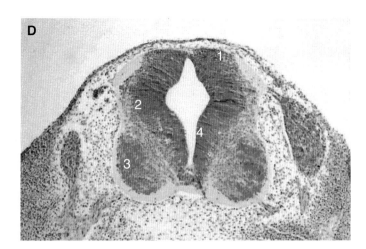

Fig. 3.22D
Human embryo aged 5 weeks. Transverse section of spinal cord immunostained with primary bcl-2 antibody. The presence of bcl-2 protein is indicated by the brown coloring in the cells' cytoplasm. ×45

1 Dorsal gray horn
2 Mantle zone
3 Ventral gray horn
4 Ventricular zone

Dr. K. Vilović US

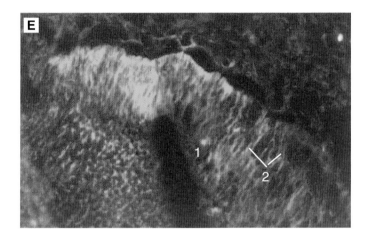

Fig. 3.22E
Cross-section of the ventral half of the spinal cord in a 7 week embryo. Intense vimentin immunostaining characterizes all layers of the spinal cord. ×250

1 Neuroepithelial cells
2 Radial glia

Professor. M. Saraga-Babić US

Summary

1. The brain and spinal cord develop from the early neural tube.
2. Three areas of brain form, which subdivide to form five main regions.
3. Brain flexures in Week 3 establish the shape of the brain.
4. The lumen of the early neural tube is retained in the brain as the ventricles.
5. Choroid plexus forms in the lateral, third and fourth ventricles.
6. The corpus striatum develops in the floor of each lateral ventricle.
7. Four layers of cerebral cortex form in the embryonic CNS.
8. The cerebellum forms from cells of the metencephalon.
9. The cranial nerves I–XII develop in weeks 5–6.
10. Meninges form from mesoderm around the neural tube.
11. The early spinal cord occupies the length of the spinal column. With development, it moves relative to the vertebral column.
12. During development, there are changing patterns of expression of various proteins.

Late Fetal and Early Postnatal Brain Development

Growth

The brain is the fastest growing organ in the fetus and infant. On average, it accounts for 12% of the body weight at birth, falling to around 2% in adults. Its growth is so rapid that it reaches 90% of its adult size by the age of 6 years. The growth rate of each part of the brain is different, so that its proportions change as development progresses. For example, the brainstem grows fastest in mid-gestation, followed by the cerebellum, and finally the cerebral hemispheres, which grow fastest after 32 weeks gestation. By 20 weeks post-conception, we have our full complement of neuronal cell bodies. The great increase in size that takes place after that date is due to the development of axons, dendrites and synapses, to the myelination of nerve fibers and to the continued formation of glial cells.

Maturation of the Cerebral Cortex

The cerebral cortex is recognizable as a distinct surface layer in the forebrain as early as 8 weeks' post-conception. By 26 weeks, it has its characteristic six-layered histological structure. At birth, it is half its adult thickness. New progenitor cells for neurons and glia migrate into the cortex from a layer known as the germinal matrix in the walls of the lateral ventricles. By 32 weeks, migration is complete and the germinal matrix disappears. A small number of undifferentiated stem cells remain in the hippocampus, along the boundaries of the dentate gyrus.

In early development, the surface of the cerebral hemisphere is smooth. Later, gyri and sulci form in an orderly sequence. When they first appear, the gyri are shallow folds and the sulci are straight, unbranched, broad and shallow grooves. The sulci gradually become deeper. The gyri become narrower and convoluted, finally branching to form secondary and tertiary gyri. The sulci also undergo branching. The lateral and central sulci are the first to appear prenatally, at 15 and 20 weeks, respectively. At around week 32, well-defined folds and some branching are present in the future primary motor and sensory cortex around the central sulcus. This is also true in the future visual areas on the medial side of the occipital lobe. After 30 weeks, the gyri develop on the lateral sides of the occipital lobes, on the parietal lobes behind the postcentral gyrus and on the posterior part of the temporal lobes. The last areas of the cortex to form are the frontal and temporal poles. There, sulcus formation starts after 32 weeks and continues after birth.

Connections and Functional Systems

Developing brain function depends on the formation and maturation of functionally specific areas in the brain and the connections between them. The first movements can be seen by ultrasound at 8 weeks, but they are too small to be felt by the mother until around 17 weeks, a process known as "quickening". They are probably involuntary at this stage because motor pathways from higher brain centers are not connected. Some aspects of sensory function are also present in the fetus well before term. Taste buds are histologically differentiated at 13 weeks, and a premature baby as young as 23 weeks will respond by pulling faces if a bitter-tasting substance is placed on its tongue.

At 5 months' gestation, the adult structure of the inner ear is established. Fetuses of this age will respond to sounds (such as music) by movements that can be seen by ultrasound and felt by the mother. Although the retina and visual pathway are not fully differentiated even at birth, fetuses respond to light at 26 weeks.

Touch receptors in the skin are present and connected to the dorsal horn of the spinal cord at 14 weeks. Ascending tracts to the developing thalamus and cerebral cortex are present at around 20 weeks' gestation.

Myelination

Fully functional maturation of the developing nervous system depends on the myelination of nerve fibers. Myelination increases the speed of impulse conduction. This is a gradual process, with some pathways continuing to myelinate well into childhood.

Myelination takes place in functional systems rather than topographical areas. In general, it occurs first, prenatally, in the brainstem and spinal cord, followed by the cerebellum, basal ganglia and thalamus. After birth, the connections to the motor and sensory cortex of the cerebral hemispheres are the first to myelinate. Connections to the cortex of the temporal lobe are the last to myelinate.

The auditory pathway myelinates slowly, between 6 months of prenatal life and 4 years postnatally. This process may parallel the progressive development of language.

The visual pathway is unmyelinated at birth, but matures rapidly afterwards. Myelin is first histologically detectable on the optic nerve at 10 weeks after birth, but not complete until about 18 months.

The development of motor pathways parallels the infant's acquisition of movement control. Sucking and swallowing movements begin prenatally and are well-developed by birth, because the cranial nerves and the pathways that control these movements are already myelinated.

The hands of a newborn baby show strong reflex grasping movements. Babies can move their arms, touch and hold objects before they can stand or walk. In the motor cortex, mature neurons appear in the areas controlling movements of the upper limb at around 1 month postnatally, but not until about 3 months for the lower limb.

Voluntary control of the anal and urethral sphincters can take as long as 18 months to appear, because of the slow myelination of the motor pathways regulating their contraction. Before this stage, the infant is incapable of continence.

Figures 3.23–3.38 were provided by Dr. M. A. Rutherford ICSM

Figures 3.23–3.26 MRI images, T2 weighting, of the brain of a premature neonate, 25 weeks gestational age, showing the early stages of cortical folding and myelination. The same labeling applies to all images in this sequence.

Fig 3.23
Parasagittal sections. **B** is closer to the midline than **A**.

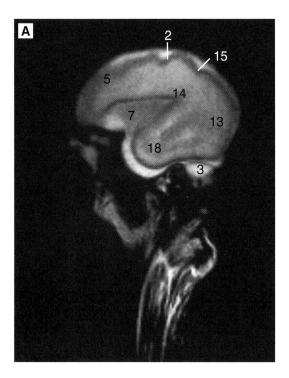
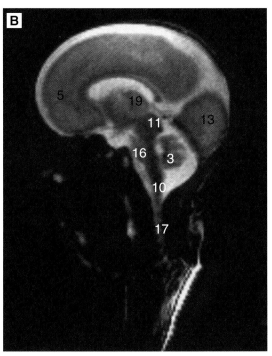

● *Brain maturation in premature neonates can be monitored by MRI scanning. Severe brain damage, such as hemorrhage due to injury at birth, may delay gyral development.*

● *In some autistic children, the brain grows faster than normal during infancy, reaching adult size by the age of 4 or 5 years.*

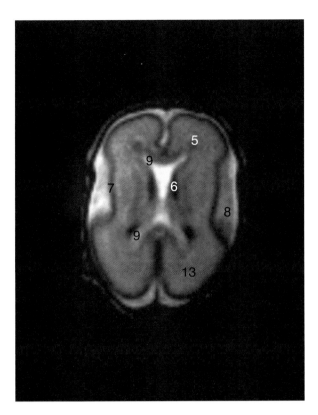

Fig. 3.24
Horizontal section through the cerebral hemispheres.

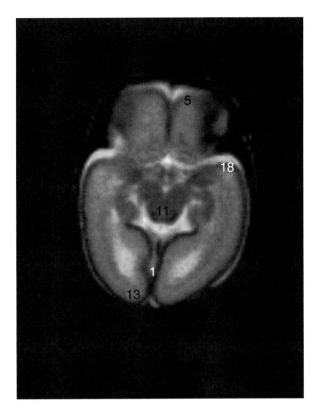

Fig. 3.25
Horizontal section at the level of the midbrain.

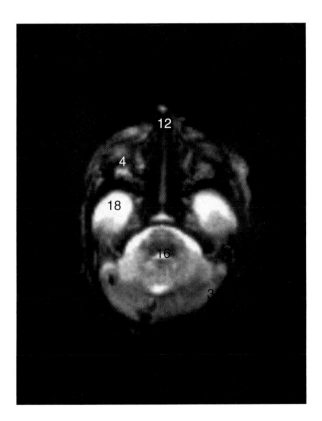

Fig. 3.26
Horizontal section through the cerebellum and lower pons. New areas of myelination appear dark in this view.

1	Calcarine sulcus	**11**	Midbrain
2	Central sulcus	**12**	Nose
3	Cerebellum	**13**	Occipital lobe
4	Eye	**14**	Parietal lobe
5	Frontal lobe	**15**	Parieto-occipital sulcus
6	Germinal matrix	**16**	Pons
7	Insula	**17**	Spinal cord
8	Lateral sulcus	**18**	Temporal lobe
9	Lateral ventricle	**19**	Thalamus
10	Medulla oblongata		

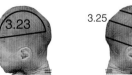
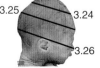

Profile views of the head of a 24 week fetus. From M. A. England (1996) *Life Before Birth* (Mosby, London), to show planes of sectioning in Figures 3.23–3.26.

Figures 3.27–3.29 Series of MRI images illustrating the progress of cortical folding and myelination in the late fetal and neonatal periods. The same labeling applies to all images in this sequence.

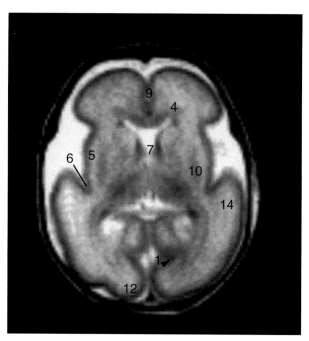

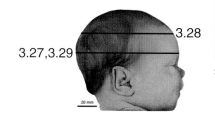

Profile view of the head of a neonate. From M. A. England (1996) *Life Before Birth* (Mosby, London), to show planes of sectioning in Figures 3.27–3.29.

1 Calcarine sulcus
2 Caudate nucleus
3 Central sulcus
4 Frontal lobe
5 Insula
6 Lateral sulcus
7 Lateral ventricle
8 Lentiform nucleus
9 Longitudinal fissure
10 Myelination in corona radiata
11 Myelination in internal capsule
12 Occipital lobe
13 Parietal lobe
14 Temporal lobe
15 Thalamus

Fig. 3.27
Horizontal T2 weighted scan of the brain of a premature infant of 30 weeks gestational age.

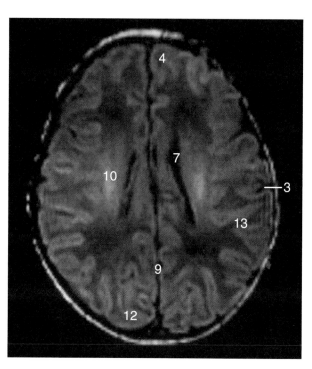

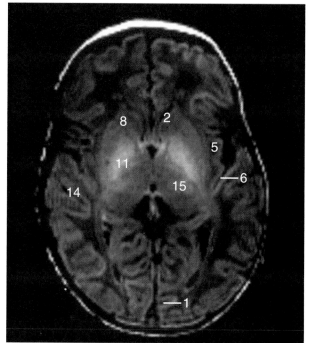

Figs 3.28 and 3.29
Horizontal T1 weighted images of the brain of a full term infant.

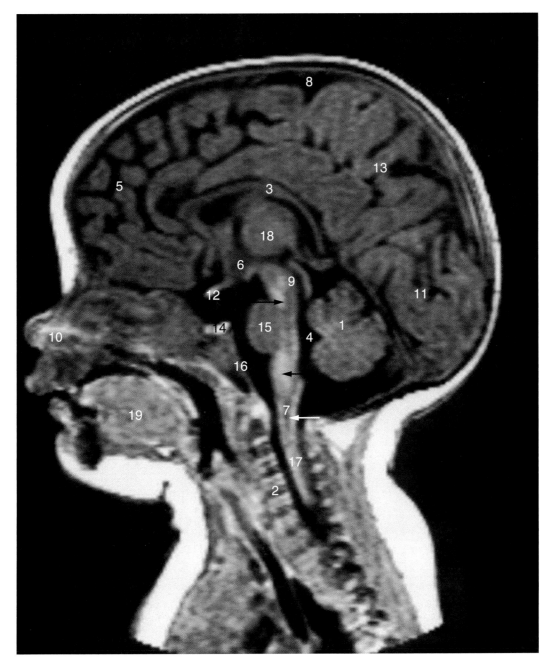

Fig. 3.30
T1 weighted MRI scan of a 2 month old infant's head, showing the development of gyri and sulci and myelination in the brainstem and optic tract. Newly myelinated white matter appears whiter than surrounding nervous tissue. It can be seen in the optic tract and also as areas (arrowed) in the brainstem. Some non-nervous tissues, e.g. fibrous tissue, may also appear white in a T1 scan because of their low water content.

1 Cerebellum	8 Meninges	14 Pituitary fossa
2 Cervical vertebrae	9 Midbrain	15 Pons
3 Corpus callosum	10 Nose	16 Sphenoid bone
4 Fourth ventricle	11 Occipital lobe	17 Spinal cord
5 Frontal lobe	12 Optic tract	18 Thalamus
6 Hypothalamus	13 Parietal lobe	19 Tongue
7 Medulla oblongata		

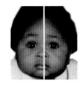

Figures 3.31–3.33 Horizontal T1 weighted MRI scans of the brain of a 6 month old infant. The development of the basal ganglia, thalamus and brainstem, and the myelination of white matter in the cerebral hemisphere and brainstem, are shown. Newly myelinated areas appear white in this view. These figures share the same labeling.

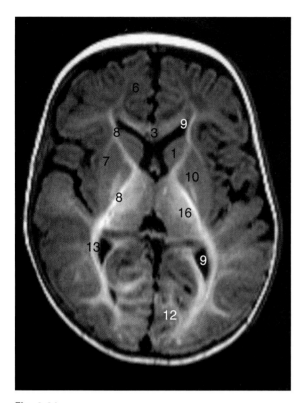

Fig. 3.31

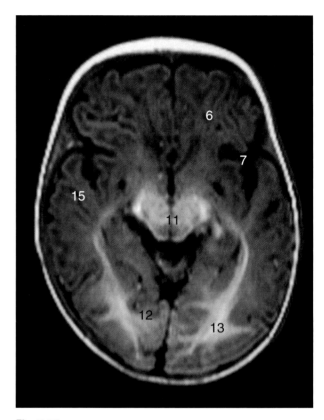

Fig. 3.32

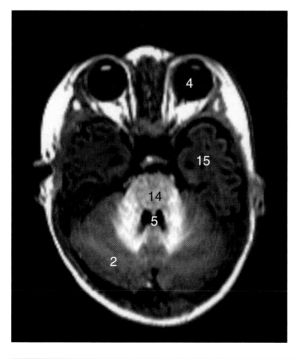

Fig. 3.33

1	Caudate nucleus	**9**	Lateral ventricle
2	Cerebellum	**10**	Lentiform nucleus
3	Corpus callosum	**11**	Midbrain
4	Eye	**12**	Occipital lobe
5	Fourth ventricle	**13**	Optic radiation
6	Frontal lobe	**14**	Pons
7	Insula	**15**	Temporal lobe
8	Internal capsule	**16**	Thalamus

Figures 3.34–3.38 T1 weighted MRI images of a 1 year old infant's head. The cerebral cortex has deep gyri, some of which are branched. Newly myelinated white matter appears whiter than surrounding nervous tissue. It can be seen throughout the corpus callosum, and also as areas (arrowed) in the fornix, diencephalon, optic nerve, brainstem, spinal cord and the arbor vitae of the cerebellum. Some non-nervous tissues, e.g. fibrous tissue, may also appear white in a T1 scan because of their low water content. The dark area in the center of the cerebral hemisphere is an artifact, caused by the plane of section of the scan just grazing the surface of the gyri. The same labeling applies to all images in this sequence.

Fig. 3.34
Sagittal section.

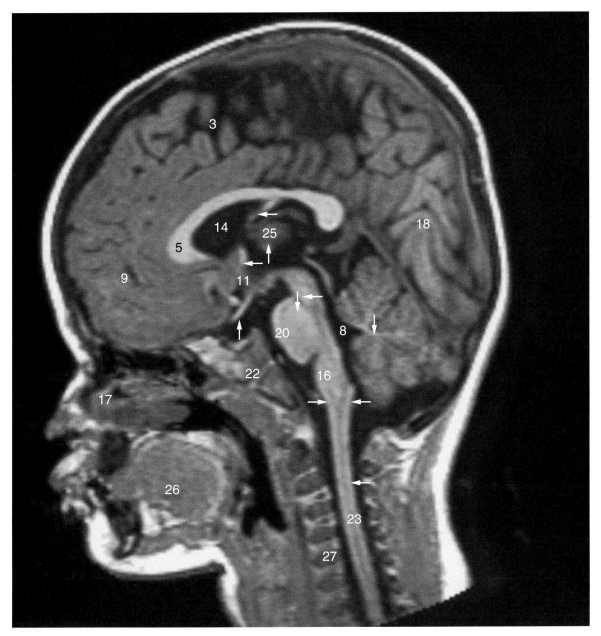

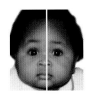

Figures 3.35–3.38 T1 weighted MRI images of the brain of a 1 year old infant. The cerebral cortex has deep gyri, some of which are branched. New myelin (white) can be seen throughout the cerebral white matter and in the cerebellum and brainstem.

Figs 3.35–3.38
Horizontal sections.

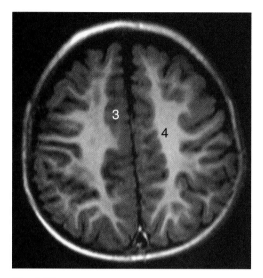

Fig. 3.35

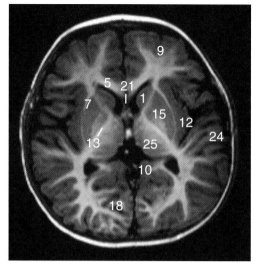

Fig. 3.36

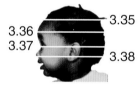

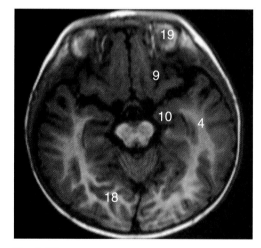

Fig. 3.37

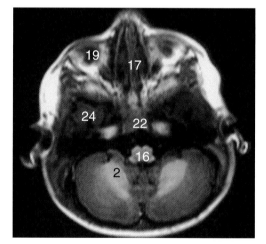

Fig. 3.38

1	Caudate nucleus	7	External capsule	14	Lateral ventricle	21	Septum pellucidum
2	Cerebellum (myelination)	8	Fourth ventricle	15	Lentiform nucleus	22	Sphenoid bone
3	Cerebral cortex	9	Frontal lobe	16	Medulla oblongata	23	Spinal cord
4	Cerebral white matter (myelination)	10	Hippocampus	17	Nose	24	Temporal lobe
5	Corpus callosum	11	Hypothalamus	18	Occipital lobe	25	Thalamus
6	Ear	12	Insula	19	Orbit	26	Tongue
		13	Internal capsule	20	Pons	27	Vertebral column

Dr M. Rutherford ICSM

Summary

1. The brain grows very rapidly during late fetal and postnatal life.
2. New cells are formed and also connections between them.
3. Myelination is a gradual process occurring prenatally and postnatally, following functional systems rather than topographical areas.
4. MRI can record the progress of brain development and maturation.

4 Cranial Cavity

The brain lies within the cranial cavity of the skull and is continuous with the spinal cord lying within the vertebral canal. The cranial cavity is an almost completely enclosed space. The only openings are the large foramen magnum in the base and several smaller foramina, which provide passages for vessels and nerves. The floor of the cranial cavity is divided into three regions separated by two descending steps.

These regions are the anterior, middle and posterior cranial fossae. The brain and spinal cord are covered with three protective layers called the meninges (see Meninges, p. 59). The outer layer, the dura mater, forms folds that project into the cranial cavity and divide it into compartments. The folds are the falx cerebri and the tentorium cerebelli.

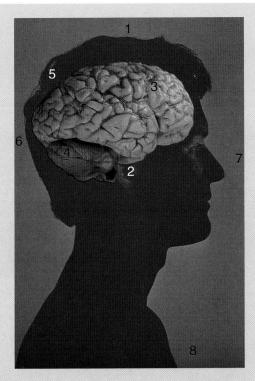

Fig. 4.1
Position of the brain *in situ* (viewed from the right side). ×0.27

1 Dorsal or superior	5 Hair
2 External acoustic meatus	6 Posterior
3 Cerebral hemisphere	7 Rostral or anterior
4 Cerebellum	8 Ventral or inferior

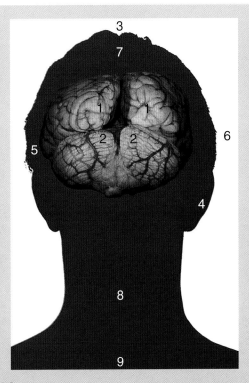

Fig. 4.2
Position of the brain *in situ* (viewed from the back). ×0.34

1 Cerebral hemisphere	6 Lateral
2 Cerebellum	7 Medial
3 Dorsal or superior	8 Neck
4 Ear	9 Ventral or inferior
5 Hair	

- *If there is swelling (edema) of the brain, excess fluid accumulation in the ventricles (hydrocephalus) or any abnormality that occupies space inside the cranial cavity, such as a tumor, the adult skull cannot expand to accommodate the extra volume. This can lead to a rise in the intracranial pressure.*

- *If the intracranial pressure rises, parts of the brain may be displaced (herniated) from one compartment to another in the cranial cavity and be compressed and damaged. The cerebellum can be pushed out through the foramen magnum, a process known as "coning".*

- *In Paget's disease there is widespread thickening of bones, including the skull. As the foramina of the skull base become constricted, the cranial nerves can be compressed and their functions impaired.*

Fig. 4.3
A transilluminated view of the base of the skull (internal aspect). ×0.6

1 Anterior cranial fossa
2 Body of sphenoid bone
3 Carotid canal
4 Foramen magnum
5 Frontal bone
6 Middle cranial fossa
7 Occipital bone
8 Parietal bone
9 Petrous temporal bone
10 Posterior cranial fossa

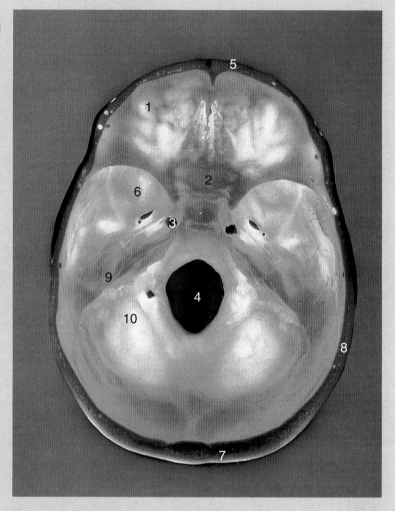

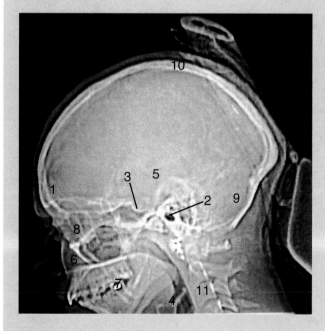

Fig. 4.4
Sagittal radiographic image electronically reconstructed from computed tomography (CT) scans to show the cranial cavity in relation to the external features of the head.

1 Anterior cranial fossa
2 External auditory meatus
3 Hypophyseal fossa
4 Larynx
5 Middle cranial fossa
6 Nasal cavity
7 Oral cavity
8 Orbit
9 Posterior cranial fossa
10 Skull vault
11 Vertebral column

Elscint Ltd

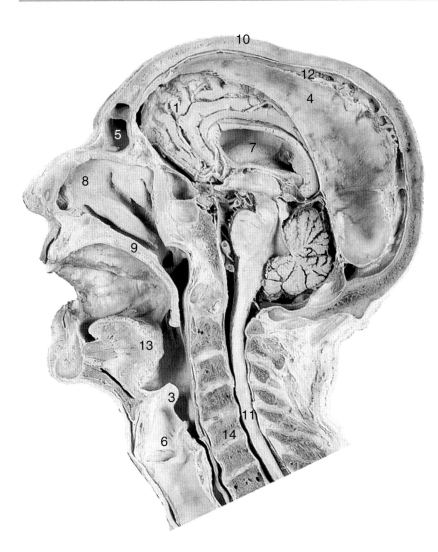

Fig. 4.5
The brain and meninges within the cranial cavity. The right half of a sagittal section. ×0.49

1 Cerebral hemisphere
2 Cerebellum
3 Epiglottis
4 Falx cerebri
5 Frontal sinus
6 Larynx
7 Lateral ventricle
8 Nasal cavity
9 Palate (hard)
10 Skull
11 Spinal cord
12 Superior sagittal sinus
13 Tongue
14 Vertebral column

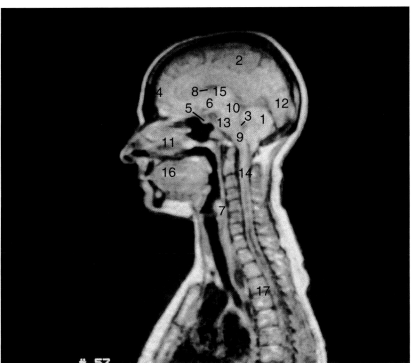

Fig. 4.6
Nuclear magnetic resonance (NMR) image of a sagittal section through the head and neck.

1 Cerebellum
2 Cerebral hemisphere
3 Fourth ventricle
4 Frontal lobe
5 Hypophysis
6 Hypothalamus
7 Larynx
8 Lateral ventricle
9 Medulla oblongata
10 Midbrain
11 Nasal cavity
12 Occipital lobe
13 Pons
14 Spinal cord
15 Thalamus
16 Tongue
17 Vertebral column

Elscint Ltd

5 External Features of the Brain

The major regions of the brain are based upon their position in the skull.

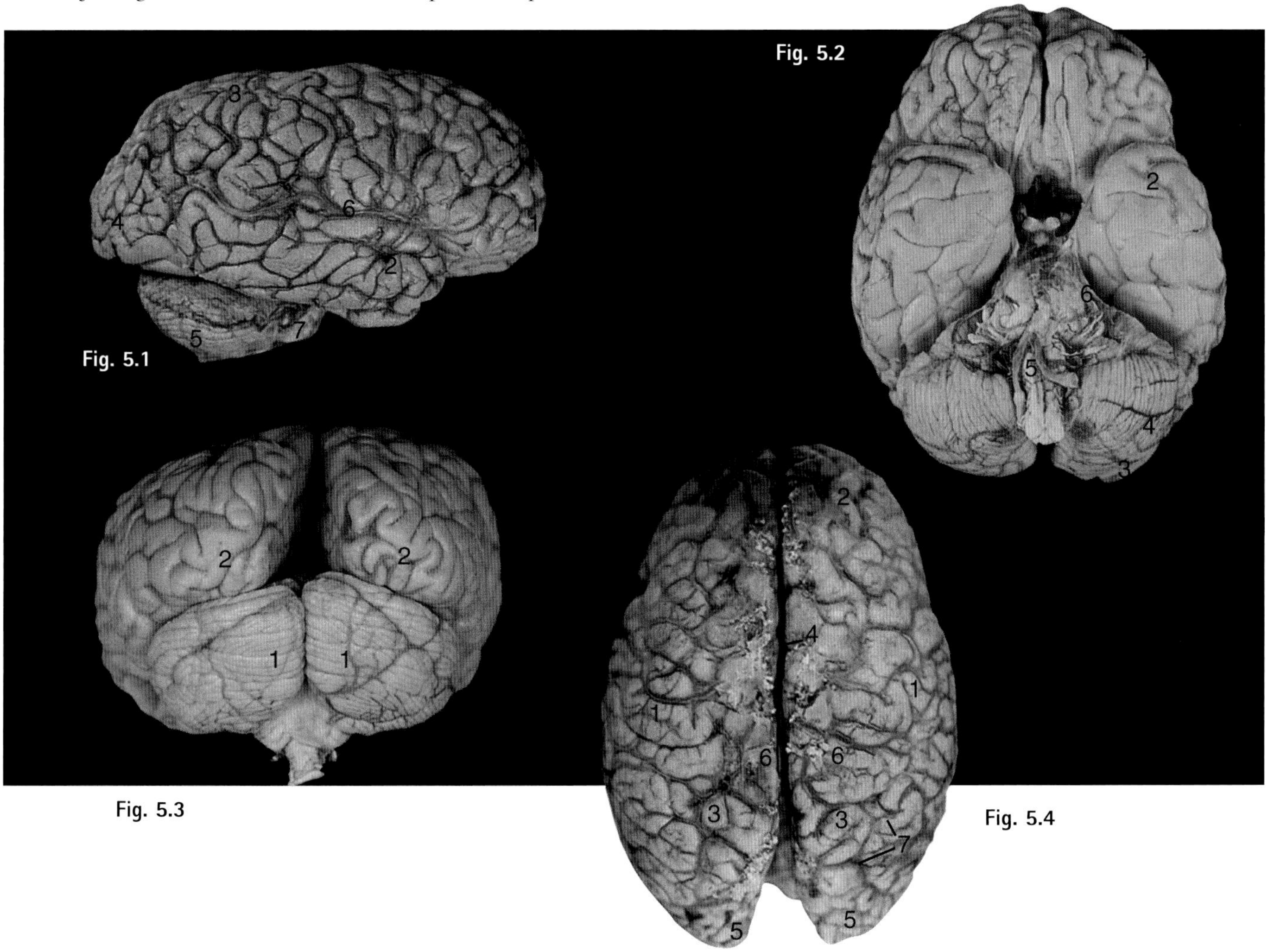

Fig. 5.2

Fig. 5.1

Fig. 5.3

Fig. 5.4

Fig. 5.1
The brain viewed from the right side with the arachnoid mater. ×0.39

1 Frontal pole	5 Cerebellar
2 Temporal lobe } Cerebral	hemisphere
3 Parietal lobe } hemisphere	6 Lateral sulcus
4 Occipital lobe	7 Medulla oblongata

Fig. 5.2
The base of the brain viewed from below. Most of the arachnoid mater and minor blood vessels have been removed. ×0.46

1 Frontal lobe } Cerebral	4 Cerebellar hemisphere
2 Temporal lobe } hemisphere	5 Medulla oblongata
3 Occipital pole	6 Pons

● *Lobe refers to an entire area, while pole refers to its extremity.*

Fig. 5.3
The back (posterior poles) of the cerebral hemispheres and cerebellum. ×0.39

1 Cerebellar hemisphere
2 Occipital lobe of cerebral hemisphere

Fig. 5.4
The brain viewed from above. ×0.46

1 Cerebral hemisphere
2 Frontal lobe of cerebral hemisphere
3 Gyri
4 Longitudinal fissure
5 Occipital lobe of cerebral hemisphere
6 Parietal lobe of cerebral hemisphere
7 Sulci

6 Internal Features of the Brain

Most brainstem structures are not visible externally. They can be seen in a sagittal section.

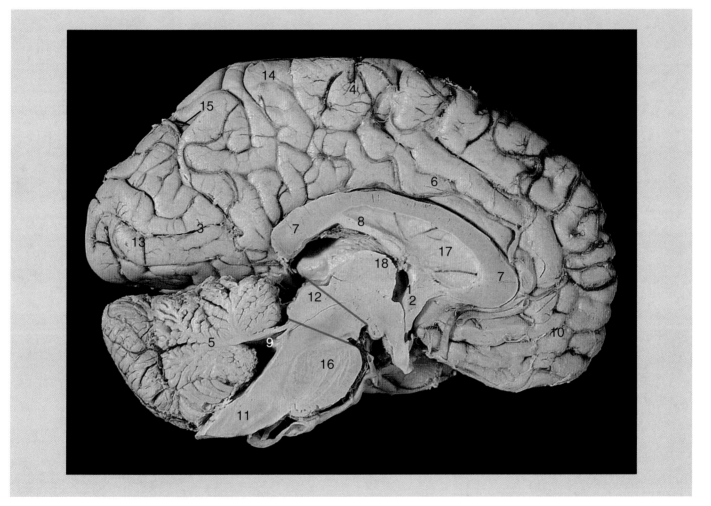

Fig. 6.1
A mid-sagittal section of the brain. ×1.1

1	Anterior column of the fornix	**6**	Cingulate gyrus	**11**	Medulla oblongata
2	Anterior commissure	**7**	Corpus callosum	**12**	Midbrain tectum*
3	Calcarine sulcus	**8**	Fornix (body)	**13**	Occipital lobe
4	Central sulcus	**9**	Fourth ventricle	**14**	Parietal lobe
5	Cerebellum	**10**	Frontal lobe	**15**	Parieto-occipital sulcus

16 Pons
17 Septum pellucidum
18 Thalamus

* The red box outlines the midbrain

- *The pineal gland and the cerebral aqueduct (of Sylvius) are not shown on this specimen (see Cerebral Hemispheres, Figure 10.3, p. 106).*

- *The brainstem comprises the midbrain, pons and medulla oblongata.*

- *The terms "medulla oblongata" and the commonly used shortened form "medulla" may be used interchangeably.*

- *The fornix and the corpus callosum are arched in shape, and their different parts have different names. The corpus callosum consists of the genu, body and splenium; the fornix comprises the columns and the body. For a more detailed nomenclature see the individual regions.*

7 Meninges

The brain and spinal cord are protected by three membranes called the meninges. The outermost is the dura mater, the middle one the arachnoid mater, and the inner one next to the nervous tissue is the pia mater. These layers have a protective function; they enclose the central nervous system and anchor it against sudden movements. They also enclose the cerebrospinal fluid, which forms a fluid cushion to protect the brain from trauma and is an intermediary in the exchange of substances between the brain and the rest of the body. The arachnoid mater is an important component of the blood–brain barrier (see p. 90), by means of which an optimal environment is created and maintained for the cells of the central nervous system.

The cranial dura mater is a double layer of tough connective tissue. Its outer layer adheres to the bones of the skull and forms their periosteum. Its inner layer, the true dura mater, lines the skull and forms sheets of tissue that dip between the cerebral hemispheres (falx cerebri), between the cerebellar hemispheres (falx cerebelli) and between the cerebellum and the cerebrum (tentorium cerebelli). At the origin of these folds and at the suture lines, the outer layer of the dura mater is particularly strongly attached to the skull. The dura mater forms a pathway for the cranial venous sinuses. There is no periosteal layer in the dura mater around the spinal cord; only the true dura mater is present.

The arachnoid mater is composed of connective tissue with flat interdigitating cells on its surface. A narrow potential space, the subdural space, lies between the arachnoid and the dura mater. It contains veins and a little serous lubricating fluid. A wider space, the subarachnoid space, separates the arachnoid from the pia mater. It is crossed by connections, the arachnoid trabeculations, which run between the arachnoid mater and the pia mater. It contains the arteries and veins of the brain and spinal cord, and the cerebrospinal fluid. The subarachnoid space is sealed off by the interdigitations and tight junctions between the cells on the arachnoid surface known as mesothelial cells. In the region of the superior sagittal sinus (see Veins, p. 82), the arachnoid mater projects through small openings in the dura mater. These projections are known as arachnoid villi. If they calcify in old age they resemble granules (arachnoid granulations). Their function is to return cerebrospinal fluid (CSF) to the blood in the superior sagittal sinus in the process of CSF circulation.

The pia mater is very thin and rich in capillaries. It is attached to the brain, closely following the contours of its folds (gyri) and fissures (sulci). It is also closely bound to the spinal cord. Additionally, the spinal pia mater forms an anchoring sheet, the denticulate ligament. Within the brain, the tela choroidea are thin areas in the roof of the third and fourth ventricles and the wall of the lateral ventricles. They consist of an adherent layer of pia mater and ependyma, and give rise to the choroid plexus.

All three layers of the meninges are continuous with the coverings of the spinal and cranial nerves. Exceptionally, the coverings of the optic nerve include an extension of the subarachnoid space.

The sensory innervation of the cranial meninges comes mainly from the mandibular division of the trigeminal nerve. These nerves are particularly sensitive to movement, and produce sensations of pain. This may explain why headaches of intracranial origin, such as migraine, are aggravated by movement.

- *The arachnoid and pia mater are collectively referred to as leptomeninges.*

- *Blood hemorrhaging between the dura mater and the skull forms an epidural (extradural) hematoma. Blood hemorrhaging between the dura mater and arachnoid mater forms a subdural hematoma, while hemorrhaging below the arachnoid is a subarachnoid hemorrhage. In a subarachnoid hemorrhage, the CSF is bloodstained, while in extradural and subdural hemorrhage it is not bloodstained.*

- *An epidural or extradural space is normally found around the spinal cord. It contains fat and veins (the epidural venous plexus) which drain the marrow spaces of the vertebral bodies and empties into the segmental veins.*

- *Meningitis is an infection of the meninges. Usually the arachnoid and pia mater are involved (leptomeningitis).*

Figures 7.1–7.3 show the dura mater and its blood supply.

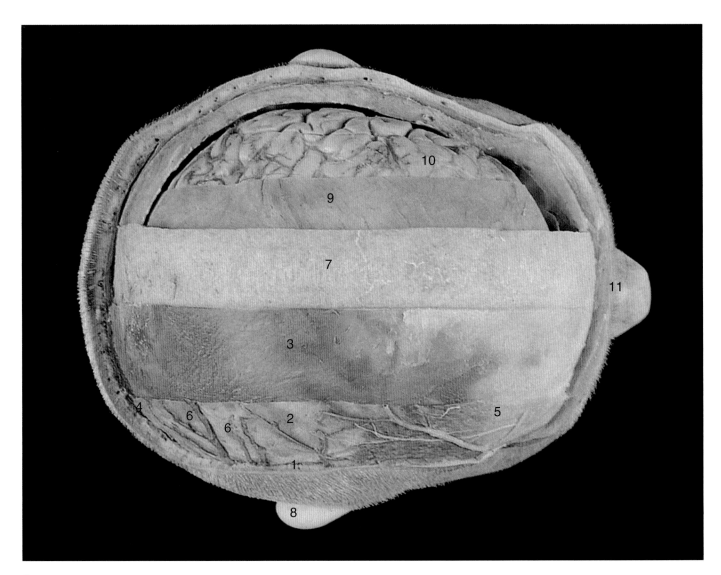

Fig. 7.1
Layered dissection of the scalp, cranial vault and its coverings viewed from above. ×0.83

1 Skin and dense subcutaneous tissue	**7** Cranial vault bone
2 Epicranial aponeurosis	**8** External ear
3 Loose connective tissue and pericranium	**9** Dura mater
4 Occipital belly of occipitofrontalis muscle	**10** Pia-arachnoid mater
5 Frontal belly of occipitofrontalis muscle	**11** Nose
6 Branches of superficial temporal artery	

1–3 } Five layers of scalp

9–10 } Meninges

Dissection by Bari M. Logan

● *Acute bacterial meningitis is a serious infection mainly affecting young people. Clusters of cases can occur in close communities such as schools and colleges. Mortality is high, ranging from 5% to 30%, often with serious consequences in those who do recover.*

Figures 7.2 and 7.3 are coronal sections through the skull and meninges.

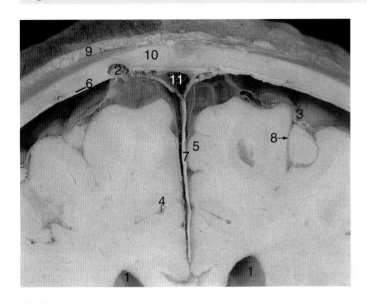

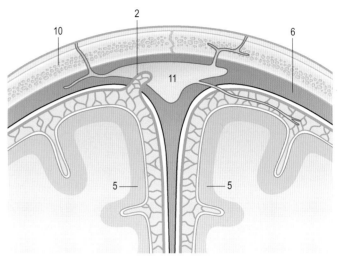

A diagram of a coronal section through the superior sagittal sinus.

Prof. G. Matsumura KUT

Fig. 7.2
A coronal section through the superior sagittal sinus. ×1.15

1	Anterior horns of lateral ventricles
2	Arachnoid granulation (villus)
3	Arachnoid mater
4	Blood vessel
5	Cerebral cortex
6	Dura mater
7	Falx cerebri
8	Pia mater (arrow)
9	Scalp (with hair roots)
10	Skull bone
11	Superior sagittal sinus

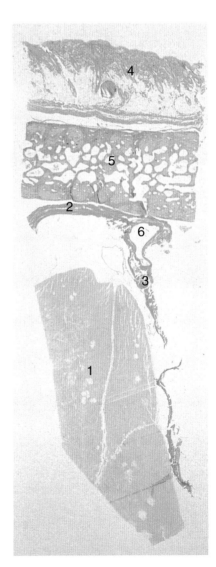

Fig. 7.3
Coronal section of the skull and meninges. Orange G and light green stain. ×4.4

1 Cerebral hemisphere
2 Dura mater
3 Falx cerebri
4 Scalp (with hair roots)
5 Skull bone
6 Superior sagittal sinus

Figures 7.4–7.7 Histological sections of the meninges.

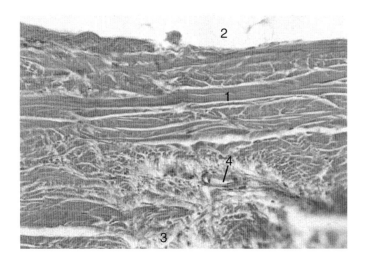

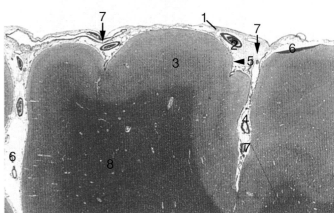

Fig. 7.4

The dura mater is composed of numerous collagen bundles. It has a rich sensory innervation. Hematoxylin and eosin stain. ×322

1 Collagen bundles
2 External aspect
3 Internal aspect
4 Small blood vessel

Fig. 7.5

Histological section showing the arachnoid mater bridging the sulci of the cerebral hemisphere. Stained with phosphotungstic acid and hematoxylin. ×4.6

1 Arachnoid mater
2 Blood vessel
3 Cerebral cortex
4 Gyri
5 Pia mater (arrowhead)
6 Subarachnoid space
7 Sulcus (bold arrows)
8 White matter

- *The outer layer of the dura mater shares a rich blood supply with the skull bones. The inner layer is more fibrous and has few blood vessels.*

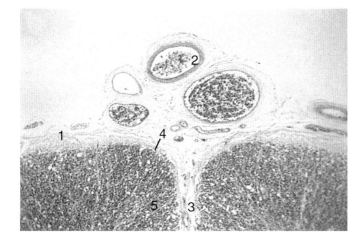

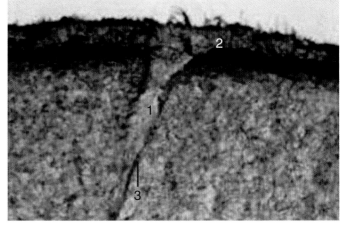

Fig. 7.6

Histological section showing the leptomeninges (the arachnoid and pia maters) investing the spinal cord. Weigert-Pal stain. ×66

1 Arachnoid mater
2 Blood vessel
3 Median fissure (of spinal cord)
4 Pia mater
5 White matter (of spinal cord)

Fig. 7.7

Histological section of the surface of the superior colliculus showing a prolongation of pia mater covering a vessel entering brain tissue. GFAP stain. ×250

1 Blood vessel
2 Pia mater
3 Prolongation of pia mater

Dr. H. Hilbig UL

Figures 7.8–7.18 Specializations of the meninges.

Figures 7.8 and 7.9 Specializations of the dura mater.

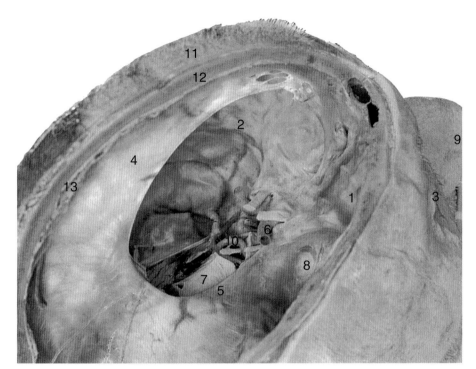

Fig. 7.8
Cranial cavity viewed from the right side and above, with the falx cerebri and tentorium cerebelli. The midbrain is *in situ*. ×0.75

  1 Anterior cranial fossa
  2 Branches of middle meningeal artery
  3 Eyelid
  4 Falx cerebri
  5 Free margin of tentorium cerebelli
  6 Internal carotid artery
  7 Midbrain
  8 Middle cranial fossa
  9 Nose
10 Posterior cerebral artery
11 Scalp
12 Skull bone
13 Superior sagittal sinus

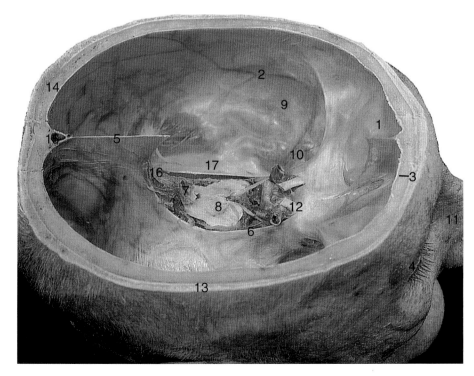

Fig. 7.9
The interior of the cranial cavity viewed from above to display the arrangement of the dura mater. Both cerebral hemispheres have been removed and the brainstem severed through the midbrain. ×0.6

  1 Anterior cranial fossa
  2 Branches of middle meningeal artery
  3 Dura mater
  4 Eyelid
  5 Falx cerebri
  6 Free edge of tentorium cerebelli
  7 Great vein (of Galen)
  8 Midbrain
  9 Middle cranial fossa
10 Middle meningeal artery
11 Nose
12 Optic nerve
13 Scalp
14 Skull bone
15 Superior sagittal sinus
16 Tentorial notch
17 Tentorium cerebelli

Figures 7.10–7.13 Specializations of the arachnoid mater.

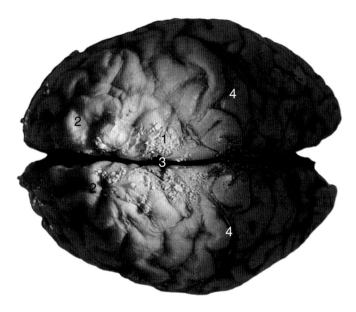

Fig. 7.10
Arachnoid granulations *in situ* on the parietal lobes of the cerebral hemispheres. ×0.57

1 Arachnoid granulations
2 Frontal lobes
3 Longitudinal cerebral fissure
4 Parietal lobes

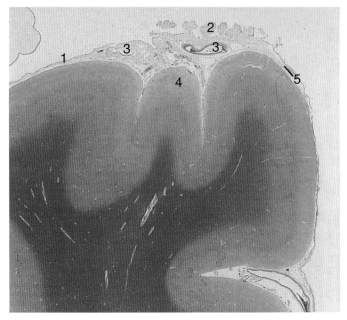

Fig. 7.11
Low-power view of a histological section showing an arachnoid granulation, stained with solochrome cyanin and nuclear fast red. ×3.3

1 Arachnoid mater	4 Cerebral cortex
2 Arachnoid granulation	5 Subarachnoid space
3 Blood vessels	

● *Arachnoid granulations consist of a group of arachnoid villi that project into the superior sagittal sinus or into venous lacunae, which drain into the sinus.*

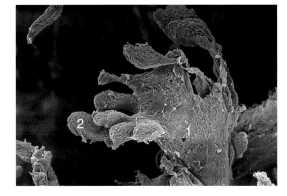

Fig. 7.12
Scanning electron micrograph showing the structure of an arachnoid granulation. ×28

1 Arachnoid granulation
2 Arachnoid villi   Mr. G. McTurk LU

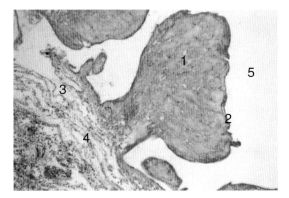

Fig. 7.13
High magnification photomicrograph illustrating the histology of an individual arachnoid villus. Hematoxylin and eosin stain. ×60

1 Arachnoid villus	4 Trabeculae
2 Mesothelial cells	5 Venous lacunae
3 Subarachnoid space	

Figures 7.14–7.17 Specializations of the pia mater (also see Ventricles, p. 93).

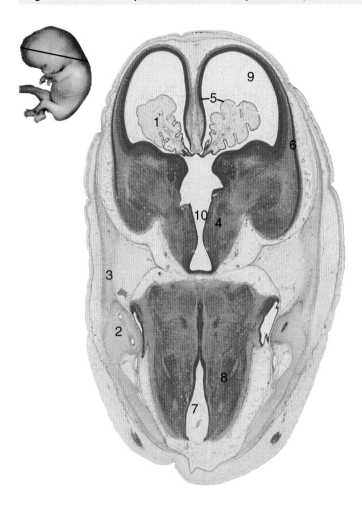

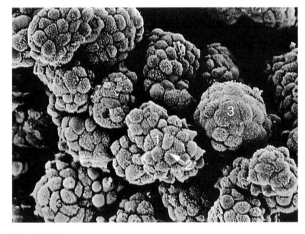

Fig. 7.14

The epithelium of the choroid plexus is a continuation of the ependymal lining of the ventricles, 27 mm CR embryo. Hematoxylin and eosin stain. ×8.45

1	Choroid plexus	6	Forebrain
2	Developing ear	7	Fourth ventricle
3	Developing skull	8	Hindbrain
4	Diencephalon	9	Lateral ventricle
5	Ependyma	10	Third ventricle MHMS

Fig. 7.16

A scanning electron micrograph showing the surface of the choroid plexus of the fourth ventricle that is bathed by cerebrospinal fluid. ×274

1	Epithelial cell	3	Villi of choroid plexus
2	Microvilli (arrow)		Mr. G .McTurk LU

- *In some cases the pia mater is so closely apposed to the underlying foot processes of the astrocytes that they are considered to be a single layer, the pia-glia.*

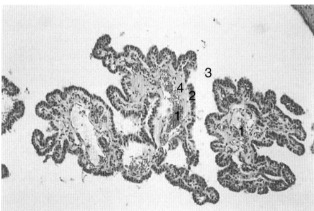

Fig. 7.15

A section of choroid plexus of the lateral ventricle. Hematoxylin and eosin stain. ×120

1 Blood vessels
2 Ependyma of choroid plexus
3 Interior of the lateral ventricle
4 Pia mater
* The line on the diagram indicates a plane of section similar to that of 7.15.

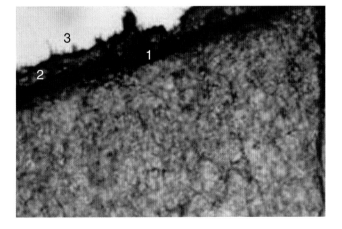

Fig. 7.17

Histological section of the superior colliculus showing the glia limitans. GFAP stain. ×250

1	Astrocyte layer	3	Subarachnoid space
2	Pia mater		Dr. H. Hilbig UL

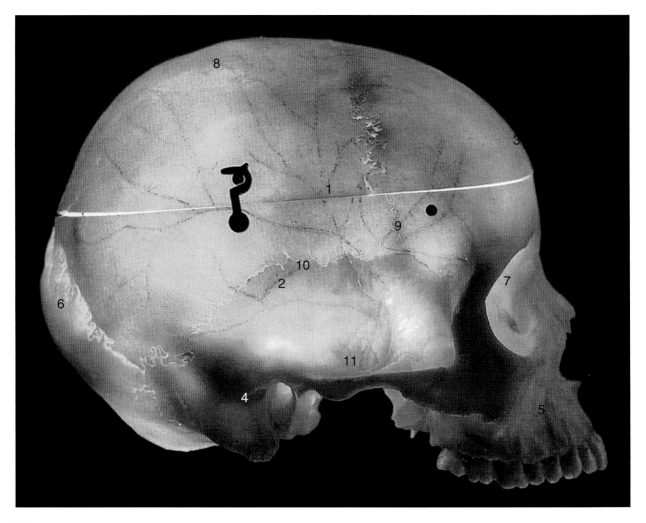

Fig. 7.18
A transilluminated adult skull illustrating the course of the middle meningeal artery in relation to the pterion. ×0.92

1 Course of the anterior branch of the middle meningeal artery and its branches
2 Course of the posterior branch of the middle meningeal artery and its branches
3 Frontal bone
4 Mastoid process
5 Maxilla
6 Occipital bone

7 Orbit
8 Parietal bone
9 Pterion
10 Squamous temporal bone
11 Zygomatic arch

Summary

1. The meninges are protective coverings of the brain and spinal cord.
2. They comprise three layers and the actual or potential spaces between them. From the outside inwards, these are the dura mater, the arachnoid mater and the pia mater.
3. The cranial dura mater is two-layered, with the venous sinuses running between the layers. In the vertebral column, the dura mater consists of one layer, and an extradural space exists between it and the bone.
4. The subarachnoid space lies between the arachnoid mater and the pia mater. It contains the cerebrospinal fluid (CSF), and the major arteries pass through it.
5. The pia mater adheres closely to the brain tissue.
6. The pia mater and arachnoid mater are continuous with the coverings of peripheral nerves.
7. Hemorrhage between the layers of the meninges can occur after head injury and may be fatal.
8. Meningitis is an infection of the meninges that can cause death or permanent disability.

8 Blood Supply to the Brain and Spinal Cord

Brain: Arteries

The brain is unable to store oxygen or glucose, but has a particularly high and constant demand for both. It receives 25% of the output of arterial blood from the heart. Brain tissue deprived of its blood supply quickly dies. The damaged and dying cells leak ions (particularly calcium) and neurotransmitters (especially glutamate) which cause further tissue damage.

1. The arteries of the brain fall into five main groups: Meningeal, ophthalmic and glandular branches;

2. Cortical branches to the surface of the brain, mostly supplying superficial gray matter;

3. Central (basal, nuclear or medullary) branches into the brain substance that supply fiber tracts and nuclear masses;

4. Choroidal branches to the choroid plexuses in the ventricles; and

5. Spinal branches.

The brain tissue is supplied by two pairs of arteries lying in the subarachnoid space: the internal carotid and the vertebral arteries. The vertebral arteries join to form the basilar artery.

These vessels, their branches and those of the other half of the brain are linked together by communicating arteries, in an anastomotic ring at the base of the brain called the arterial circle (circle of Willis). Large cortical branches (anterior, middle and posterior cerebral arteries), radiating from the circle, supply the surface and fine, penetrating branches, for example the striate arteries, supply the interior of the brain. The cerebral arteries anastomose on the surface of the cerebral hemispheres. Once arteries have penetrated the brain substance they become end arteries, communicating only at capillary level.

The brainstem and cerebellum are supplied by the basilar and vertebral arteries.

The most powerful cerebral vasodilator is carbon dioxide. During sleep there is normally cerebral vasodilation but no increase in blood flow during anxiety or intellectual activity.

A diagram showing the arterial circle (circle of Willis).

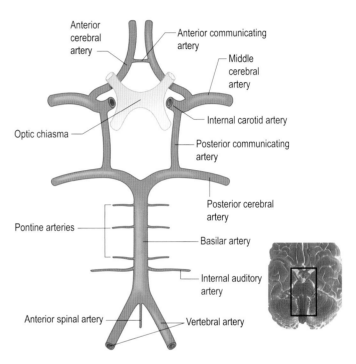

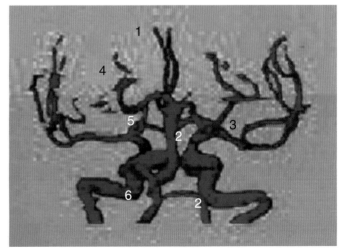

Fig. 8.1
Computer reconstruction of a combined MRI and angiogram showing a posterior view of the arterial circle of Willis.

1 Anterior cerebral artery
2 Internal carotid artery
3 Middle cerebral artery
4 Posterior cerebral artery
5 Posterior communicating artery
6 Vertebral artery

Prof. F. W. Zonneveld UUH

● A "stroke" or cerebrovascular accident (CVA) is a sudden loss of the blood supply to brain tissue, usually following occlusion of, or hemorrhage from, an artery. An infarct is an area of dead tissue resulting from loss of blood supply.

● Thomas Willis (1621–1675) was one of the founders of the Royal Society who made extensive studies of the human brain and its blood supply.

● The circle of Willis is a frequent site of aneurysm.

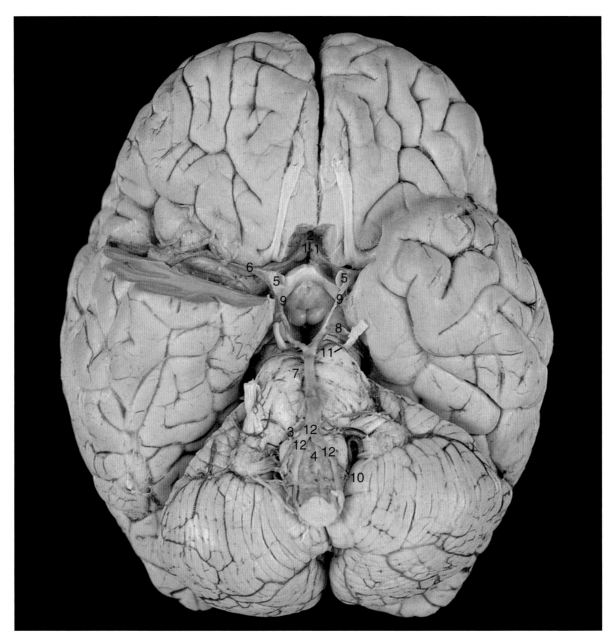

Fig. 8.2
The arterial circle (circle of Willis) on the base of the brain. ×1.05

1 Anterior cerebral artery	**7** Pontine branches of basilar artery
2 Anterior communicating artery	**8** Posterior cerebral artery
3 Anterior inferior cerebellar artery	**9** Posterior communicating artery
4 Anterior spinal artery	**10** Posterior inferior cerebellar artery
5 Internal carotid artery	**11** Superior cerebellar artery
6 Middle cerebral artery	**12** Vertebral arteries joining to form basilar artery

1 Meningeal, ophthalmic and glandular branches

The meningeal branches are illustrated in the chapter on Meninges (p. 59). The blood supply to the eye is illustrated in the section on the visual system (p. 241). The glandular branches (e.g. hypophysis [pituitary]) are not within the scope of this book.

Superior hypophyseal branches of the internal carotid artery supply capillary beds in the hypothalamus and hypophyseal stalk. These capillary networks drain into long and short portal veins along the hypophyseal stalk. The portal veins form a second bed of sinusoidal capillaries between the endocrine cells of the adenohypophysis (anterior lobe of the pituitary gland, see Diencephalon p. 141). These in turn drain into the cavernous sinus (see Veins p. 82). Inferior hypophyseal arteries from the internal carotid artery supply the neurohypophysis (posterior or neural lobe of the pituitary gland).

2 Cortical branches

The cortical branches of the cerebrum and cerebellum arise from larger vessels. They pass along the sulci to penetrate the gray matter. They are covered by a sleeve of pia mater.

Fig. 8.3
The superior cerebral arteries and veins supplying the substance of the hemispheres follow the gyri and sulci. ×1.15

1 Blood vessels	**4** Sulci
2 Corpus callosum	**5** Superior cerebral surface
3 Gyri	

Fig. 8.4
Carmine-injected blood vessels on the surface of the cerebellum giving off fine branches into the substance of the gray matter. *c.* 1860. ×5.6.

Wellcome Museum

Fig. 8.5
Carmine-injected specimen of the cerebral cortex to demonstrate that the gray matter has a richer blood supply than the white matter. *c.* 1860. ×5.6

1 Blood vessels	**4** Gray matter
2 Cerebellar cortex (Fig. 8.4 only)	**5** White matter
3 Cerebral cortex (Fig. 8.5 only)	

Wellcome Museum

Fig. 8.6
Scanning electron micrograph of a cast of the intracortical vascularization. ×32

1 Intracortical artery	**3** Intracortical vein
2 Intracortical capillaries	**4** Subcortical vessels

Prof. H. Duvernoy UFC

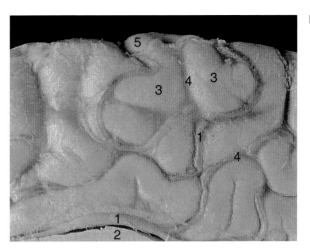

Fig. 8.3

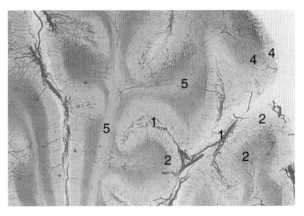

Fig. 8.4

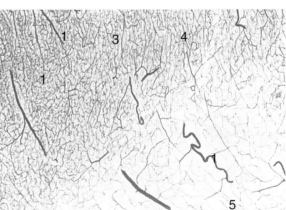

Fig. 8.5

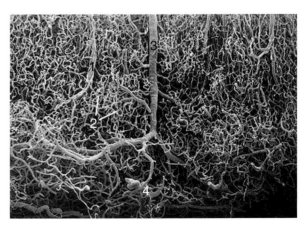

Fig. 8.6

Cerebrum

Figures 8.7 and 8.8 The areas supplied by the anterior, middle and posterior cerebral arteries. Lateral view (Fig. 8.7) and medial view (Fig. 8.8) share the same labels.

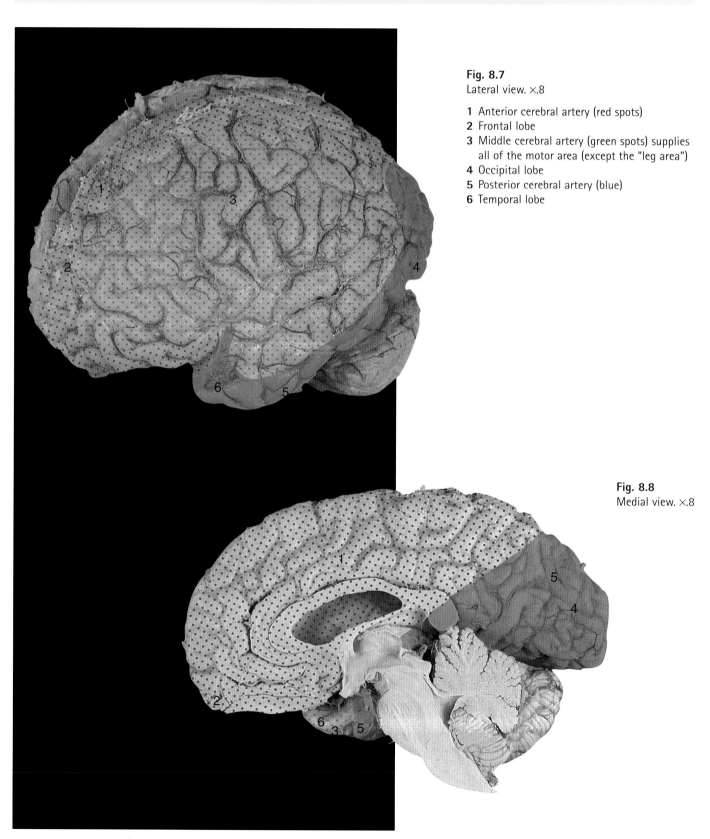

Fig. 8.7
Lateral view. ×.8

1 Anterior cerebral artery (red spots)
2 Frontal lobe
3 Middle cerebral artery (green spots) supplies all of the motor area (except the "leg area")
4 Occipital lobe
5 Posterior cerebral artery (blue)
6 Temporal lobe

Fig. 8.8
Medial view. ×.8

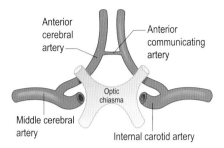

A diagram illustrating this region.

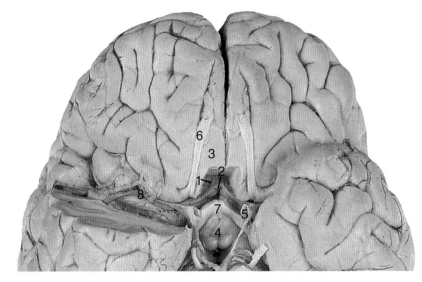

Fig. 8.9
The anterior cerebral artery supplies the medial aspect of the frontal and parietal lobes (except the cuneus). Base of brain showing the anterior cerebral artery arising from the arterial circle (circle of Willis). ×.85

1 Anterior cerebral artery
2 Anterior communicating artery
3 Gyrus rectus
4 Hypothalamus
5 Internal carotid artery
6 Olfactory tract
7 Optic chiasma
8 Middle cerebral artery

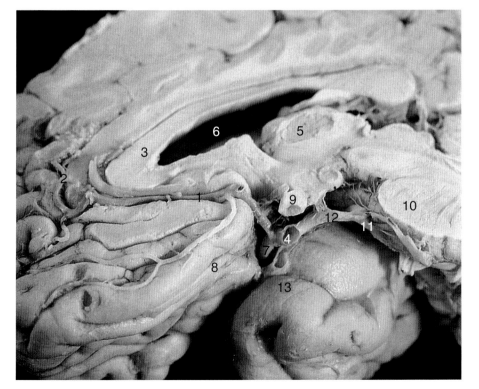

Fig. 8.10
The anterior cerebral artery viewed from the medial surface of the frontal lobe. ×1.1

1 Anterior cerebral artery
2 Branches of anterior cerebral artery
3 Corpus callosum
4 Internal carotid artery
5 Interthalamic connection
6 Lateral ventricle
7 Middle cerebral artery
8 Olfactory tract
9 Optic chiasma
10 Pons
11 Posterior cerebral artery
12 Posterior communicating artery
13 Temporal lobe

● *The anterior cerebral artery is a branch of the internal carotid artery.*

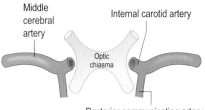

A diagram illustrating this region.

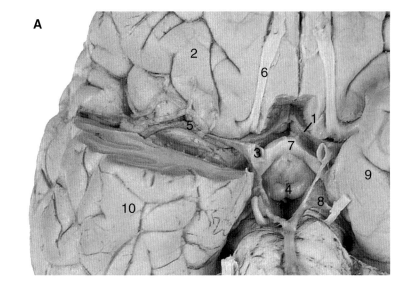

Fig. 8.11 A and B
The middle cerebral artery runs in the lateral sulcus.
Inferior view of the cerebral hemispheres.

  A ×1.16
  B ×1.3
  1 Anterior cerebral artery
  2 Frontal lobe
  3 Internal carotid artery
  4 Mamillary bodies
  5 Middle cerebral artery
  6 Olfactory tract
  7 Optic chiasma
  8 Posterior cerebral artery
  9 Temporal lobe
10 Temporal lobe (removed on the left side of photograph)

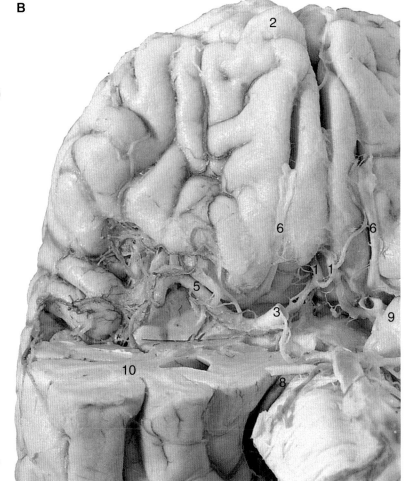

● *The middle cerebral artery is the largest branch of the internal carotid artery.*

● *The internal carotid artery is divided into four parts: cervical, intrapetrosal, intracavernous and supraclinoid. The latter two are referred to as the "carotid siphon".*

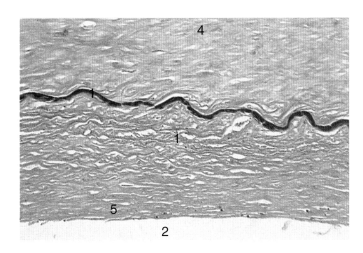

Fig. 8.12
A transverse section of the internal carotid artery. Elastin stain. ×257

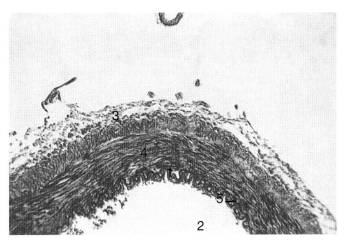

Fig. 8.13
A transverse section of the middle cerebral artery to show it contains a substantial amount of elastic tissue. Phosphotungstic acid and hematoxylin stain. ×103

1 Elastin
2 Lumen of vessel
3 Tunica adventitia
4 Tunica media
5 Tunica intima

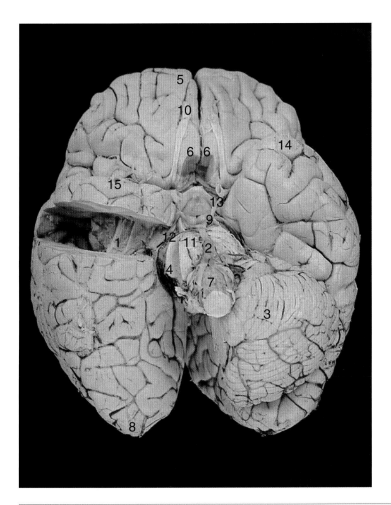

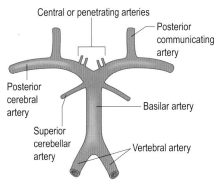

A diagram of the posterior cerebral artery, basilar artery and vertebral arteries.

Fig. 8.14
The posterior cerebral artery supplies the occipital lobe and some of the inferior surface of the temporal lobe. ×0.7

 1 Basal ganglia (temporal lobe removed)
 2 Basilar artery
 3 Cerebellum
 4 Cerebellum (removed)
 5 Frontal lobe
 6 Gyrus rectus (partly removed)
 7 Medulla oblongata
 8 Occipital lobe
 9 Oculomotor nerve
10 Olfactory bulb
11 Pons
12 Posterior cerebral artery
13 Posterior communicating artery
14 Temporal lobe
15 Temporal lobe (removed)

Cerebellum

Each half of the cerebellum is supplied by three arteries: the superior cerebellar, anterior inferior cerebellar, and posterior inferior cerebellar. The posterior inferior cerebellar also supplies the adjacent portion of the medulla oblongata.

A diagram to illustrate the three cerebellar arteries.

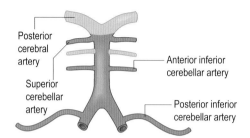

Posterior cerebral artery

Superior cerebellar artery

Anterior inferior cerebellar artery

Posterior inferior cerebellar artery

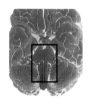

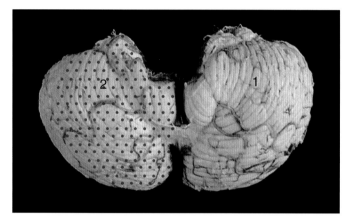

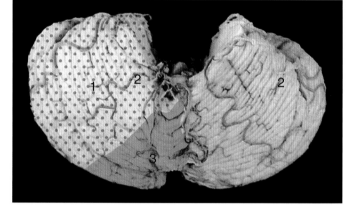

Fig. 8.15
The superior cerebellar arteries are on the superior surface of the cerebellar hemispheres (areas of supply in red spots). The brainstem has been removed. ×0.76

1 Cerebellum
2 Superior cerebellar artery

Fig. 8.16
The anterior inferior cerebellar (area of supply in green spots) and posterior inferior cerebellar (area of supply in blue) arteries are on the inferior surface of the cerebellar hemispheres. The brainstem has been removed. ×0.83

1 Anterior inferior cerebellar artery
2 Cerebellum
3 Posterior inferior cerebellar artery

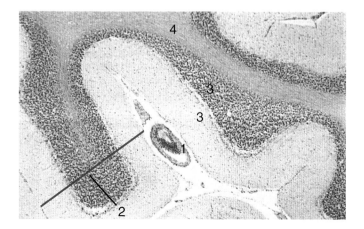

Fig. 8.17
A small artery and vein on the cerebellar surface showing that they run between the folia. Bodian stain and neutral red stain. ×37

1 Blood vessel
2 Folium (indicated by red line)
3 Gray matter
4 White matter

3 Central branches

These small vessels are branches of larger vessels, and pass into the brain. Three areas with a very rich supply are the anterior perforated substance (striate or lenticulostriate arteries), the internal and external capsules (branches of the anterior and middle cerebral arteries and anterior and posterior communicating arteries), and the posterior perforated substance (branches of basilar and posterior cerebral arteries). The central branches supply the basal ganglia, brainstem, cerebellum, thalamus and hypothalamus.

● *The striate arteries are frequently the site of cerebrovascular accidents (CVA).*

A diagram to illustrate the striate arteries.

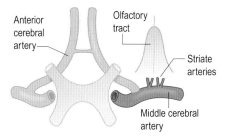

Figures 8.18 and 8.19 Anterior perforated substance.

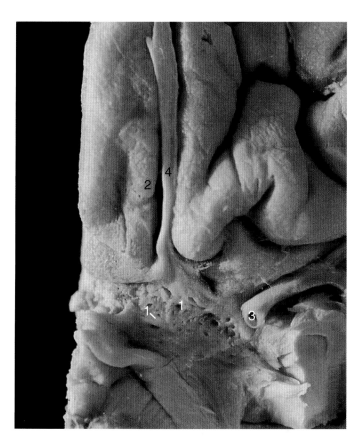

Fig. 8.18 A and B
Radiographs of fixed brain injected with radio-opaque material to show the deep branches of the middle cerebral artery supplying the basal ganglia.

A Lateral view   **B** Frontal view

1 Anterior perforated substance   5 Occipital lobe
2 Cerebellum   6 Temporal lobe
3 Frontal lobe   7 Parietal lobe
4 Middle cerebral artery   8 Position of basal ganglia and
                                        internal capsule

Dr. Harry A. Kaplan and Dr. M. B. Carpenter

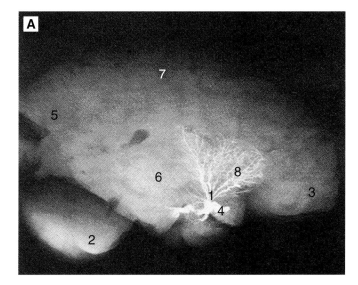

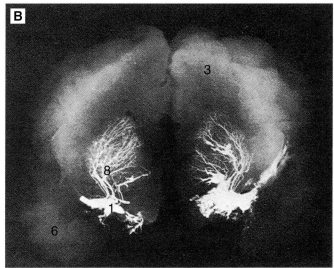

Fig. 8.19
The frontal lobe viewed from below. The temporal lobe has been partially removed to show the anterior perforated substance. ×6.5

1 Anterior perforated substance (with openings for striate arteries)
2 Gyrus rectus
3 Middle cerebral artery
4 Olfactory tract

● *The posterior perforated substance lies in the midbrain between the cerebral peduncles.*

4 Choroidal branches

The branches supplying the choroid plexus of the ventricles are:

Location of choroid plexus	Blood supply
Lateral ventricle	Anterior choroidal (a branch of internal carotid artery) Posterior choroidal (a branch of posterior cerebral artery)
Third ventricle	Posterior choroidal
Fourth ventricle	A branch of posterior inferior cerebellar artery

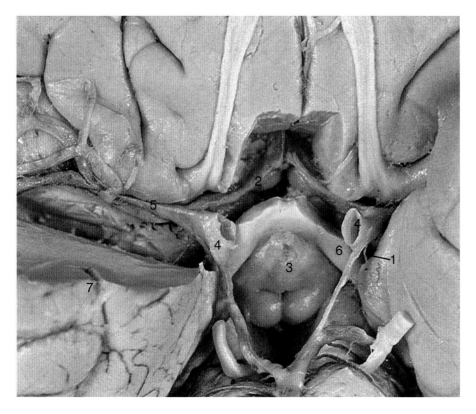

Fig. 8.20
The origin of the anterior choroidal artery
from the internal carotid artery. ×2.2

1 Anterior choroidal artery
2 Anterior cerebral artery
3 Hypothalamus
4 Internal carotid artery
5 Middle cerebral artery
6 Optic tract
7 Temporal lobe

5 Brainstem and spinal branches

Brainstem

The basilar artery supplies almost all of the brainstem and cerebellum. It bifurcates to form the posterior cerebral arteries supplying blood to the occipital lobe.

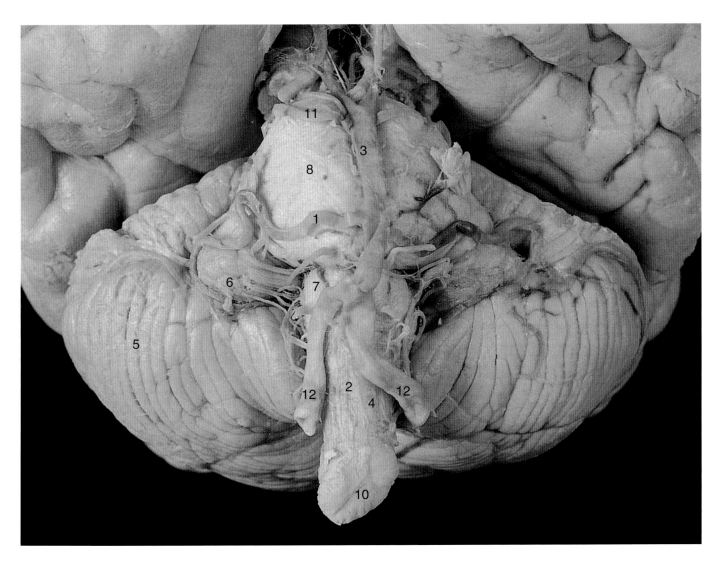

Fig. 8.21
Blood supply to the brainstem. ×1.85

1 Anterior inferior cerebellar artery
2 Anterior spinal artery
3 Basilar artery
4 Brainstem
5 Cerebellum

6 Choroid plexus in the lateral aperture of the fourth ventricle
7 Medulla oblongata
8 Pons
9 Posterior inferior cerebellar artery

10 Spinal cord
11 Superior cerebellar artery
12 Vertebral artery

- *Nuclei consisting of cell bodies have a greater density of blood supply than tracts that consist of fibers.*

- *The medial medullary syndrome is caused by interruption to the supply in the anterior group of arteries.*

- *The lateral medullary syndrome is caused by interruption to the supply in the lateral arteries.*

- *The posterior inferior cerebellar artery is one of the commonest sites for occlusion by thrombus.*

Figures 8.22–8.24 Territories of arterial supply (shown by outlines) of the medulla oblongata and pons. They share the same labels.

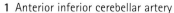

1 Anterior inferior cerebellar artery
2 Anterior spinal artery
3 Long circumferential branches (basilar artery)
4 Medulla oblongata
5 Paramedian branches (basilar artery)
6 Posterior inferior cerebellar artery
7 Posterior spinal artery
8 Short circumferential branches (basilar artery)
9 Vertebral artery

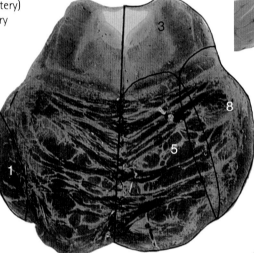
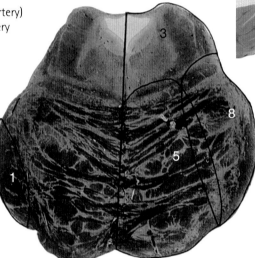

Fig. 8.22
Pons. Weigert stain. ×3.1

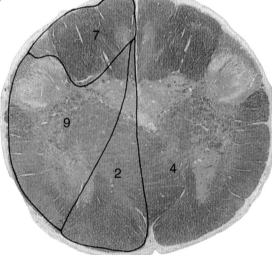

Fig. 8.23
Medulla oblongata at the level of the inferior olivary nuclear complex. Mulligan stain. ×2

Fig. 8.24
Medulla oblongata at the level of the posterior column nuclei. Weigert stain. ×2.3

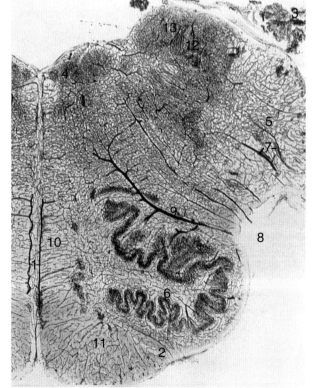
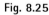

Fig. 8.25
A cleared section of the medulla oblongata at the level of the inferior olivary nucleus. It was injected with a mixture of gelatine and India ink to show the internal distribution of the anterior spinal, vertebral and posterior inferior cerebellar arteries. ×7.3

1 Anterior group of arteries (from anterior spinal artery)
2 Anterolateral group of arteries (from vertebral artery)
3 Choroid plexus of the fourth ventricle
4 Hypoglossal nucleus
5 Inferior cerebellar peduncle
6 Inferior olivary nucleus
7 Lateral group of arteries (from vertebral and posterior inferior cerebellar arteries)
8 Lateral medullary fossa
9 Lateral medullary vein
10 Medial lemniscus
11 Medullary pyramid
12 Posterior group of arteries (from posterior inferior cerebellar artery)
13 Vestibular nuclei

Prof. H. Duvernoy UFC

Spinal branches

The spinal cord is supplied by two branches from each vertebral artery that descend to supply the cord. Additionally, the cord receives an arterial supply from small branches (radicular arteries) that are derived from segmental branches of the aorta and from the vertebral arteries.

● *The posterior spinal artery may be a branch from the vertebral artery.*

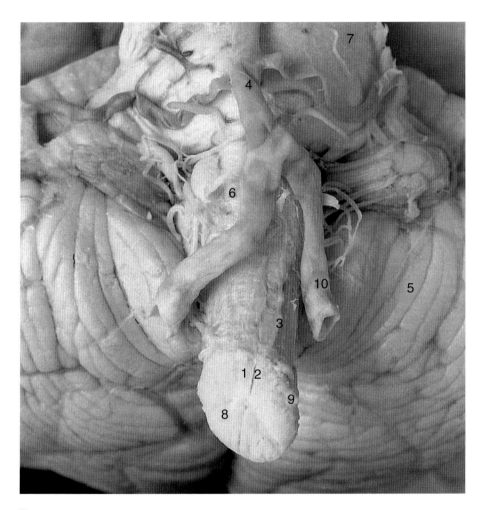

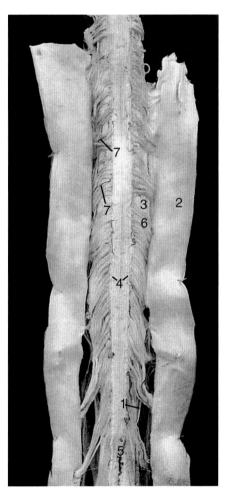

Fig. 8.26
The anterior spinal artery descends in the anterior median fissure of the cord. View of the base of the brain and upper cervical cord. ×2.16

1 Anterior (ventral) horn
2 Anterior median fissure
3 Anterior spinal artery
4 Basilar artery
5 Cerebellum
6 Medulla oblongata
7 Pons
8 Posterior (dorsal) horn
9 Spinal cord
10 Vertebral artery

Fig. 8.27
The posterior spinal artery descends in two branches, one on each side of the posterior (dorsal) spinal nerve roots. View of part of the spinal cord from the posterior surface. ×0.83

1 Denticulate ligament
2 Dura mater
3 Pia mater
4 Posterior (dorsal) columns
5 Posterior (dorsal) spinal artery
6 Posterior spinal nerve roots
7 Radicular vessels

UN

Cerebral angiography

Figures 8.28–8.31 Cerebral angiograms demonstrating the blood supply to the brain and skull. An angiogram is produced by introducing a radio-opaque substance into a blood vessel. Angiograms of the carotid and vertebral arteries demonstrate their territories in the head, neck and brain.

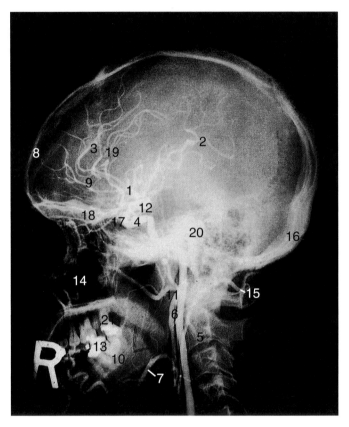

Fig. 8.28
A carotid arterial angiogram in lateral view.

1	Anterior cerebral artery	12	Middle cerebral artery
2	Branches of middle cerebral artery	13	Mouth
3	Callosomarginal artery	14	Nasal cavity
4	Carotid siphon	15	Occipital artery
5	Cervical vertebra	16	Occiput
6	External carotid artery	17	Ophthalmic artery
7	Facial artery	18	Orbitofrontal arteries
8	Frontal bone	19	Pericallosal artery
9	Frontopolar arteries	20	Petrous temporal bone
10	Mandible	21	Teeth
11	Maxillary artery		

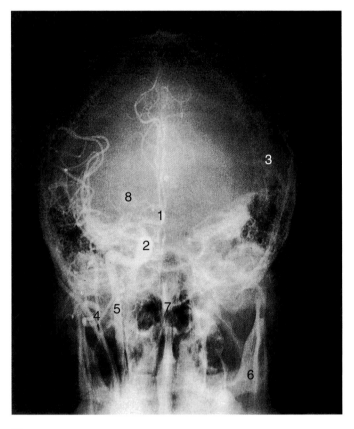

Fig. 8.29
A frontal view of a carotid angiogram.

1 Anterior cerebral artery
2 Carotid siphon
3 Coronal suture
4 External carotid artery
5 Internal carotid artery
6 Mandible
7 Nose
8 Striate arteries

● *The convoluted course of the internal carotid artery through the base of the skull is known as the carotid siphon.*

● *Branches of the middle cerebral artery crossing the insula form loops.*

● *A tumor in the hypophyseal (pituitary) fossa may cause the curves of the carotid siphon to straighten.*

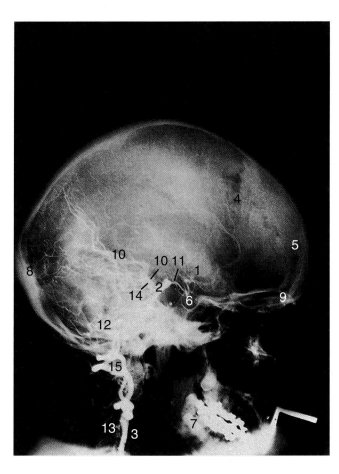

Fig. 8.30
A vertebral artery angiogram in lateral view.

1 Arteries to thalamus
2 Basilar artery
3 Body of a cervical vertebra
4 Coronal suture
5 Frontal bone
6 Hypophyseal fossa
7 Mandible
8 Occiput
9 Orbit
10 Posterior cerebral artery
11 Posterior communicating artery
12 Posterior inferior cerebellar artery
13 Spine of a cervical vertebra
14 Superior cerebellar artery
15 Vertebral artery

● *In this individual, some filling of the posterior communicating and anterior cerebral arteries has occurred, showing the continuity of the arterial circle (circle of Willis).*

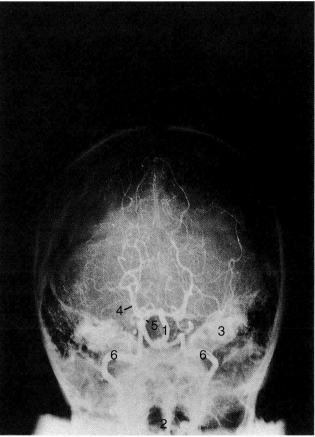

Fig. 8.31
A frontal view of a vertebral artery angiogram.

1 Basilar artery
2 Nose
3 Petrous temporal bone
4 Posterior cerebral artery
5 Superior cerebellar artery
6 Vertebral artery

Figs. 8.28–8.31 Dr. D. James LRI

Brain: Veins

Cerebrum

Most veins throughout the body with diameters of between 1 and 10 mm have a thick tunica media containing bundles of smooth muscle cells. They also possess valves to direct blood flow towards the heart. Cerebral veins are unusual because they have neither valves nor muscular tissue. Blood drains from deep in the substance of the brain into large superficial veins which cross the subarachnoid space and drain into large venous sinuses of the dura mater.

The veins may be divided into two groups: those draining the cerebrum and those of the cerebellum and brainstem.

Those of the cerebrum are further divided into external and internal vessels. The external veins drain the surface of the cerebrum. The superolateral surface of each hemisphere is drained by 8–12 superior superficial veins which pass upward and forward to end in the superior sagittal sinus. Some veins from the medial aspect also drain into this sinus.

Other veins on the superolateral surface drain into the superficial middle cerebral vein, which lies in the lateral sulcus and joins the cavernous sinus. Anastomotic vessels drain from it inferolaterally into the transverse sinus and superiorly into the superior sagittal sinus.

The superficial middle cerebral vein is connected to the superior sagittal sinus by the superior anastomotic vein, and to the transverse sinus by the inferior anastomotic vein.

The surface of the insula is drained by the deep middle cerebral vein. The anterior cerebral vein accompanies the anterior cerebral artery and drains the territory supplied by the artery. The anterior cerebral and the deep middle cerebral vein join with striate veins (internal cerebral veins which emerge through the anterior perforated substance) to form the basal vein. The basal vein on each side ultimately joins the great cerebral vein (of Galen) which drains the inside of the brain. The great cerebral vein is formed by the union of two internal cerebral veins under the splenium of the corpus callosum. The internal cerebral veins receive the thalamostriate veins (also known as venae terminales) from the corpus striatum and the choroidal veins of each lateral ventricle.

The inferior surface of each cerebral hemisphere is drained by inferior superficial cerebral veins. They drain into the transverse sinus, inferior cerebral veins, superior petrosal sinus, cavernous sinus, middle cerebral veins and basal vein of their own side.

Cerebellum

There are two main groups of cerebellar veins: the superior and inferior veins. The superior veins drain into the straight sinus, the internal cerebral veins, and the transverse and superior petrosal sinuses.

The inferior veins drain into the inferior petrosal, sigmoid and occipital sinuses.

Brainstem

Veins of the brainstem form a superficial venous plexus, deep to the arteries, within which larger venous channels can be distinguished.

1. Midbrain. Veins from the midbrain drain into the great cerebral vein, and some, along with those of the area around the interpeduncular fossa, also drain into the basal veins.
2. Pons. The pontine veins drain into the basal vein, cerebellar veins, and the superior and inferior petrosal and transverse sinuses. Sometimes a median pontine vein is present, and a distinct lateral venous channel is usually present on either side.
3. Medulla oblongata. Some veins on the anterior surface drain into a midline anterior median vein which is continuous with a vein of the same name on the anterior surface of the spinal cord. On the posterior surface, the veins drain into a posterior median vein which is continuous with a vein of the same name on the posterior surface of the spinal cord. This vein drains into the inferior petrosal and basilar venous sinuses.

Radicular veins (associated with the last four cranial nerve rootlets) drain into the petrosal sinus, occipital sinuses or internal jugular vein.

A lateral vein similar to that found in the pons may be present on each side, draining into the petrosal or transverse sinus.

Venous sinuses of the dura mater

There are several large sinuses lying externally to the brain in the dural folds. These are the superior sagittal sinus, inferior sagittal sinus and straight sinus; the blood from these sinuses and from the great cerebral vein meets at the confluence of the sinuses, where venous blood then flows into the bilateral transverse sinuses. They eventually pass from the skull as the internal jugular veins through the jugular foramina.

The cavernous sinuses, lying on each side of the body of the sphenoid bone, connect with the other intracranial sinuses (for example, superior petrosal, sigmoid, occipital). Blood may flow in any direction in this sinus. It also connects with the superficial middle cerebral veins draining the lateral surfaces of the brain, and with veins in the pharyngeal, pterygoid and orbital regions. Left and right cavernous sinuses communicate with each other behind the pituitary fossa.

Blood from the great cerebral vein (of Galen) joins the straight sinus at the junction with the inferior sagittal sinus.

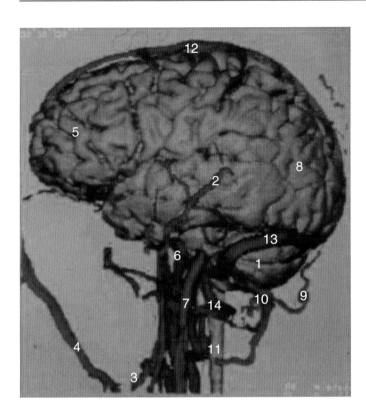

Fig. 8.32
Computer reconstruction of a combined MRI/angiogram showing the dural venous sinuses.

 1 Cerebellum
 2 Cerebral veins
 3 External jugular vein
 4 Facial vein
 5 Frontal lobe
 6 Internal carotid artery
 7 Internal jugular vein
 8 Occipital lobe
 9 Occipital veins
10 Sigmoid sinus
11 Spinal cord
12 Superior sagittal sinus
13 Transverse sinus
14 Vertebral artery

Prof. F. W. Zonneveld UUH

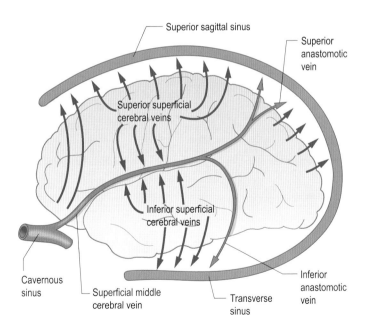

Venous drainage of the superior and lateral surfaces of the cerebrum.

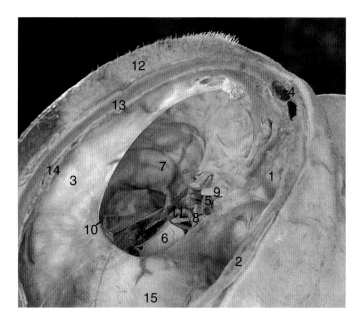

Fig. 8.33
The superior and inferior sagittal sinuses. ×0.56

 1 Anterior cranial fossa
 2 Diploë
 3 Falx cerebri
 4 Frontal sinus
 5 Internal carotid artery
 6 Midbrain
 7 Middle cranial fossa
 8 Oculomotor nerve
 9 Optic nerve
10 Position of inferior sagittal sinus
11 Posterior cerebral artery
12 Scalp
13 Skull vault
14 Superior sagittal sinus
15 Tentorium cerebelli

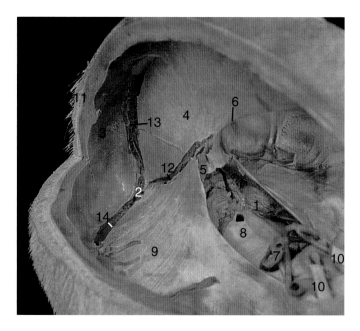

Fig. 8.34
The dural venous sinuses. ×0.56

 1 Cerebellum
 2 Confluence of the sinuses
 3 Dura mater
 4 Falx cerebri
 5 Great cerebral vein (of Galen)
 6 Inferior sagittal sinus (position of)
 7 Internal carotid artery
 8 Midbrain
 9 Tentorium cerebelli
10 Optic nerve
11 Scalp
12 Straight sinus
13 Superior sagittal sinus
14 Transverse sinus

● *If the infant's head is hyperextended in a difficult birth, hemorrhage can occur at the junction of the great cerebral vein and the straight sinus.*

● *Claudius Galen (AD 130–200) was a Roman physician to the gladiators, who became the accepted authority on human anatomy until the Renaissance.*

● *The direction of blood flow can vary in valveless veins.*

● *Blood seeping from a ruptured vein may collect between the dura and arachnoid mater to form a subdural hematoma. Elderly individuals have fragile veins; a slight blow to the head may lead to a subdural hematoma.*

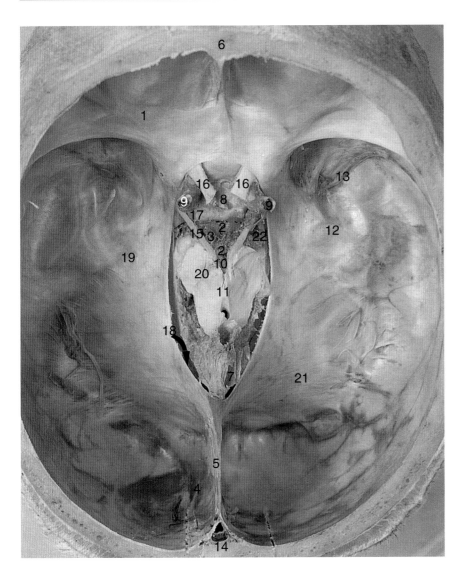

Fig. 8.35
The floor of the cranial cavity viewed from above
to demonstrate the relationships of the cavernous
sinus. ×0.82

1 Anterior cranial fossa
2 Basilar venous plexus
3 Cavernous sinus
4 Confluence of the sinuses (position of)
5 Falx cerebri
6 Frontal bone
7 Great cerebral vein
8 Hypophyseal fossa
9 Internal carotid artery
10 Interpeduncular fossa
11 Midbrain
12 Middle cranial fossa
13 Middle meningeal vessels
14 Occipital bone
15 Oculomotor nerve
16 Optic nerve
17 Posterior clinoid process
18 Posterior cranial fossa
19 Superior petrosal sinus (position of)
20 Substantia nigra
21 Tentorium cerebelli
22 Wall of cavernous sinus (cut edge)

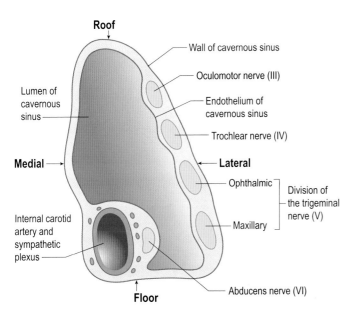

A diagram showing the structures running in the walls of the
cavernous sinus.

- *If the internal carotid artery is ruptured in the cavernous
  sinus, arteriovenous communication results. Arterial
  blood is pumped into the sinus and its communicating
  veins, especially the ophthalmic veins. The eye on the
  affected side bulges and pulsates in time with the radial
  pulse (pulsating exophthalmos).*

- *The oculomotor, trochlear and abducens nerves and the
  ophthalmic and maxillary divisions of the trigeminal
  nerve may all be compressed together in the cavernous
  sinus by aneurysms of the internal carotid artery or
  tumors of the pituitary gland. This can cause a
  combination of facial pain (V), eye muscle paralysis (III,
  IV, VI) and loss of the corneal reflex (V and VII).*

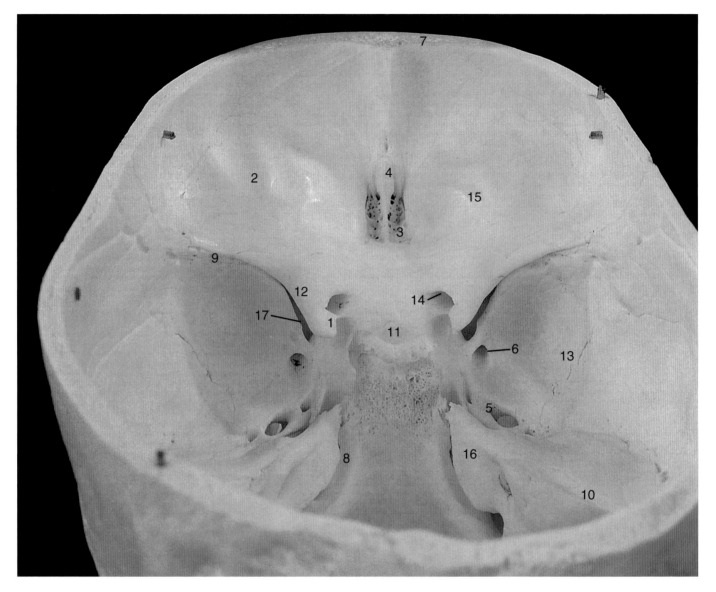

Fig. 8.36
The positions of the petrosal and sphenoparietal sinuses. The floor of the cranial cavity viewed from behind. The cranial vault has been removed. ×1.5

1 Anterior clinoid process
2 Anterior cranial fossa
3 Cribriform plate of ethmoid bone
4 Crista galli
5 Foramen ovale
6 Foramen rotundum
7 Frontal bone
8 Groove for inferior petrosal sinus
9 Groove for sphenoparietal sinus

10 Groove for superior petrosal sinus
11 Hypophyseal fossa
12 Lesser wing of sphenoid
13 Middle cranial fossa
14 Optic canal
15 Orbital part of frontal bone
16 Petrous temporal bone
17 Superior orbital fissure

● *The abducens nerve (VI) has the longest intracranial course of all the cranial nerves. As it runs from the brainstem to the cavernous sinus it passes over the sharp apex of the petrous temporal bone. If intracranial pressure is raised, the nerve can be stretched over the bone, causing paralysis of the lateral rectus muscle of the eye, and diplopia (double vision).*

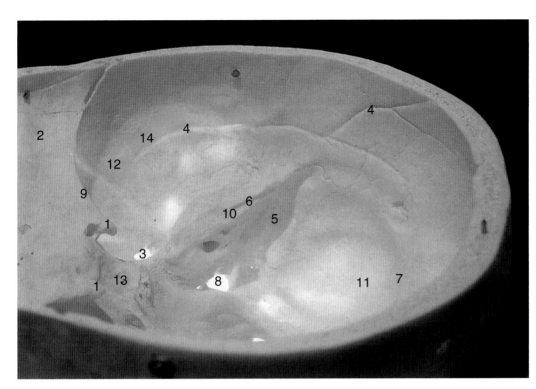

Fig. 8.37
The middle cranial fossa and the groove for the sigmoid sinus viewed from the side. The cranial vault has been removed. ×0.93

1 Anterior clinoid process
2 Anterior cranial fossa
3 Foramen ovale
4 Groove for middle meningeal artery
5 Groove for sigmoid sinus
6 Groove for superior petrosal sinus
7 Groove for transverse sinus
8 Jugular foramen
9 Lesser wing of sphenoid bone
10 Petrous part of temporal bone
11 Posterior cranial fossa
12 Pterion
13 Sella turcica (hypophyseal fossa)
14 Squamous part of temporal bone

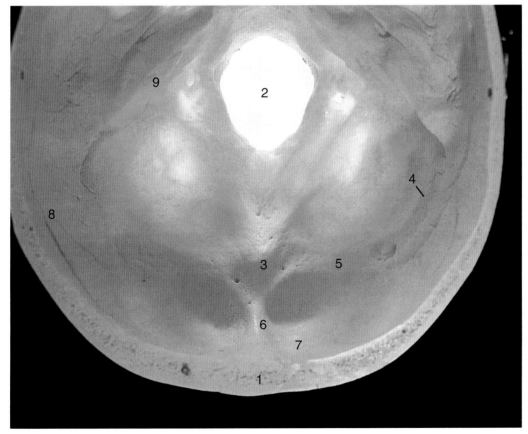

Fig. 8.38
The posterior cranial fossa and the grooves for its associated sinuses viewed from above. The vault has been removed. Note the density of the occipital bone. ×0.93

1 Diploë of the skull
2 Foramen magnum
3 Groove for confluence of the sinuses
4 Groove for sigmoid sinus
5 Groove for transverse sinus
6 Internal occipital protuberance
7 Occipital bone
8 Parietal bone
9 Petrous part of temporal bone

● *Note the thin parts of the squamous temporal, greater wing of sphenoid, and frontal and parietal bones. This position is called the pterion. The branches of the middle meningeal artery can easily be injured at this site.*

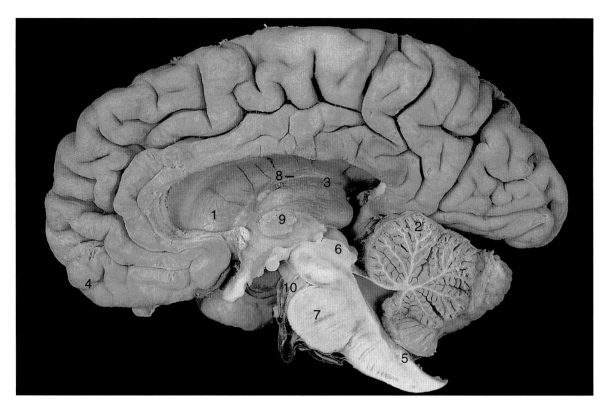

Fig. 8.39
The deep venous drainage of the caudate nucleus and thalamus. ×0.88

1 Caudate nucleus
2 Cerebellum
3 Choroid plexus of lateral ventricle
4 Frontal pole
5 Medulla oblongata

6 Midbrain (tectum)
7 Pons
8 Thalamostriate vein (drains into the internal cerebral vein)
9 Thalamus
10 Vessels on surface of brainstem

● *The two internal cerebral veins join together to form the great cerebral vein (of Galen).*

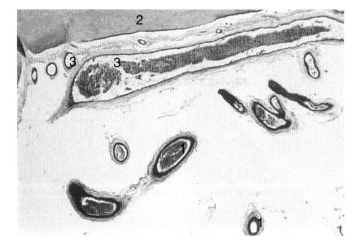

Fig. 8.40
Vessels on the surface of the medulla oblongata form a plexus with veins lying deep to the arteries. Van Gieson stain. ×38

1 Artery
2 Medulla oblongata (surface)
3 Vein

Mr. D. Adams

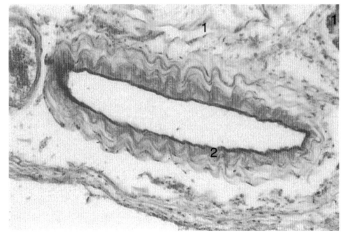

Fig. 8.41
A transverse section adjacent to the medulla oblongata demonstrating the lack of muscle in the vein wall. Van Gieson stain. ×194

1 Medulla oblongata
2 Vein

Mr. D. Adams

Summary

1. The arterial supply of the brain is derived from two sources: branches of the two internal carotid arteries and branches of the two vertebral arteries.
2. The major arteries form an anastomosis beneath the base of the brain known as the circle of Willis.
3. From the circle of Willis and its main branches, cortical arteries spread over the brain surface in the subarachnoid space, and deep arteries penetrate into the brain substance.
4. Small arteries inside brain tissue are end arteries.
5. A stroke is the loss of the arterial supply to an area of the brain, resulting in neuronal death, loss of brain function, and disability or death of the patient. Obstruction of a vein causes only a transient edema of the surrounding tissue.
6. The venous drainage of the brain passes into the venous sinuses of the dura mater.

Blood–Brain and Blood–CSF Barriers

Neuronal function requires a micro-environment that is precisely controlled. Several mechanisms exist in the nervous system to isolate the brain and spinal cord from changes elsewhere in the body that might have an adverse effect. Collectively, these mechanisms constitute the blood–brain barrier and the blood–CSF barrier. These barriers have six major functions:

A) Large molecules, for example plasma proteins present in the blood, are excluded from the CSF and nervous tissue.

B) The ionic composition and glucose concentration of the extracellular fluid in the nervous system is controlled at levels appropriate for neuronal function but not necessarily the same as those elsewhere in the body.

C) The brain and spinal cord are protected from the effect of neurotransmitters in the blood, for example epinephrine (adrenaline) from the adrenal gland.

D) Neurotransmitters produced in the CNS are prevented from leaking into the general circulation.

E) Toxins are excluded either because of their molecular size or because of their solubility. Only substances soluble in water and cell-membrane lipids can pass these barriers.

F) Most micro-organisms are unable to cross the barrier and infect brain tissue.

Anatomically, the blood–brain barrier resides in the capillaries in the nervous tissue. Their endothelia have restricted permeability. The cells are attached to each other by tight (occluding) junctions which prevent large molecules, for example proteins, passing between the cells, effectively sealing off the lumen of the vessel from the extracellular space outside it. In addition, the endothelium has few of the vesicles found in other capillary endothelia which are responsible for the transport of macromolecules across the cell. Outside the capillary endothelium, a second barrier is created by an encirclement of cell processes from the astrocytes (see Glial cells, p. 13).

The blood–CSF barrier exists in the choroid plexuses and in the arachnoid mater. Choroid plexus capillaries are fenestrated and highly permeable. However, the epithelial cells are attached to each other by tight junctions so that substances cannot pass between the epithelial cells into the CSF in the ventricles but have to be transported by the cells. Choroid plexus epithelial cells have active transport mechanisms for ions, glucose and amino acids but large molecules are unable to pass.

The subarachnoid space is sealed against free exchange of substances between the CSF in the space and blood in the vessels passing in or beside the space. A layer of flat, interdigitating cells, attached to each other by tight junctions, covers the outside of the arachnoid, and the vessels crossing the subarachnoid space have endothelia with occluding tight junctions between the cells, sealing the lumen.

No barrier exists between the CSF in the ventricles or subarachnoid space and the nervous tissue because neither the astrocytes at the glia limitans nor the ependymal cells at the ventricular lumen have tight junctions. Water and electrolytes produced by metabolism pass freely between the brain and the CSF and are removed when the CSF is recirculated back to the blood via the arachnoid granulations. The CSF is performing the same function here that lymphatics do for other tissues. The CNS is devoid of lymphatic capillaries. A blood–CSF barrier exists in the choroid plexus, where the epithelial cells are attached to one another by tight junctions, and in the arachnoid mater between the outermost arachnoid cells (arachnoid barrier layer).

- *The pineal gland and the median eminence of the hypothalamus have fenestrated capillaries. In the hypothalamus these allow hypothalamic neurosecretions to enter the circulation (see Diencephalon, p. 141).*

- *The blood–brain barrier is not fully developed at birth and albumin is present in the CSF.*

- *The blood–brain barrier was first discovered by observing that India ink injected into the blood vessels of brain tissue did not pass through their walls.*

- *The subfornical organ (under the fornix), the area postrema (in the floor of the fourth ventricle) and the organum vasculosum of the lamina terminalis are areas with no blood–brain barrier. They are chemoreceptor areas containing specific sense organs for blood-borne substances. The area postrema detects circulating toxins and induces vomiting in an attempt to eliminate them from the body.*

- *Alcohol and opiates can cross the blood–brain barrier.*

- *Most antibiotics do not cross the blood–brain barrier.*

- *Fluid accumulation (edema) can occur in brain tissue, causing it to swell if the blood–brain barrier breaks down and the ionic balance of the brain is disturbed. Ischemia, acidosis and hemorrhage can all cause edema in this way.*

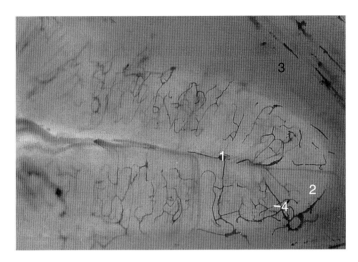
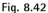

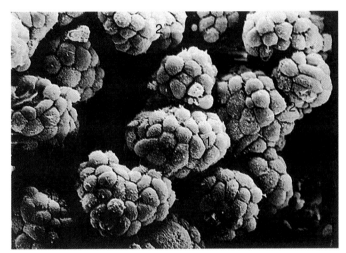

Fig. 8.42
A low power photomicrograph to show blood vessels entering the cerebellum as an example of the small blood vessels supplying the brain tissue. Golgi-Cox stain. ×63

1 Blood vessel on surface of cerebellum
2 Cerebellar cortex
3 Cerebellar white matter
4 Penetrating vessels

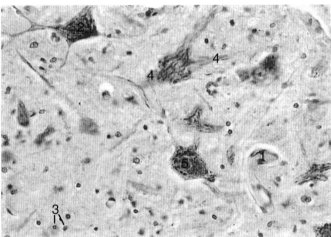

Fig. 8.43
A histological section showing a capillary in the brainstem surrounded by multipolar neurons and nerve fibers. Cresyl violet stain. ×746

1 Capillary
2 Cell body of neuron
3 Neuroglial cell nuclei
4 Neuronal processes or nerve fibers
5 Nucleus of neuron

A blood–CSF barrier exists in the choroid plexus, where the epithelial cells are attached to one another by tight junctions, and in the arachnoid mater between the outermost arachnoid cells (arachnoid barrier layer).

Fig. 8.44
Scanning electron micrograph showing the epithelium of the choroid plexus that would be in contact with the cerebrospinal fluid. ×470

1 Epithelial cell
2 Villi

Fig. 8.45
A histological section to show the arachnoid mater and the subarachnoid space. Solochrome cyanin and light green stain. ×4

1 Arachnoid mater
2 Blood vessels in subarachnoid space
3 Gray matter of cerebral cortex
4 Subarachnoid space
5 Surface of arachnoid mater (arrow)

Fig. 8.44

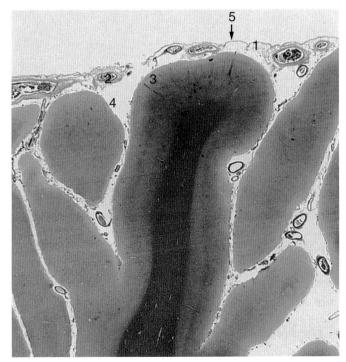

Fig. 8.45

Summary

1. The blood–brain barrier is formed by specializations in the structure of the capillaries in brain tissue.
2. Blood–CSF barriers exist in the choroid plexus and the arachnoid mater.
3. Blood–brain and blood–CSF barriers maintain the optimal physiological conditions for brain function.
4. The blood–brain barrier breaks down in damaged tissue.

9 Ventricles

Deep inside the forebrain, midbrain and hindbrain is a series of connecting chambers (ventricles) lined with an epithelium called the ependyma. There are two large lateral ventricles inside the cerebral hemispheres (forebrain), each of which connects in the midline through the interventricular foramen (of Monro) which leads into the midline third ventricle. This connects through the narrow cerebral aqueduct (of Sylvius) in the midbrain to the midline fourth ventricle in the pons and medulla oblongata (hindbrain).

Projecting into each ventricle is a structure called the choroid plexus which produces cerebrospinal fluid (CSF). It consists of tufts of capillaries covered by an epithelium, the ependyma. CSF is produced by a combination of filtration from the blood and active secretion by the epithelium. The active secretory mechanism results in differences in its chemical composition from that of blood plasma. As CSF is constantly produced it percolates through and fills all of the ventricles. It leaves the system by flowing out of three openings. In the hindbrain roof above the fourth ventricle is a midline median aperture (foramen of Magendie) and two lateral apertures (foramina of Luschka) which open from the sides of the fourth ventricle. CSF flows into and completely fills the subarachnoid space around the brain and spinal cord. Areas where the arachnoid and pia mater are widely separated are referred to as cisterns or cisternae.

Finally, CSF then leaves the ventricular system through small openings in the superior sagittal sinus. These openings, found in the dura mater, have small projections of arachnoid bulging through them (arachnoid granulations). The CSF passes through the granulations and is carried away in the dural venous blood.

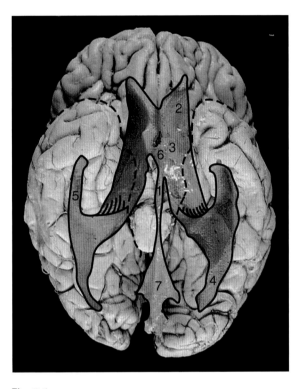

Fig. 9.1
A cast of the ventricles of the adult brain superimposed on the base of a brain to illustrate their position internally. ×0.64

1 Cerebral aqueduct ⎫
2 Anterior horn ⎪
3 Body ⎬ Lateral ventricle
4 Posterior horn ⎪
5 Inferior horn ⎭
6 Third ventricle
7 Fourth ventricle   RCS

Solid outline = ventricles
Dashed outline = medial border of the temporal lobe

● *CSF cushions the brain and spinal cord by absorbing shocks.*

● *A lumbar puncture or spinal tap is made to measure the pressure of the intracranial CSF, to take a sample of spinal fluid, to introduce dyes and radio-opaque contrast media for diagnostic purposes and to administer anesthetics and other drugs.*

● *CSF is a clear fluid similar to lymph and does not normally contain blood, pus or bacteria. In a spinal tap the levels of sugar, chloride and protein are measured. Any cells are counted and identified. In bacterial meningitis, polymorphs appear and the glucose content of the CSF falls. If the infection is viral, the glucose level is normal and lymphocytes increase in number.*

● *One cause of hydrocephalus in newborn infants is an accumulation of CSF caused by an obstruction in the ventricular system. CSF is unable to flow out and accumulates in the ventricles.*

Fig. 9.2
The ventricles viewed from the medial aspect of a sagittal section. Septum pellucidum has been removed. ×0.63

1 Anterior horn of lateral ventricle
2 Body of lateral ventricle
3 Choroid plexus
4 Corpus callosum
5 Diencephalon
6 Frontal lobe
7 Inferior horn of lateral ventricle
8 Occipital lobe
9 Parietal lobe
10 Posterior horn of lateral ventricle
11 Temporal lobe

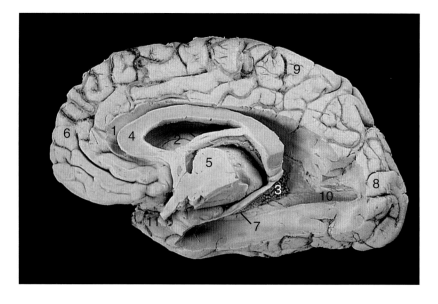

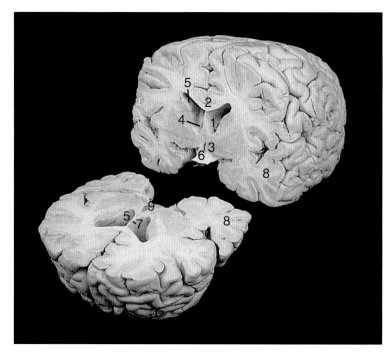

Fig. 9.3
A coronal section through the cerebral hemispheres and diencephalon to illustrate the position of the interventricular foramen between the lateral and third ventricles. ×0.55

1 Choroid plexus
2 Corpus callosum
3 Hypothalamus
4 Interventricular foramen
5 Lateral ventricle
6 Optic chiasma
7 Septum pellucidum
8 Temporal lobe
9 Third ventricle

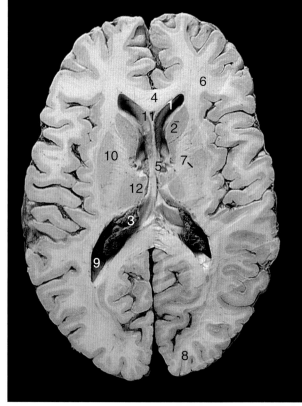

Fig. 9.4
A horizontal section through the brain to show the anterior and posterior horns of the lateral ventricles. ×0.62

1 Anterior horn of lateral ventricle
2 Caudate nucleus
3 Choroid plexus
4 Corpus callosum
5 Fornix
6 Frontal lobe
7 Globus pallidus
8 Occipital lobe
9 Posterior horn of lateral ventricle
10 Putamen
11 Septum pellucidum
12 Thalamus

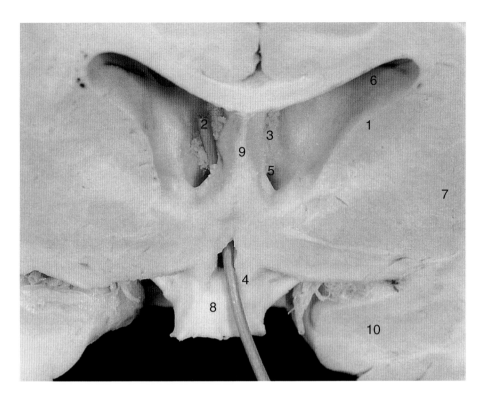

Fig. 9.5
A coronal section through the diencephalon to illustrate the relationship between the interventricular foramen and the third ventricle. ×1.95

1 Caudate nucleus
2 Connection between lateral and third ventricle (shown by the position of a red wire)
3 Choroid plexus
4 Hypothalamus
5 Interventricular foramen
6 Lateral ventricle
7 Lentiform nucleus
8 Optic chiasma
9 Septum pellucidum
10 Temporal lobe

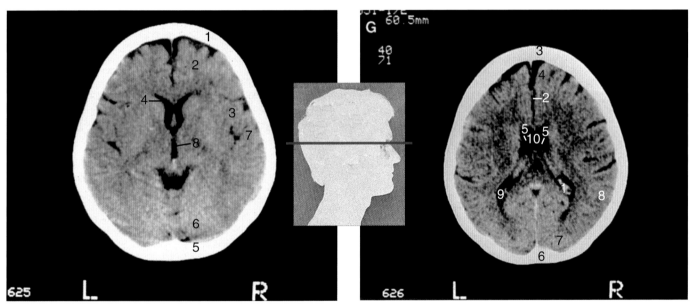

Fig. 9.6
Computed axial tomography (CAT) scan image to show the third and lateral ventricles.

1 Frontal bone
2 Frontal lobe
3 Insula
4 Lateral ventricle
5 Occipital bone
6 Occipital lobe
7 Temporal lobe
8 Third ventricle

Elscint Ltd

Fig. 9.7
CAT scan image to show posterior horn of the lateral ventricle.

1 Choroid plexus (shows calcification in this instance)
2 Falx cerebri
3 Frontal bone
4 Frontal lobe
5 Lateral ventricle
6 Occipital bone
7 Occipital lobe
8 Parietal lobe
9 Posterior horn of ventricle
10 Septum pellucidum

Elscint Ltd

● *In chronic alcoholism there is atrophy of the cerebral cortex and an apparent increase in the size of the ventricles.*

Fig. 9.8
The choroid plexus of the lateral ventricle viewed *in situ* from the lateral surface. ×0.7

1 Choroid plexus
2 Frontal lobe
3 Insula
4 Lateral ventricle
5 Parietal lobe
6 Occipital lobe
7 Temporal lobe

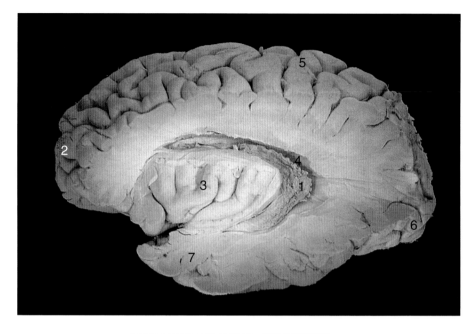

Fig. 9.9
A histological section to show the choroid plexus of the lateral ventricle, stained with phosphotungstic acid and hematoxylin. ×5.6

1 Caudate nucleus
2 Choroid plexus
3 Corpus callosum
4 Lateral ventricle
5 Thalamus

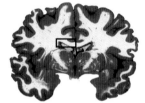

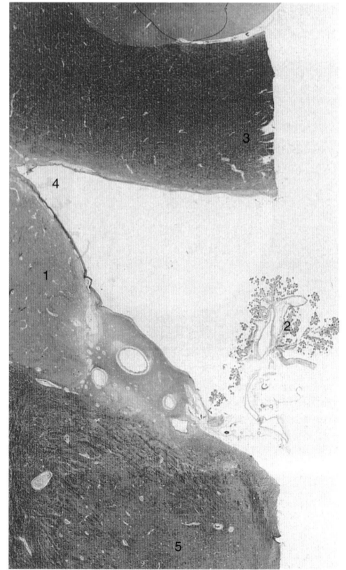

The density of capillary meshworks in the choroid plexus provides a large surface area for filtration of blood in CSF formation. Their complex three-dimensional organization is best appreciated in a cast, prepared by injecting a liquid plastic medium into the vessels and allowing it to set. The tissue is then removed leaving a replica of the vessels.

Figures 9.10 and 9.11 Casts of the vessels of the choroid plexus. Capillaries of the choroid plexus form either dichotomous or glomerular formations.

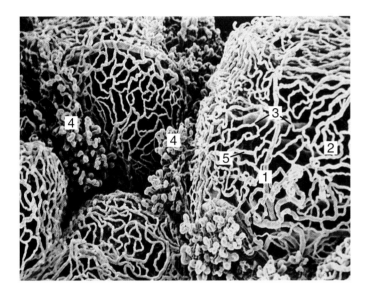

Fig. 9.10
Scanning electron micrograph of a cast of the capillary network in the choroid plexus. ×84

Dr. E. Motti

1 Artery
2 Capillary
3 Dichotomous branching
4 Glomerular formation
5 Vein

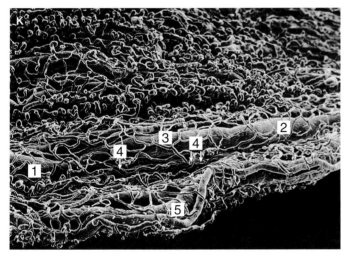

Fig. 9.11
A cast of an artery and a vein surrounded by capillary meshes. ×84

Dr. E. Motti

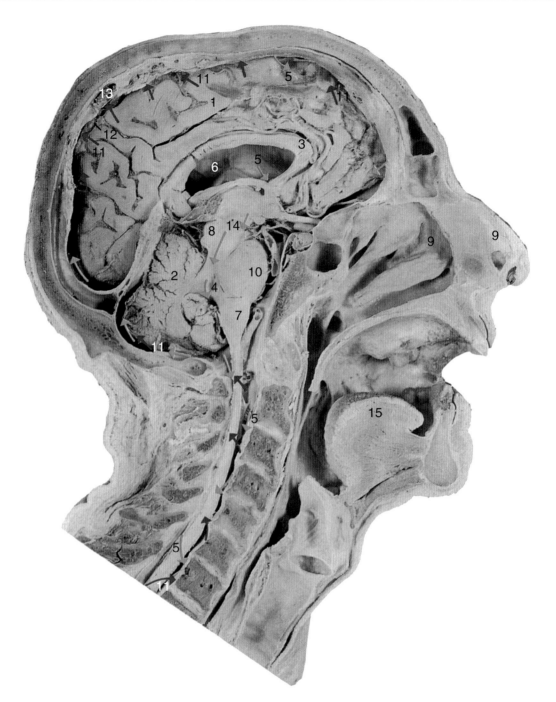

Fig. 9.12
Sagittal section of a head to illustrate the circulation of cerebrospinal fluid through the ventricles and subarachnoid space and its return to the blood circulation. ×0.65

1 Cerebral hemisphere
2 Cerebellum
3 Corpus callosum
4 Fourth ventricle
5 Green arrows (circulation of CSF)
6 Lateral ventricle
7 Medulla oblongata
8 Midbrain

9 Nose
10 Pons
11 Red arrows (return of CSF to blood circulation)
12 Subarachnoid space
13 Superior sagittal sinus
14 Third ventricle
15 Tongue

● *A spinal tap should be avoided if the intracranial pressure is raised. There is a risk of displacing part of the cerebellum into the foramen magnum and fatally compressing the brainstem, a process known as coning.*

Figures 9.13 and 9.14 Foramina of the fourth ventricle.

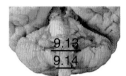

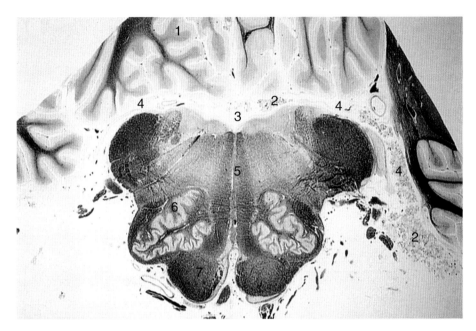

Fig. 9.13
Transverse histological section of medulla and cerebellum passing through the lateral apertures of the fourth ventricle. Weigert stain. ×3.3

1 Cerebellum
2 Choroid plexus of fourth ventricle
3 Fourth ventricle
4 Lateral aperture (foramen of Luschka)
5 Medulla oblongata
6 Olive
7 Pyramid

MHMS

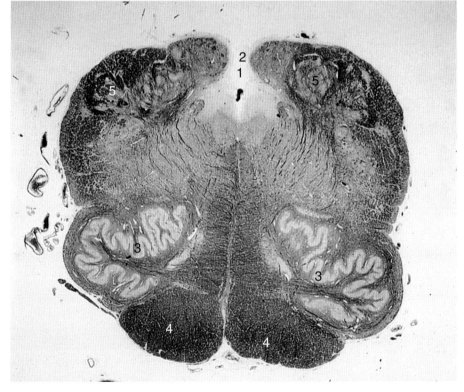

Fig. 9.14
Transverse section of medulla oblongata passing through the median aperture of the fourth ventricle. Myelin stain. ×6.3

1 Fourth ventricle
2 Median aperture (foramen of Magendie)
3 Olive
4 Pyramid
5 Posterior (dorsal) column nuclei

MHMS

● *The lateral aperture is a gap between the cerebellum and medulla rather than a well-defined opening. The choroid plexus protrudes through it, into the subarachnoid space.*

Figures 9.15–9.17 The subarachnoid space.

Fig. 9.15
The subarachnoid space on the parietal lobe (opened by removing the arachnoid mater). ×0.66

1 Arachnoid granulations
2 Arachnoid mater
3 Gyri
4 Frontal lobe
5 Longitudinal fissure
6 Occipital lobe
7 Parietal lobe
8 Subarachnoid space (arrow: space between pia mater investing the brain and the arachnoid mater)

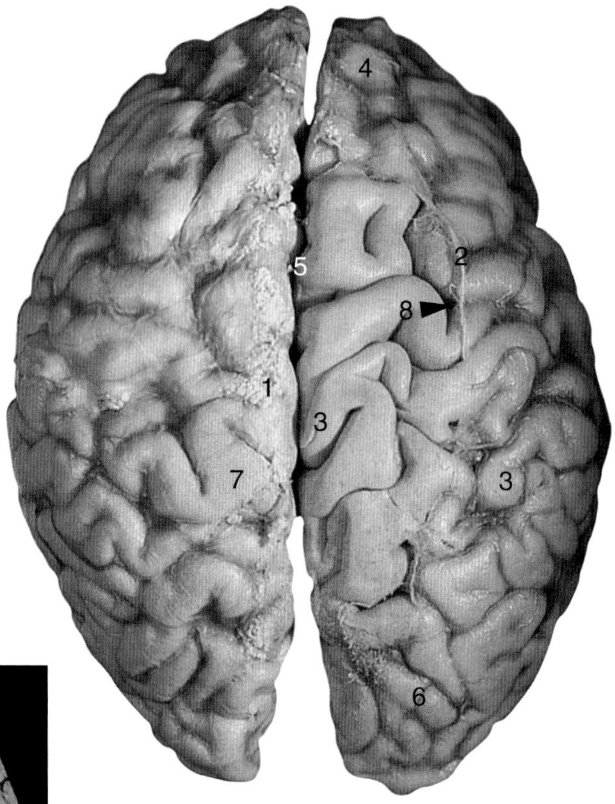

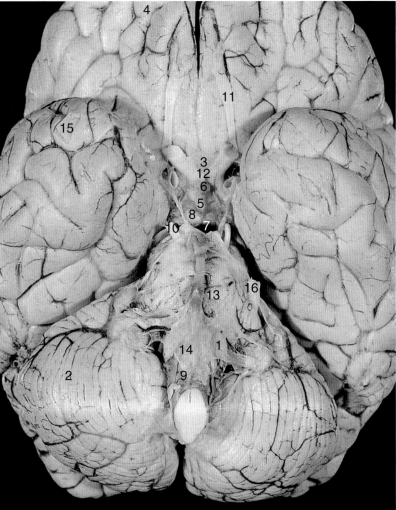

Fig. 9.16
The base of the brain with the arachnoid mater *in situ* to show the major cisternae associated with the ventral aspect of the brainstem. The interpeduncular cisterna has been partly opened to reveal the hypothalamus. ×1.6

1 Arachnoid mater
2 Cerebellum
3 Cisterna of the optic chiasma
4 Frontal lobe
5 Hypothalamus
6 Infundibulum
7 Interpeduncular cisterna
8 Mamillary body
9 Medulla oblongata
10 Oculomotor nerve
11 Olfactory tract
12 Optic chiasma
13 Pons
14 Pontine cisterna
15 Temporal lobe
16 Trigeminal nerve

All the cisternae shown on this picture are intracranial.

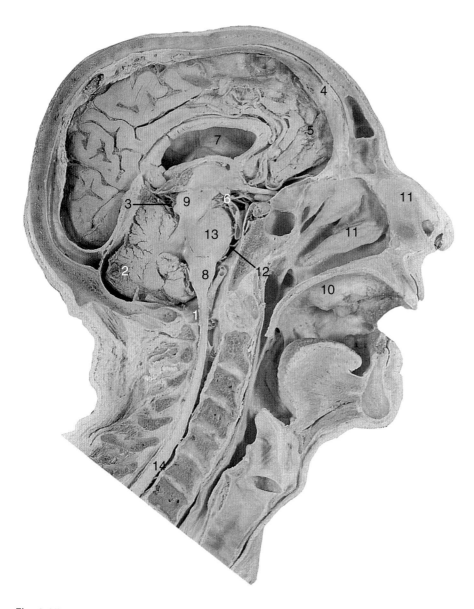

Fig. 9.17
A sagittal section of the head to illustrate the cisternae. ×0.56

1 Cerebello-medullary cisterna
2 Cerebellum
3 Cisterna of the great cerebral vein (of Galen) (or cisterna ambiens)
4 Falx cerebri
5 Frontal lobe
6 Interpeduncular cisterna
7 Lateral ventricle
8 Medulla oblongata
9 Midbrain
10 Mouth
11 Nose
12 Pontine cisterna
13 Pons
14 Spinal cord

● *All the ventricles are lined by an epithelium called the ependyma.*

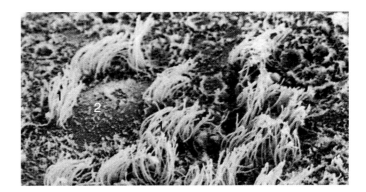

Fig. 9.18
Scanning electron micrograph of the ependyma lining the fourth ventricle.

1 Cilia
2 Ependyma

Prof. J. S. Lowe QMC

● *The composition of CSF is broadly similar to that of blood plasma, with important differences. CSF contains only two-thirds the concentration of glucose and one two-hundredth as much protein as is found in the plasma.*

● *In bacterial meningitis the glucose content of CSF falls because the bacteria consume the glucose. Viruses do not utilize glucose; in viral meningitis the concentration does not fall.*

Summary

1. The ventricles comprise an interconnecting system of spaces: a lateral ventricle in each cerebral hemisphere, a single midline third ventricle in the diencephalon, the cerebral aqueduct (of Sylvius) in the midbrain and the fourth ventricle in the hindbrain.

2. Cerebrospinal fluid (CSF) fills the ventricles and also fills the subarachnoid space around the brain and spinal cord.

3. CSF is produced by choroid plexuses in the two lateral, and the third and fourth ventricles.

4. CSF passes from the ventricles into the subarachnoid space via the median and two lateral apertures (the foramina of Magendie and Luschka).

5. Arachnoid granulations return CSF to the circulation via the dural venous sinuses.

6. Diagnostic samples of CSF can be taken in a lumbar puncture.

10 Cerebral Hemispheres and Basal Ganglia

The two cerebral hemispheres are the largest part of the brain and cover many other structures. The right and left cerebral hemispheres are connected to one another medially by a band of transversely running white fibers called the corpus callosum. Each hemisphere has four lobes named after their position in the skull, i.e. frontal, parietal, temporal and occipital. Inside, each cerebral hemisphere has a C-shaped lateral ventricle. In the floor and medial walls of the hemispheres are collections of grey matter, (basal ganglia or nuclei) and nerve fibers.

Many functions have been localized to specific regions of the brain. For example, the frontal lobe is generally concerned with personality and higher centers for voluntary motor activities. The temporal lobe deals with sensations of smell, taste and hearing; the parietal lobe is concerned with the peripheral sensations and the occipital lobe with vision. Speech is associated with the frontal and temporal lobes in the major or dominant hemisphere i.e. the left hemisphere in right-handed individuals.

The surface of each hemisphere is covered by broad folds of grey matter (gyri) and spaces or furrows (sulci) between the gyri. Many of the gyri and sulci are variable in position but a small number are constant due to their development and are important functionally.

Buried immediately below the lateral sulcus is an island of cerebral cortex called the insula. This was buried during embryonic development when adjoining cortical areas overgrew this region.

The grey matter (cortex) covering the surface of the hemispheres is composed of neuronal cell bodies, their proximal neurites, blood vessels and supporting neuroglial cells. The neurons are of various types and some areas contain a concentration of certain types of multipolar neurons. Predominantly sensory (afferent) areas (postcentral gyrus) contain more stellate neurons while motor (efferent) areas (precentral gyrus) contain a greater proportion of the larger type of pyramidal cells. In the phylogenetically older areas of cortex in the temporal lobe (areas with a longer evolutionary history), three layers are distinguishable; while in the newer areas (neocortex), which include most of the cerebral cortex, there are six layers.

The white matter consists of myelinated nerve fibers (axons) embedded in neuroglia. The nerve fibers in the white matter form nerve tracts which connect different areas of the same hemisphere (short and long association fibers) or connect one hemisphere with the other hemisphere (commissural fibers) or are afferent and efferent fibers (projection fibers) which pass from and to the brain stem or spinal cord, sometimes via masses of grey matter (basal nuclei) buried inside the cerebral hemisphere.

The two cerebral hemispheres, however, are not identical. Left/right asymmetries appear in fetal development and persist into childhood and adulthood. They may lead to hand preference and cerebral dominance for language.

The lateral ventricle is larger on the left and the left lateral sulcus is longer and straighter than the right. In many right handers the right frontal lobe is larger than the left and the left temporal and occipital lobes are larger than the right. The corpus callosum is larger in left-handed and ambidextrous people, reflecting a greater interconnectedness of the two hemispheres.

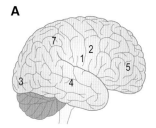
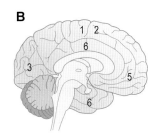

A   **B**

Diagrams showing a lateral (A) and a medial (B) view of the brain, labelled to illustrate the classical concept of functional localization in the cerebral cortex.

1 Somatic sensory	**5** Higher functions (cognitive)
2 Motor	**6** Limbic system
3 Visual	**7** Sensory association
4 Auditory	

- Lesions involving the frontal lobe produce motor and autonomic disturbances and alteration in character and behavior are apparent. Certain types of pain are no longer perceivable.

- Lesions involving the temporal lobe may produce disturbances in hearing, memory and in emotional behavior.

- Lesions in the parietal lobe produce a disturbance or loss of function in perception of shape, size and texture (agnosia), and are associated with difficulties in writing and talking (sensory aphasia) and memory.

- Destruction of the cortical visual areas of the occipital lobes produces blindness, although the pupillary reactions to light persist.

- Specific speech areas are located in the frontal, parietal and temporal lobes. Lesions in these areas affect the use of language.

Gyri and Sulci

Maps of the brain are based on the positions of constant gyri (folds) and sulci (furrows). Some of the gyri have specific functions. Areas of cortex adjacent to these are called association areas if they are related in function. Often they are concerned with interpretation which is called gnosis (to know). The entire brain surface is further subdivided into numbered areas which can be referred to for position of functions. Several different systems exist; Brodmann's is useful for localizing function (see pp. 108–115), while von Economo's is based on wider cellular differences between the layers (see p. 115), and Bailey and von Bonin's is based on the distribution of fibers spreading out from the thalamus into the cortex (see p. 115).

If certain areas are damaged on the dominant side of the brain, normal functioning is impaired.

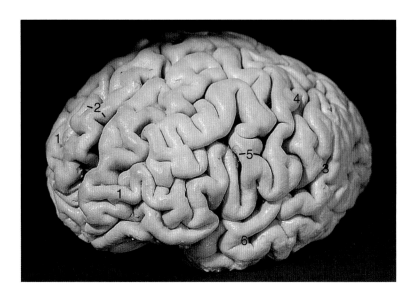

Fig. 10.1
Gyri and sulci on a lateral view of the brain. (The dura mater and arachnoid mater have been removed.) ×.52

1 Frontal lobe
2 Gyri
3 Occipital lobe
4 Parietal lobe
5 Sulci
6 Temporal lobe

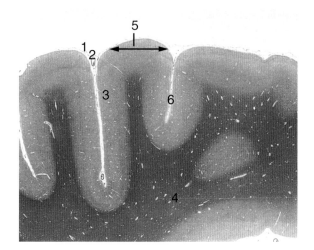

Fig. 10.2
Histological section to show gyri and sulci of the temporal lobe, stained with Solochrome cyanin and nuclear fast red. ×2.8

1 Arachnoid mater
2 Blood vessel
3 Cerebral cortex (gray matter)
4 Cerebral white matter
5 Gyrus
6 Sulcus

● *The existence of gender differences in the pattern of cortical gyri and sulci is controversial. Individual differences between persons of the same sex may be greater than any overall differences between males and females. However, in structures connected with reproductive functions, distinct sexual dimorphism has been demonstrated in laboratory mammals and there is reason to believe that differences also exist in humans.*

Functional Localization in the Sensory and Motor Cortex

The precentral gyrus of the frontal lobe is described as the primary motor cortex because of its function in controlling voluntary movement (see p. 108). Similarly, the postcentral gyrus is called the primary sensory or somatosensory cortex because it processes the somatic senses of touch, pain and temperature, as well as some aspects of proprioception (see p. 207). Each region of the body is served by a specific area of motor and somatosensory cortex. These areas are arranged in sequence along the pre- and postcentral gyri. The face is represented on the lateral aspect of the hemisphere and the legs and feet on the medial side. The term used to describe this pattern of innervation is "somatotopic". It occurs widely in the nervous system.

Structures that make fine complex movements or have an especially rich sensory innervation are served by larger areas of cerebral cortex than those that make large movements or have sparse sensory innervation. For example, the hand is served by a larger area of cortex than the back. This pattern can be represented as a distorted body image, projected on the surface of the cortex like a film on a screen, known as the "homunculus". For illustrations see the diagram below and p. 288.

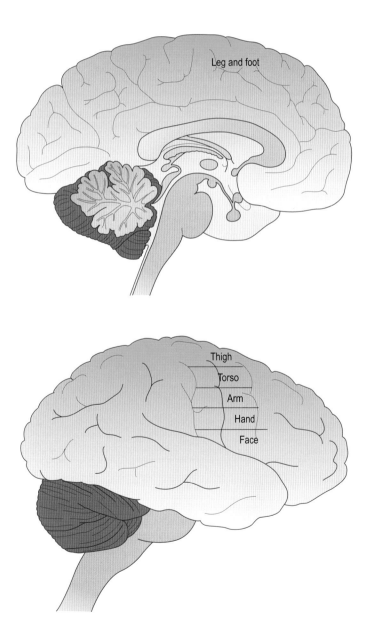

Figures 10.3–10.5 Gyri and sulci have relatively constant locations on every brain.

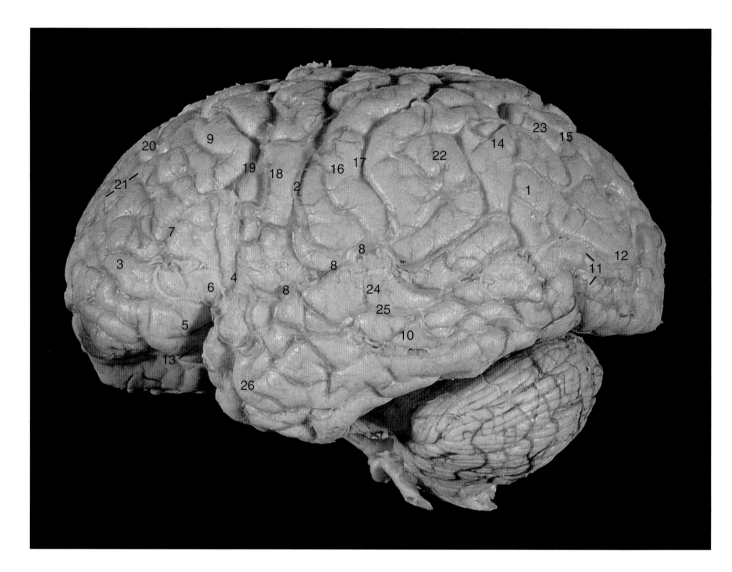

Fig. 10.3
The lateral surface of the brain. ×1.1

1 Angular gyrus
2 Central sulcus
3 Frontal lobe
4 Pars opercularis
5 Pars orbitalis
6 Pars triangularis
7 Inferior frontal sulcus
8 Lateral fissure (Sylvian fissure)
9 Middle frontal gyrus
10 Middle temporal gyrus
11 Occipital gyri
12 Occipital lobe
13 Orbital gyri

14 Parietal lobe
15 Parieto-occipital sulcus
16 Postcentral gyrus
17 Postcentral sulcus
18 Precentral gyrus
19 Precentral sulcus
20 Superior frontal gyrus
21 Superior frontal sulcus
22 Supramarginal gyrus
23 Superior parietal lobule
24 Superior temporal gyrus
25 Superior temporal sulcus
26 Temporal pole

● *The pars opercularis, pars orbitalis and pars triangularis are all parts of the inferior frontal gyrus.*

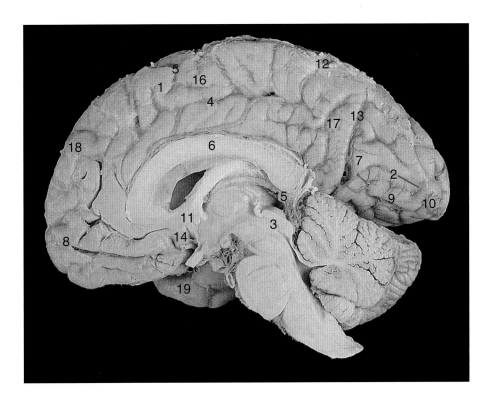

Fig. 10.4
The medial surface of the brain. ×0.79

 1 Anterior paracentral lobule
 2 Calcarine sulcus
 3 Cerebral aqueduct
 4 Cingulate sulcus
 5 Central sulcus
 6 Corpus callosum
 7 Cuneate gyrus
 8 Frontal lobe
 9 Lingual gyrus
10 Occipital lobe
11 Paraterminal gyri
12 Parietal lobe
13 Parieto-occipital sulcus
14 Paraolfactory gyri
15 Pineal gland (body)
16 Posterior paracentral lobule
17 Precuneate gyrus
18 Superior frontal gyrus
19 Temporal lobe

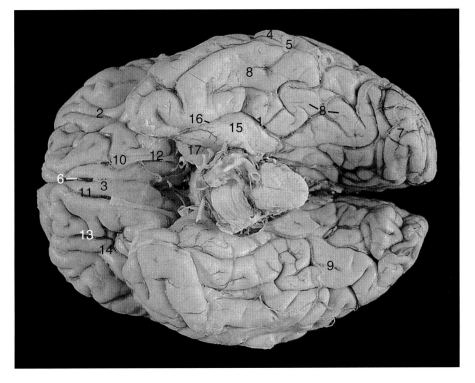

Fig. 10.5
The base of the hemispheres. ×0.69

 1 Collateral sulcus
 2 Frontal lobe
 3 Gyrus rectus
 4 Inferior temporal gyrus
 5 Inferior temporal sulcus
 6 Longitudinal fissure
 7 Occipital lobe
 8 Occipitotemporal gyri
 9 Occipitotemporal sulcus
10 Olfactory bulb
11 Olfactory sulcus
12 Olfactory tract
13 Orbital gyri
14 Orbital sulcus
15 Parahippocampal gyrus
16 Rhinal sulcus
17 Uncus

Pioneering studies by Brodmann (1904) originally described 47 areas with distinct boundaries in the six-layered neocortex of the brain. These areas were based on minute histological variations. Many of these have since been ascribed functions and are designated below as motor, sensory (including touch, taste and sight), speech and hearing, and the limbic system (including mood, behavior and smell). The remaining numbered areas are indeterminate functionally and appear on page 113.

This method of describing the brain was once thought to be outdated, but recent work in cellular neuroanatomy and neurophysiology, particularly the use of functional imaging techniques such as positron emission tomography (PET) and functional magnetic resonance imaging (fMRI), have re-emphasized the importance of a detailed knowledge of cellular arrangements (cytoarchitectonics) for an understanding of cortical function.

PET scanning uses radioactive tracers, such as glucose, to identify sites of enhanced blood flow at regions of high activity in the living brain. It creates an image in which different colors indicate different activity levels, and so can be used to localize functional areas in the brain.

Anatomical detail is poor, but it may be combined with the accurate topography revealed by MRI scanning to produce a functional brain map for any chosen activity, for example vision or movement. This method is known as fMRI scanning. These studies have confirmed the validity of Brodmann's original concept.

Figure 10.6–10.14 demonstrate Brodmann's areas related to function.

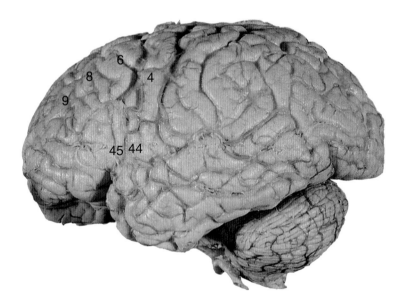

Fig. 10.6
Brodmann's areas with motor functions (lateral view). ×0.64

4 Precentral gyrus (performance of movements).
6, 8, 9 "Pre-motor" (planning of movements, connections to basal ganglia, and controls eye movements).
44, 45 Broca's area (parts of these areas control speech movements; also see Hearing and Language below).

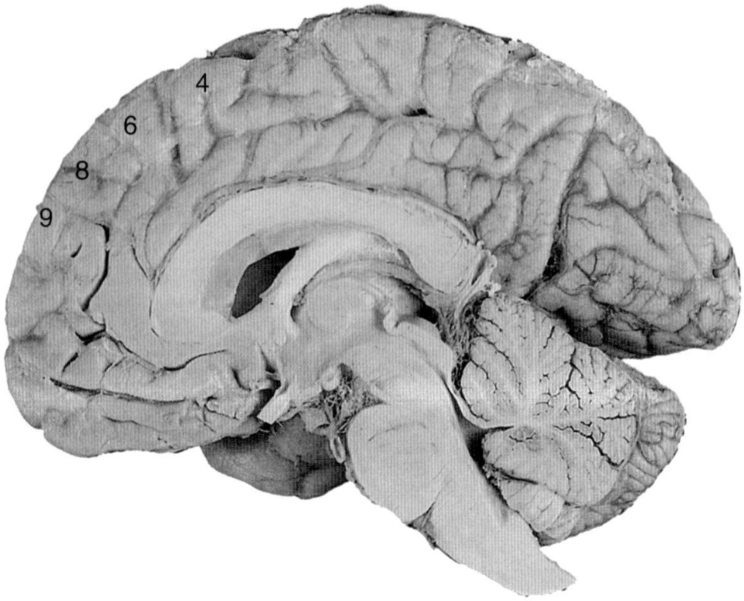

Fig. 10.7
Brodmann's areas with motor functions (medial view). ×0.64

4 Precentral gyrus (leg and foot movements).
6, 8, 9 "Pre-motor" (planning of movements, connections to basal ganglia).

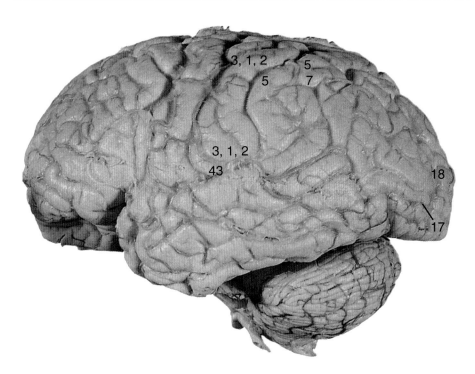

Fig. 10.8
Brodmann's areas with sensory functions (touch, taste, sight, balance) (lateral view). ×0.75

1, 2, 3 Postcentral gyrus (touch, pain, temperature, conscious proprioception, balance).

5,7 Parietal lobe (sensory association cortex: interpretation of senses perceived in areas 1, 2 and 3). 7 particularly associated with spatial perception.

17 Lips of the calcarine sulcus (vision).

18 Remainder of occipital lobe (visual association for interpretation of visual information).

43 Adjacent to the most inferior part of postcentral gyrus, 1, 2 and 3 (taste).

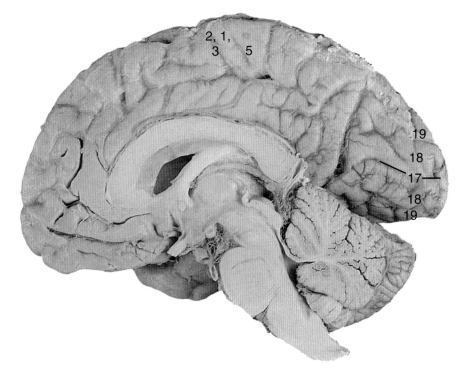

Fig. 10.9
Brodmann's areas with sensory functions (touch and sight) (medial view). ×0.75

1, 2, 3 Postcentral gyrus (touch, pain, temperature, conscious proprioception, balance).
5 Parietal lobe (sensory association cortex: interpretation of senses perceived in areas 1, 2 and 3).
17 Lips of calcarine sulcus (vision).
18, 19 Remainder of occipital lobe (visual association for interpretation of visual information).

● *For Hearing see p. 112.*

Figures 10.10 and 10.11 Brodmann's areas concerned with emotion, mood and behavior, including the limbic system.

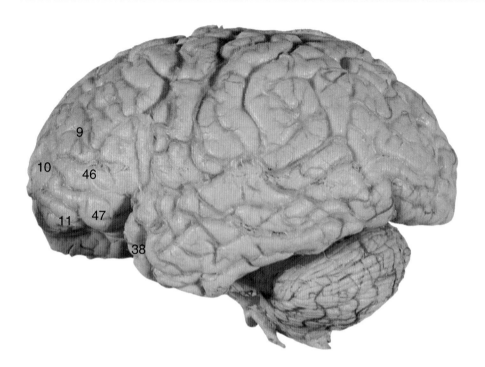

Fig. 10.10
Lateral view. ×0.75

9, 10   Superior, middle and inferior gyri of frontal lobe. The "higher" intellectual functions.

11, 46, 47 Anterior frontal cortex.

38   Anterior pole of temporal lobe. Complex memory and imaginative processes.

● *Areas 9, 10, 11, 46 and 47 are sometimes grouped together as the "prefrontal cortex", especially in imaging studies of brain function.*

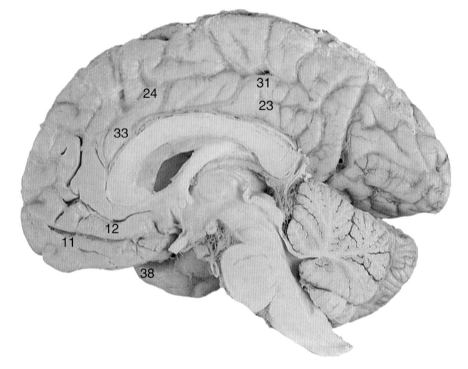

Fig. 10.11
Medial view. ×0.75

11, 12   Orbital region of frontal lobe. May have an inhibitory effect on expression of emotions.

23, 24, 31, 33 Cingulate gyrus. May add emotional "tone" to sensory experience, including pain. Area 33 is specifically activated by heat- or cold-induced pain (see Limbic System).

38   Anterior pole of temporal lobe. Complex memory and imaginative processes.

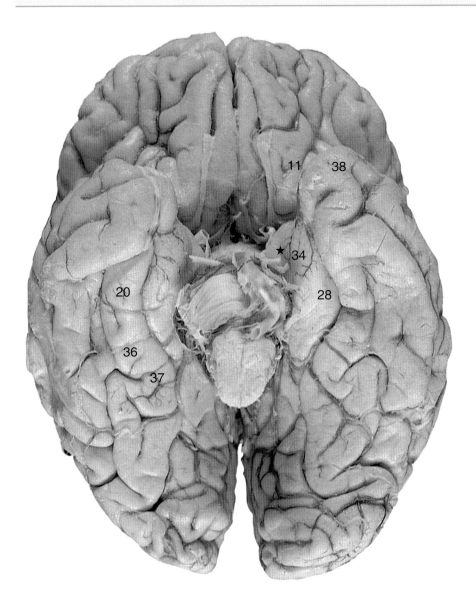

Fig. 10.12
Brodmann's areas concerned with olfactory functions and those concerned with emotion, mood and behavior, including the limbic system, and with object recognition (basal view). ×0.93

11	Posterior end of orbital gyri of frontal lobe. Olfactory.
28	Parahippocampal gyrus (anterior part). Olfactory and memory.
34	Adjacent to uncus. Olfactory.
38	Anterior pole of temporal lobe. Complex memory and imaginative processes.
20, 36, 37	Occipitotemporal or fusiform gyrus. Recognition of objects, faces and colors.

- *The occipitotemporal (fusiform) gyrus is concerned with object recognition. It includes Brodmann's areas 20, 36 and 37. Lesions at the anterior end, including area 20, cause prosopagnosia, the inability to recognize faces. Lesions in area 37 cause achromatopsia, or "cortical color blindness", the inability to recognize colors.*

- *The uncus (marked by a star in Fig. 10.12) is not included in Brodmann's map because it is not formed from six-layered neocortex. It is the primary olfactory cortex. The posterior end of area 11, and areas 28 and 38, form the olfactory association cortex involved in the interpretation of olfactory sensations (see Smell, p. 275).*

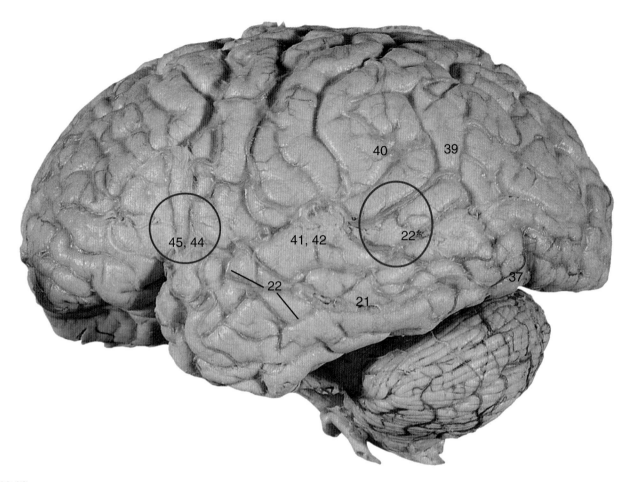

Fig. 10.13
Brodmann's areas concerned with hearing and language (lateral view). ×1.2

21 Middle temporal gyrus. Auditory and visual memory.

22 Superior temporal gyrus and part of the middle temporal gyrus. Auditory association cortex for interpretation of sound including speech (see **22*** below).

22* Posterior end of the superior temporal gyrus. Wernicke's area or sensory speech area. Perception and comprehension of speech and formulation of speech content (blue circle).

37 On border between temporal and occipital lobes. Mainly visual memory (possibly including written language) and color recognition.

39 Angular gyrus. Important in reading.

40 Supramarginal gyrus. Comprehension and ability to repeat speech.

41, 42 Middle of superior temporal gyrus. Primary auditory cortex. Perception of sound.

44, 45 Part of pars triangularis and pars opercularis of inferior frontal gyrus. Broca's area for control of speech movements and speech production (red circle).

● *Language involves listening, comprehension and production of speech sounds. In most people, the left hemisphere is dominant in language functions, although the right is important for the emotional "tone" and expression of spoken words. Left-sided dominance has also been demonstrated in deaf people using sign language.*

● *Aphasia is the inability to understand or express language in symbols. Damage to Brodmann's area 39 (angular gyrus) produces a sensory (receptor) aphasia called alexia or visual aphasia, "word blindness". The printed word is meaningless. Damage to area 22 (sensory) produces auditory aphasia or word deafness. Damage to areas 44 and 45 (Broca's area) produces a motor aphasia in which the patient cannot convert thoughts into speech sounds. Damage to the left prefrontal cortex produces grammatical aphasia, the inability to construct sentences.*

● *Agraphia is the loss of the ability to write.*

● *Apraxia is the inability to carry out learned voluntary acts, which may include speech movements.*

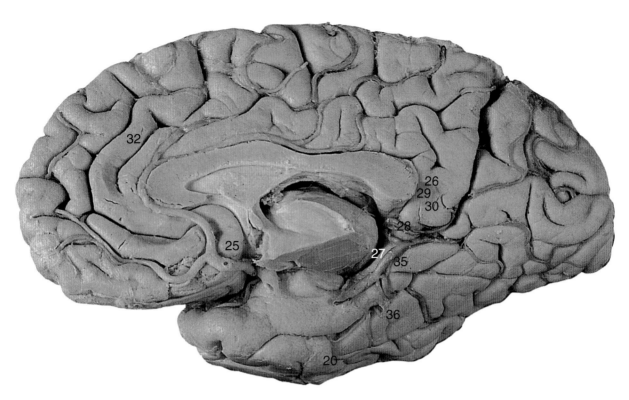

Fig. 10.14
Brodmann's areas that have no clearly determined function (indeterminate), and those that have complex cognitive functions (inferomedial view). ×0.89

13, 14, 15, 16	Areas ascribed to the insula on the grounds of comparative anatomy (not seen in this view).
25	Frontal lobe adjacent to olfactory tract and part of **32**, medial side of frontal lobe above cingulate gyrus. Emotional responses to complex situations, e.g. social situations.
26, 27, 28, 29, 35	Behind the splenium of the corpus callosum. Connect cingulate and parahippocampal gyri.
30	Medial side, behind corpus callosum. Interpretation of facial expression.
20	Inferior temporal gyrus.
32	(part of) Medial side of frontal lobe. Direction of attention.
36	Occipitotemporal gyrus.

Functional localization studies appear to present the cerebral cortex as a mosaic of discrete areas with separate functions. However, any complex behavior needs the cooperation of several areas, linked by the association pathways described on page 122. An example of this is seen in fMRI studies of chess players. During the game, activity can be seen in areas 17, 18 and 19 (vision), 4 (motor), 6 and 8 (eye movements), 7 (sensory association cortex for spatial perception), the inferior temporal lobe (memory) and cognitive areas in the prefrontal cortex.

Another example of functional cooperation is seen in the recognition of words and pictures. This process utilizes many of the same areas in the occipital, temporal and parietal lobes. Because of this link, it has been suggested that an object recognition system already existing in the primate brain was adapted to a new use when human language evolved.

Fig. 10.15
A fMRI scan showing active language processing areas in the left frontal and parietal lobes as red and yellow pixels. These results confirm the areas 22, 39 and 40, and 44 and 45 as defined by Brodmann. The image is a composite of results from five right-handed males, all asked to think of any word beginning with the letter "U".

1 Frontal lobe
2 Occipital lobe
3 Parietal lobe
4 Temporal lobe

Dr. S. C. R. Williams IP

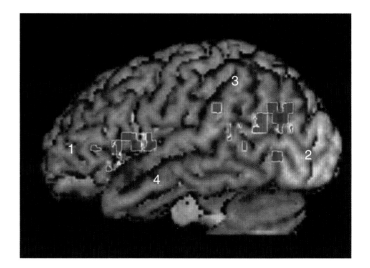

● *Functional imaging methods also show some evidence of human sex differences. For example, areas in the frontal lobe that control movements dependent on spatial skills, such as following a map, have been shown to be more active in men than in women given the same task to do. Conversely, the brains of women showed more widespread activity than those of men in a test involving the interpretation of words.*

Alternative systems to Brodmann's areas

Alternatives to Brodmann's methods for anatomical mapping of the cerebral cortex place less emphasis on small local variations in histology (cytoarchitecture).

The Bailey and von Bonin system divides the cortex into nine sections according to their afferent connections with the thalamus.

The von Economo system, not illustrated here, recognizes five types of six-layered neocortex based on variation in the relative thickness of the cellular layers.

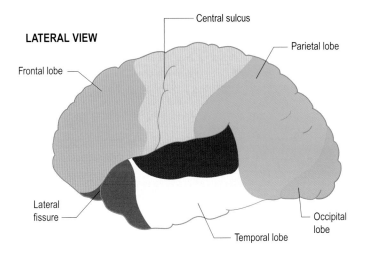

Maps of the cerebral cortex based on the distribution of fibers from the thalamus, according to Bailey and von Bonin. It is useful to compare these diagrams with that of the thalamic peduncles (see p. 145).

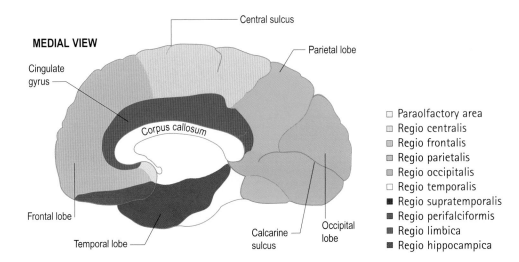

- ☐ Paraolfactory area
- ☐ Regio centralis
- ▨ Regio frontalis
- ▨ Regio parietalis
- ▨ Regio occipitalis
- ☐ Regio temporalis
- ■ Regio supratemporalis
- ■ Regio perifalciformis
- ■ Regio limbica
- ■ Regio hippocampica

Summary

1. Each cerebral hemisphere consists of four lobes, the frontal, parietal, occipital and temporal lobes.
2. Its surface is covered by gray matter, the cerebral cortex.
3. Inside the hemisphere lie the basal ganglia and tracts of white matter.
4. The cortex is folded into a pattern of gyri and sulci.
5. Functions may be "mapped"onto the cerebral cortex by observing the effects of disease, and by imaging methods such as PET and fMRI scanning.
6. Some functional localizations correspond to the histological variations described by Brodmann.

Histology of the Cerebral Cortex

Most parts of the cerebral hemisphere are covered by cortex comprising six layers of neurons. This type of cortex is known as neocortex, or isocortex. Modified forms of cortex are found in cortical areas associated with the limbic system; the cortex of the hippocampal formation, the parahippocampal gyrus and uncus is three-layered (allocortex); that of the insula and cingulate gyrus has six indistinct layers (mesocortex). The cortex of the cerebellum also has three layers (see p. 207). In neocortex, while the layers run parallel to the cortical surface, functionally the cells are associated in columns at right angles to the cortical surface, spanning all the layers. Cortical cells form synapses with each other. They also connect with association and projection fibers entering the cortex from the cerebral white matter and project fibers into the white matter.

Within the basic six-layer pattern different parts of the cortex show minor variations in their cellular arrangements (cytoarchitecture) and fiber distribution (myeloarchitecture). Some of these can be correlated with the localization of specific cortical functions (see Brodmann's areas).

Layer I contains some small cells but consists mainly of intracortical fibers.

Layer II contains small, mainly stellate, cells connected in local circuits.

Layer III cells are predominantly pyramidal in shape and give rise to commissural and association fibers.

Layer IV is well developed in cortical areas with a sensory function (for example, Brodmann's areas 1, 2, 3 [somatic sensory], 41 and 42 [hearing], and 17 [vision]) and poorly represented in motor cortex (for example, area 4). Its cells are granular in form and it receives many projection fibers from thalamic nuclei which are components of specific sensory pathways.

Layer V cells are mostly pyramidal and give off projection fibers to the basal ganglia, brainstem and spinal cord. This is the predominant layer in motor cortex.

Layer VI cells are variable in shape and send fibers to the thalamus.

Some pyramidal cells are present in all layers except layer I.

Using specific cytochemical techniques, a variety of neurotransmitters and their receptors can be identified in the cortical cells and fibers. Pyramidal cells are excitatory in function and contain glutamate. Non-pyramidal cells predominantly use gamma-aminobutyric acid (GABA). Some cells contain neuropeptide transmitters either alone or co-localized with GABA. These are not confined to any one layer. Fibers entering the cortex from subcortical structures may be noradrenergic (transmitter noradrenaline), serotonergic (transmitter serotonin), dopaminergic (transmitter dopamine) or cholinergic (transmitter acetylcholine). In addition, there are corticopetal fibers (from the thalamus and the basal ganglia) for which the transmitters are unknown.

Fig. 10.16
A low power view of part of an histological section of cerebral hemisphere to differentiate the gray matter of the cortex on its surface from the white matter inside. Solochrome cyanin and light green stain. ×4

1 Arachnoid mater
2 Blood vessel
3 Cortex
4 Gyrus
5 Sulcus
6 White matter

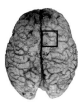

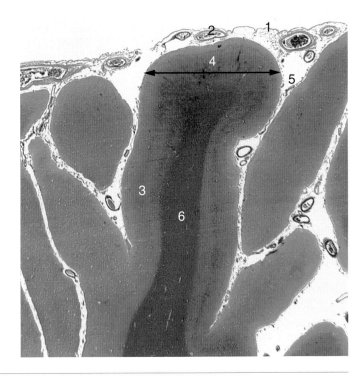

● *In Alzheimer's disease, there is a loss of cholinergic axons to the cortex from the basal forebrain, particularly the nucleus of Meynert (see p. 119).*

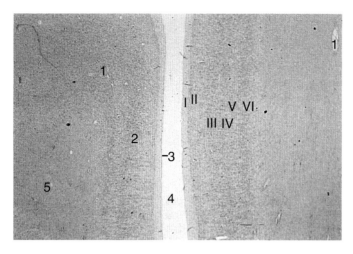

Fig. 10.17
Section through the cortex of the frontal lobe to show the six-layered structure of neocortex. Cresyl violet stain. ×7

1 Blood vessel
2 Cerebral cortex (the layers are numbered I–VI)
3 Pia mater
4 Sulcus
5 White matter

OXF

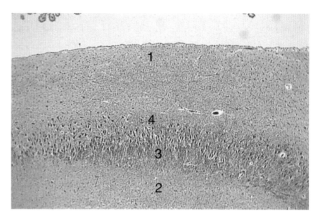

Fig. 10.18
An histological section to show the three layers of cells in the cortex of Ammon's horn, part of the hippocampus. Cresyl violet stain. ×56

1 Alveus (fibers)
2 Molecular layer (stratum radiatum)
3 Pyramidal cell layer
4 Stratum oriens or polymorphic cell layer

CAM

● *Unlike other parts of the cerebral cortex, small numbers of new cells can be formed in the hippocampus throughout life.*

Fig. 10.19
A paraffin wax section through layers I to IV of the primary visual cortex of the occipital lobe to show neurons and fibers. Myelin stain. ×65

1 Blood vessel
2 Intracortical fibers of layer I
3 Layer I
4 Layer II
5 Layer III
6 Layer IV
7 Neuronal cell body
8 Outer band of Baillarger
9 Projection fibers

CAM

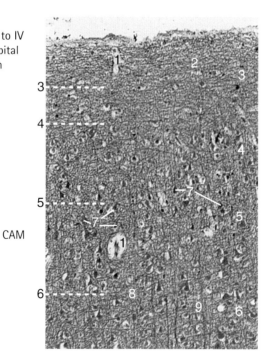

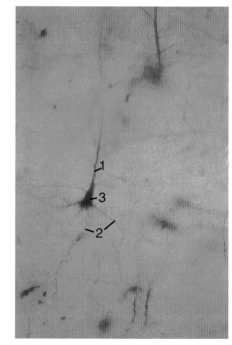

Fig. 10.20
A pyramidal cell from layer V of the temporal lobe cortex. Golgi-Cox stain. ×267

1 Apical dendrite
2 Basal processes
3 Cell body

● *The outer band of Baillarger is formed by thalamic afferent fibers entering layer IV. It is, therefore, well developed in sensory areas of cortex. In the visual cortex, it is especially prominent and known as the stria of Gennari (see Fig. 19.21, p. 253).*

Figures 10.21–10.23 Examples of the use of specific immunocytochemical staining methods to demonstrate the presence of neuropeptides in neurons of the cerebral neocortex.

Neuropeptides, of which neuropeptide Y and somatostatin are examples, are a group of substances that may act as modulators of the sensitivity of neurons to other transmitters rather than as transmitters in their own right. They may coexist in the same cell with other transmitter substances.

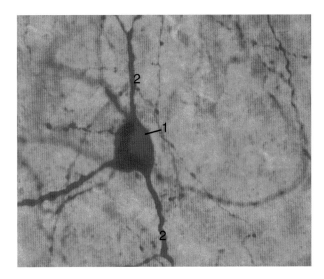

Fig. 10.21
A neuropeptide Y-containing neuron in the normal temporal neocortex, from a surgical specimen. The dark staining demonstrates the presence of neuropeptide Y in this cell. ×1100

1 Cell body   2 Cell processes

Dr. Victoria Chan-Palay

Fig. 10.22
Somatostatin-immunoreactive non-pyramidal neuron from layer V of the frontal cortex. ×733

1 Cell body   3 Thin axon-like process
2 Cell processes   Dr. Eva Braak

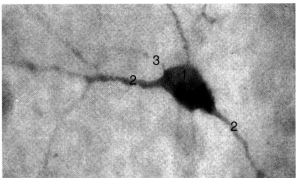

Fig. 10.23
Somatostatin-immunoreactive non-pyramidal neuron from layer VI of the frontal neocortex. Surrounding non-reactive cells are demonstrated by gallocyaninchromalum counterstain. ×760

1 Non-reactive cells
2 Somatostatin-immunoreactive cell

Dr. Eva Braak

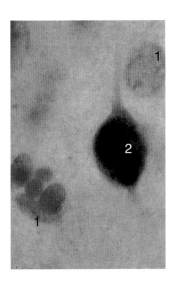

Fig. 10.24
A coronal section of one cerebral hemisphere to show the position of the substriatal gray matter, in which the nucleus of Meynert is situated. Phosphotungstic acid and hematoxylin stain. ×0.98

1 Amygdaloid nucleus	6 Extreme capsule	11 Lateral ventricle
2 Caudate nucleus	7 Globus pallidus	12 Putamen
3 Claustrum	8 Hypothalamus	13 Substriatal gray matter
4 Corpus callosum	9 Insula	14 Temporal lobe
5 External capsule	10 Internal capsule	

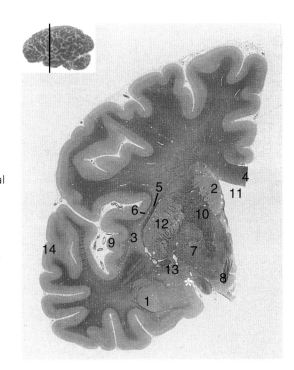

The white asterisk indicates the nucleus of Meynert. From its neurons, cholinergic nerve fibers spread out to all parts of the cerebral cortex and to the amygdaloid nucleus. They play an important role in regulating the activity of the cortex, especially in relation to sleeping and waking.

Figures 10.25–10.29 Histological sections to show the variety of neuronal shapes in the cerebral cortex. Hematoxylin and eosin stain.

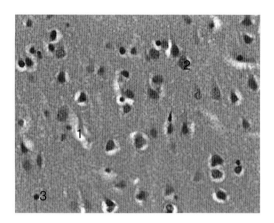

Fig. 10.25
An area of cortex from layer II. Most of the cells are stellate. ×300

Figures 10.25–10.27 share the following labels:

1 Blood vessel
2 Neuron
3 Nucleus of glial cell

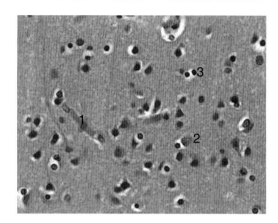

Fig. 10.26
An area of cortex from layer IV. Most of the cells are small and granular. ×300

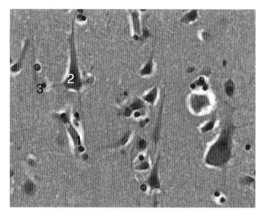

Fig. 10.27
An area of cortex from layer V. Most of the cells are pyramidal. ×300

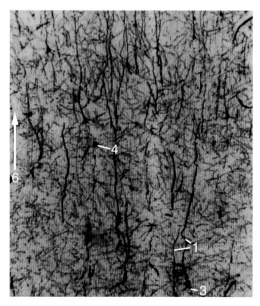

Fig. 10.28
Golgi-Cox stain. ×110   Dr. M. Rossi WCNN

Figures 10.28 and 10.29 demonstrate an area of cortex from the cingulate gyrus, showing a number of pyramidal neurons. Their dendrites are highly orientated relative to the surface of the cortex. Synapses are formed at dendritic spines along the length of the dendrite. Both figures have been electronically color-enhanced. Figures 10.28 and 10.29 share the following labels:

1 Apical dendrite
2 Axon
3 Basal processes
4 Cell body
5 Dendritic spines
6 Toward the surface of the cortex

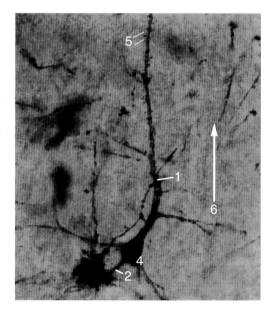

Fig. 10.29
A pyramidal cell to show the dendritic spines. ×400
Dr. M. Rossi WCNN

● *In adolescence, some loss of axons occurs in the cerebral cortex. This is known as "pruning" and is a normal developmental process.*

● *In people with schizophrenia and bipolar mood disorder, the pyramidal cells of the prefrontal cortex and hippocampus are smaller and have fewer dendritic spines than normal.*

Fig. 10.30
Myelin-stained autoradiographic images of the same area showing the cholinergic muscarinic receptors for the transmitter acetylcholine in the visual cortex of the occipital lobe. The highest receptor density is seen in the primary visual cortex (VI), identified in the myelin-stained section (**A**) by the presence of the stria of Gennari. In section **B**, the receptor molecules on the neurons have been stained with the radioactive tracer molecule [³H]oxotremorine. The image has then been computer enhanced to indicate the intensity of staining by a color code. Red indicates an area of cells with a high cholinergic receptor density; green or blue areas have fewer receptors.

Prof. K. Zilles UD

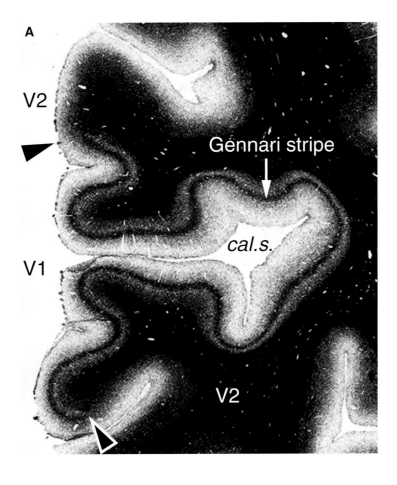

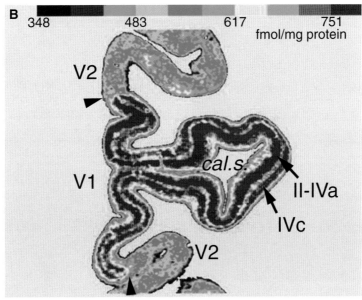

Short and Long Association Fibers

Association fibers connect different areas in the same hemisphere. They are divided into short and long groups. The short fibers connect adjacent gyri and dip below the floor of the intervening sulcus. The long fibers connect different lobes. There are four main deep bundles of long fibers: the uncinate fasciculus, the superior longitudinal fasciculus (including the arcuate fasciculus), the inferior longitudinal fasciculus, and the cingulum. The first two are found laterally in the brain.

The uncinate fasciculus connects parts of the orbital, middle and inferior frontal gyri with anterior portions of the temporal lobe. A deeply placed part also connects the frontal

and occipital lobes. The inferior longitudinal fasciculus connects the occipital lobe to the temporal lobe.

The superior longitudinal fasciculus connects the frontal to the occipital, temporal and parietal lobes. The fronto-occipital fasciculus connects the frontal lobe to the occipital and temporal lobes. The arcuate fasciculus, sometimes described as part of this fasciculus, connects the middle frontal gyri to parts of the temporal lobe.

The cingulum is the principal, medially placed long association bundle. It connects regions of the frontal and parietal lobes with the parahippocampal area and adjacent temporal region.

Short association fibers

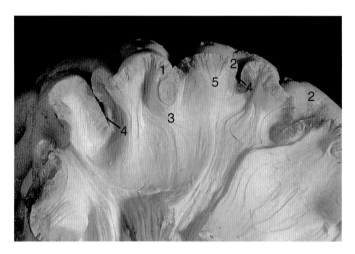

Fig. 10.31
Short association fibers between gyri in the frontal lobe. ×1.4

1 Gray matter   **4** Sulci
2 Gyri   **5** White matter
3 Short association fibers

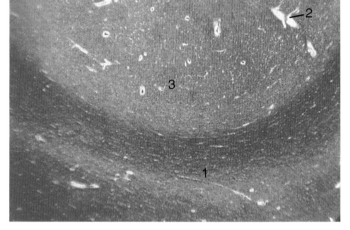

Fig. 10.32
Histological section of short association fibers between gyri of the frontal lobe. Solochrome cyanin and nuclear fast red stain. ×26

1 Association fibers   **3** Cortex
2 Blood vessel

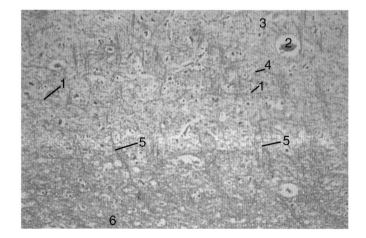

Fig. 10.33
Higher magnification view of an histological section through the transition between the gray matter of the cerebral cortex and the white matter. Projection fibers (see p. 125), which enter and leave the cortex, run at right angles to the cortical surface, while the association fibers run parallel to it. Luxol fast blue and cresyl violet stain. ×400

1 Association fibers
2 Blood vessel
3 Gray matter
4 Neuronal cell body
5 Projection fibers
6 White matter

Long association fibers

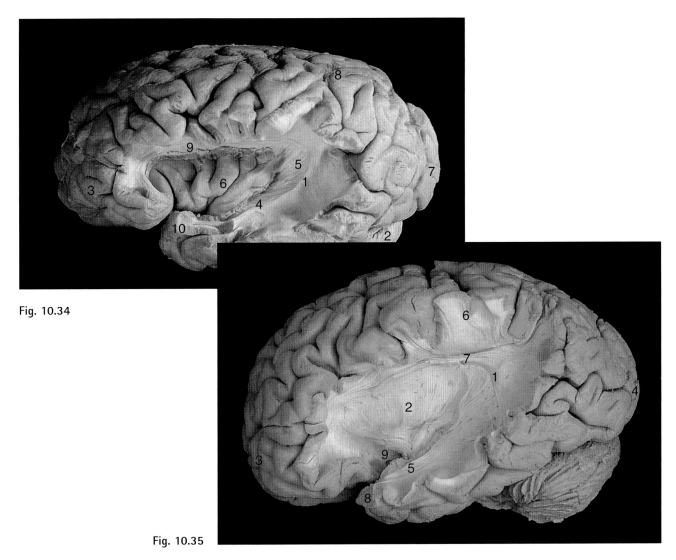

Fig. 10.34

Fig. 10.35

Fig. 10.34
The bundle of long association fibers called the superior longitudinal fasciculus lies immediately deep to the gyri and sulci laterally. ×0.69

1 Arcuate fasciculus
2 Cerebellum
3 Frontal lobe
4 Inferior longitudinal fasciculus
5 Inferior occipitofrontal fasciculus
6 Insula
7 Occipital lobe
8 Parietal lobe
9 Superior longitudinal fasciculus
10 Temporal lobe

Fig. 10.35
Association fibers located immediately deep to the gyri and sulci on the lateral surface (including those of the insula). ×0.68

1 Arcuate fasciculus
2 Extreme capsule
3 Frontal pole
4 Occipital pole
5 Inferior longitudinal fasciculus
6 Short association fibers
7 Superior longitudinal fasciculus
8 Temporal pole
9 Uncinate fasciculus

The freezing and thawing technique used to prepare this specimen produces a color change. Brains may become yellow.

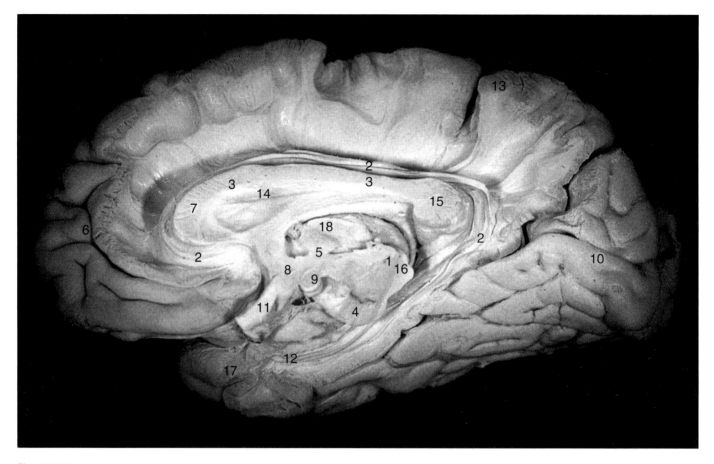

Fig. 10.36
The long association fibres in the cingulate and hippocampal gyri are known as the cingulum. Medial aspect of the brain with the cortex of the cingulate gyrus removed to reveal the cingulum. ×1

1 Cerebral aqueduct	**7** Genu (of corpus callosum)	**13** Parietal lobe
2 Cingulum	**8** Hypothalamus	**14** Septum pellucidum
3 Corpus callosum	**9** Mamillary body	**15** Splenium (of corpus callosum)
4 Corpus cerebri	**10** Occipital lobe	**16** Tectum of midbrain
5 Diencephalon	**11** Optic nerve	**17** Temporal lobe
6 Frontal lobe	**12** Parahippocampal gyrus	**18** Thalamus

Projection Fibers

Projection fibers, which are both afferent and efferent, connect the spinal cord, brainstem, diencephalon and deep telencephalic nuclei with the cerebral cortex. Within the cerebral hemisphere, the projection fibers are "fan-shaped", the internal capsule forming the handle of the "fan", as the fibers pass between the gray nuclear masses (the basal ganglia) lying in the floor of each cerebral hemisphere (see p. 130). Immediately above the nuclear masses, the fibers radiate vertically to the cerebral cortex, forming the "fan" itself, the corona radiata. Most of these fibers lie deep to the association fibers and intersect the commissural fibers. They include all the major ascending (sensory) and descending (motor) pathways. The internal capsule is supplied by central branches of the middle and anterior cerebral arteries.

As the internal capsule passes between the nuclear masses, it conforms to the shapes of their outlines and is divided into an anterior and a posterior limb which are joined at the genu.

The anterior limb contains the frontopontine and thalamocortical fibers. The genu contains corticonuclear fibers. The anterior one-half to two-thirds of the posterior limb contains thalamocortical fibers (general somatic sensory pathway) and corticospinal fibers.

The most posterior of the internal capsule fibers are "retrolentiform" as they lie posterior to one of the nuclear masses (the lentiform nucleus). The retrolentiform region contains fibers of the auditory and optic radiations. Lesions in the internal capsule cause widespread neurological defects due to interruptions of a variety of nervous pathways.

The external capsule lies superficial to the basal ganglia. It also contains projection fibers. Its composition is incompletely known but it contains corticostriate fibers ending in the putamen and corticoreticular connections to the reticular formation. These also run in the internal capsule.

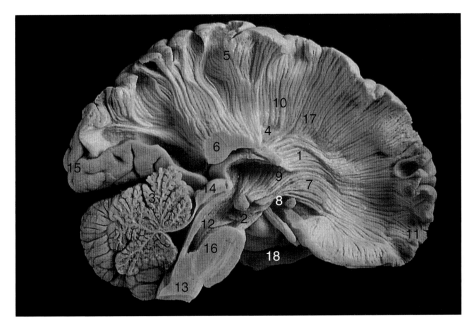

Fig. 10.37
Projection fibers of the left cerebral hemisphere viewed from the medial aspect. ×.5

 1 Anterior thalamic peduncle (or radiation)
 2 Basis pedunculi
 3 Cerebellum
 4 Caudate nucleus
 5 Corona radiata
 6 Corpus callosum
 7 Corticohypothalamic fibers in the internal capsule
 8 Corticonigral tract
 9 Corticorubral tract
 10 Corticostriate fibers
 11 Frontal lobe
 12 Medial lemniscus
 13 Medulla
 14 Midbrain
 15 Occipital lobe
 16 Pons
 17 Superior thalamic peduncle (or radiation)
 18 Temporal lobe

Prof. N. Gluhbegovic

● *The name of a nervous pathway indicates its origin and destination, e.g. corticospinal fibers run from the cerebral cortex to the spinal cord, corticohypothalamic fibers run from the cerebral cortex to the hypothalamus. Corticohypothalamic, corticonigral, corticorubral and corticostriate fibers are descending pathways. The thalamic peduncles are ascending pathways.*

● *In addition to the grouping of nerve fibers by function in the internal capsule, described above, there is also a somatotopic grouping in the posterior limb of the capsule. Corticospinal and corticonuclear (corticobulbar) motor pathways controlling movement in the head and neck lie most anteriorly, next to the genu. Behind them in sequence lie the pathways for the upper limb, torso and lower limb.*

Fig. 10.38
Horizontal section of brain showing the relationship between internal, external and extreme capsules, the thalamus and the basal ganglia. Mulligan stain. ×0.8

1 Anterior limb of internal capsule
2 Caudate nucleus
3 Cerebellum
4 Claustrum
5 Corpus callosum
6 External capsule
7 Extreme capsule
8 Fornix
9 Frontal lobe
10 Genu of internal capsule
11 Insula
12 Lateral ventricle
13 Lentiform nucleus
14 Posterior limb of internal capsule (lenticulothalamic portion)
15 Retrolentiform part of posterior limb of the internal capsule
16 Thalamus
17 Third ventricle

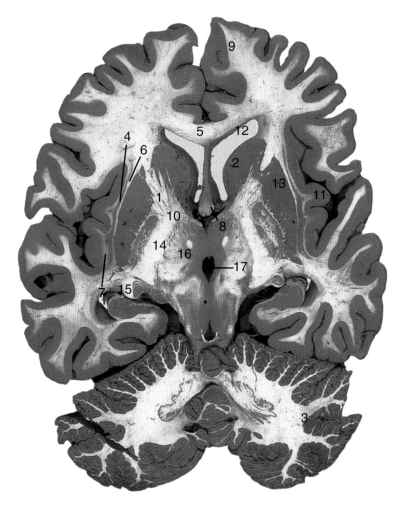

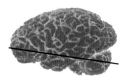

Fig. 10.39
Thick section of brain to show the passage of the projection fibers between the brainstem through the internal capsule into the cerebral hemisphere. Mulligan stain. ×0.86

1 Cerebral white matter
2 Corpus callosum
3 Crus cerebri (cerebral peduncle)
4 Fornix
5 Frontal lobe
6 Hippocampal formation
7 Internal capsule (posterior limb)
8 Lateral ventricle
9 Midbrain
10 Pons
11 Substantia nigra
12 Temporal lobe
13 Thalamus

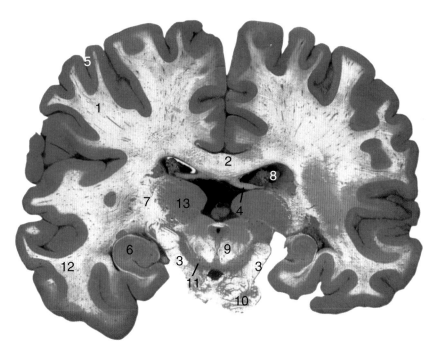

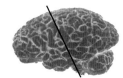

Fig. 10.40
A paraffin wax coronal section passing through one cerebral hemisphere, the caudal end of the diencephalon, the midbrain and the pons, showing the sublenticular portion of the posterior limb of the internal capsule. Solochrome cyanin and nuclear fast red stain. ×1.6

1 Caudate nucleus
2 Cerebral aqueduct
3 Cerebral peduncle
4 Cingulate gyrus
5 Claustrum
6 Corona radiata
7 Corpus callosum
8 Decussation of the superior cerebellar peduncle
9 External capsule
10 Extreme capsule
11 Fornix
12 Habenular nuclei and stria medullaris thalami
13 Hippocampus

14 Insula
15 Internal capsule (posterior limb)
16 Internal capsule (sublenticular portion)
17 Lateral geniculate body
18 Lateral posterior nucleus of thalamus
19 Lateral ventricle
20 Midbrain
21 Pons
22 Putamen
23 Temporal lobe
24 Ventral posterior thalamic nuclei
25 Visual (optic) radiation

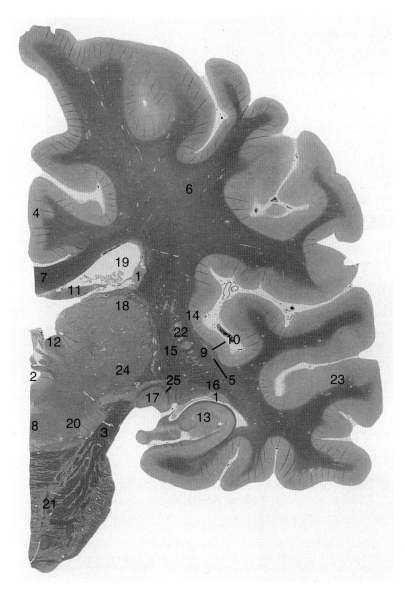

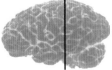

Insula

The insula is an area of cerebral cortex buried deep to the lateral sulcus. It is not visible unless the two gyri adjacent to the lateral sulcus are separated.

Histologically, the anterior part of the insula is granular and the posterior part is agranular. The insula is believed to be associated with visceral functions such as autonomic and emotional responses to external stimuli, though many of its fiber connections are unknown. It is recognized that the anterior part of the insula is connected to the olfactory and taste areas of the cerebral cortex. The posterior part is connected to the auditory cortex and to a somatic sensory area of the parietal operculum known as SII because it is secondary to the main somatic sensory area.

Immediately deep (medial) to the insula are the external capsule and the lentiform nucleus.

Figures 10.41 and 10.42 show the position of the insula.

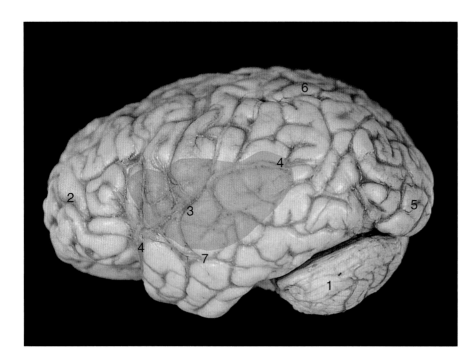

Fig. 10.41
A lateral view of the brain with a colored overlay to indicate the position of the insula buried below the surface. ×0.58

1 Cerebellum
2 Frontal lobe
3 Insula (colored overlay)
4 Lateral sulcus
5 Occipital lobe
6 Parietal lobe
7 Temporal lobe

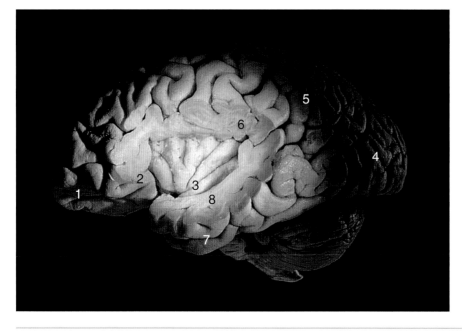

Fig. 10.42
Cerebral hemisphere dissected from the lateral side to reveal the insula. ×0.62

1 Frontal lobe
2 Frontal operculum (cut)
3 Insula
4 Occipital lobe
5 Parietal lobe
6 Parietal operculum (cut)
7 Temporal lobe
8 Temporal operculum (cut)

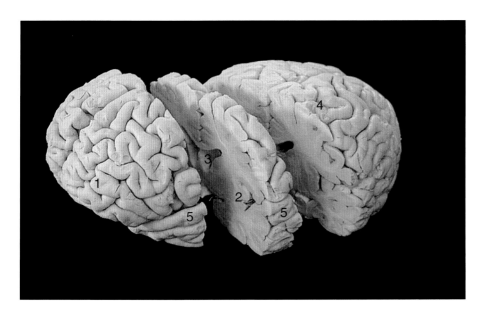

Fig. 10.43
A coronal section through the insula. ×0.5

1 Frontal lobe
2 Insula
3 Lateral ventricle
4 Parietal lobe
5 Temporal lobe

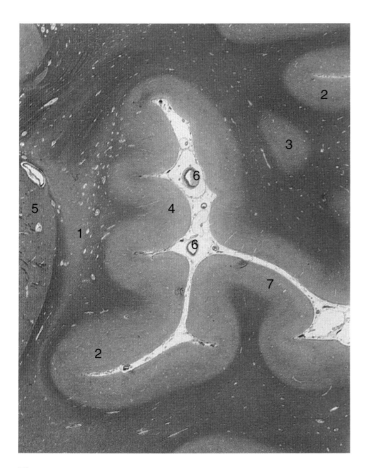

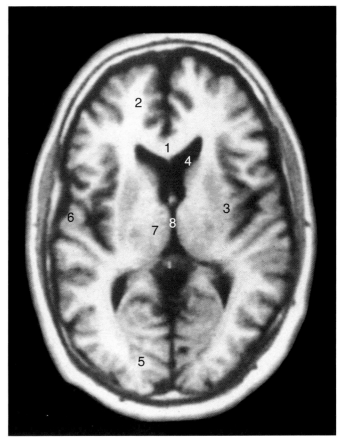

Fig. 10.44
Histological section to show the insula and the middle cerebral vessels. Section stained with solochrome cyanin and nuclear fast red. ×3

1 Claustrum
2 Cortex
3 Frontal operculum
4 Insula
5 Lentiform nucleus
6 Middle cerebral artery
7 Temporal operculum

Fig. 10.45
Transverse image of the normal adult brain as seen by the nuclear magnetic resonance (NMR) technique.

1 Corpus callosum
2 Frontal lobe
3 Insula
4 Lateral ventricle
5 Occipital lobe
6 Temporal lobe
7 Thalamus
8 Third ventricle

Dr. G. Bydder

129

Basal Ganglia or Basal Nuclei

The basal nuclei are well-defined masses of gray matter that are grouped together, embedded in the subcortical white matter of the telencephalon around the lateral ventricle. They can be seen only when the brain has been sectioned or dissected. Anatomically, the basal ganglia comprise the corpus striatum, amygdaloid nucleus and claustrum. Functionally, the corpus striatum and claustrum are both concerned with motor functions, but the amygdaloid nucleus is not (see Limbic System). A functional definition of the basal ganglia includes the subthalamic nucleus and the substantia nigra with the corpus striatum and claustrum in a system for movement control and coordination.

The corpus striatum is divided into two parts, the caudate nucleus and the lentiform nucleus, by a band of white matter called the internal capsule.

The caudate nucleus forms a "C" shape closely applied to the contours of the lateral ventricle (along the floor of the anterior horn and body, and the roof of the inferior horn). It ends anteriorly in apparent continuity with the amygdaloid nucleus (or "amygdala").

The lentiform (lens-shaped) nucleus lies deep to the insula, and is divided by a vertical sheet of white matter into a dark, large lateral portion (putamen) and an inner, paler portion (globus pallidus).

The amygdaloid nucleus is concerned with olfactory reflexes and is part of the limbic system concerned with aggressive and sexual behavior.

The claustrum is a thin sheet of gray matter whose function is unknown.

There are afferent and efferent connections between the corpus striatum and the cerebral cortex, thalamus, subthalamus and brainstem (see Movement control, p. 299).

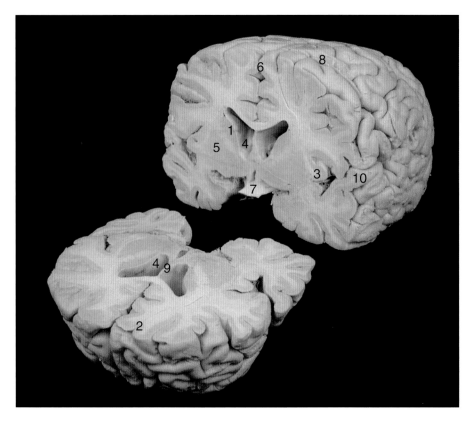

Fig. 10.46
Coronal section through the cerebral hemispheres and the diencephalon to illustrate the position of the caudate and lentiform nuclei. ×0.65

1 Caudate nucleus
2 Frontal lobe
3 Insula
4 Lateral ventricle
5 Lentiform nucleus
6 Longitudinal fissure
7 Optic chiasma
8 Parietal lobe
9 Septum pellucidum
10 Temporal lobe

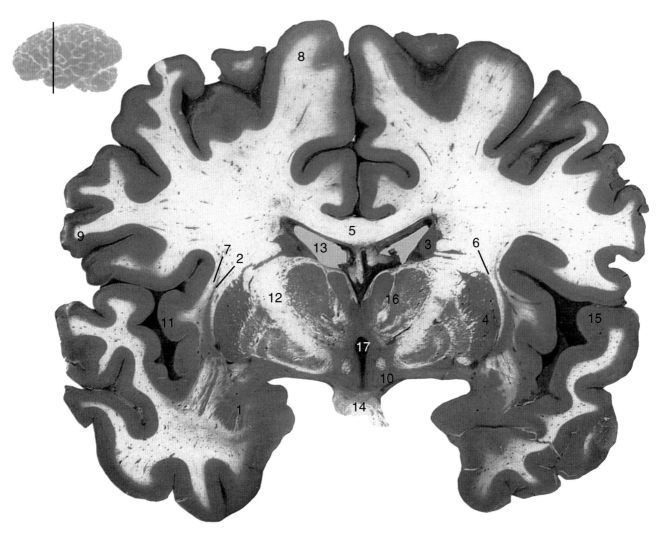

Fig. 10.47
Stained thick coronal slice through both cerebral hemispheres at the level of the optic chiasma to show the caudate, lentiform and amygdaloid nuclei. Mulligan stain. ×1.2

1 Amygdaloid nucleus (amygdala)
2 Claustrum
3 Caudate nucleus ⎫
4 Lentiform nucleus ⎭ Corpus striatum
5 Corpus callosum
6 External capsule

7 Extreme capsule
8 Frontal lobe
9 Frontal operculum
10 Hypothalamus
11 Insula
12 Internal capsule

13 Lateral ventricle
14 Optic chiasma
15 Temporal lobe
16 Thalamus
17 Third ventricle

Figures 10.48–10.53 If the brain is dissected from the lateral side, the caudate and lentiform nuclei and associated white matter are revealed in sequence.

Fig. 10.48
The extreme capsule lies immediately deep to the gyri and sulci of the insula. ×0.68

1 Corona radiata
2 Extreme capsule
3 Frontal lobe
4 Occipital lobe
5 Parietal lobe

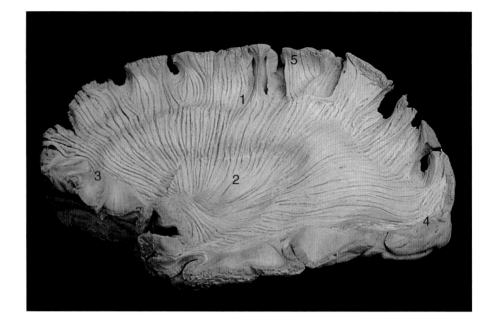

Fig. 10.49
The brain dissected from the lateral surface to show the claustrum. ×0.66

1 Claustrum
2 Corona radiata
3 External capsule
4 Frontal lobe
5 Inferior longitudinal fasciculus
6 Occipital lobe
7 Parietal lobe
8 Temporal lobe
9 Uncinate fasciculus

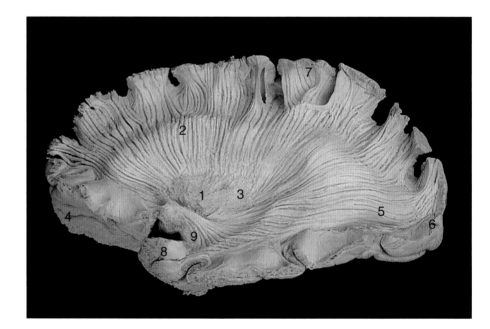

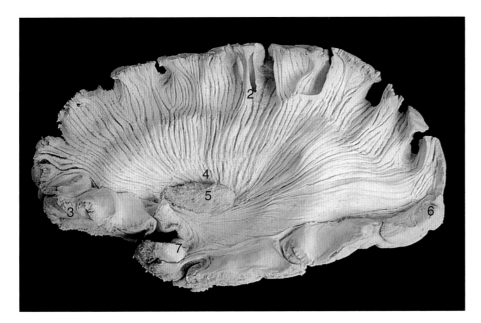

Fig. 10.50
The brain dissected deeper than in Fig. 10.48 to show the most lateral part of the lentiform nucleus. ×0.6

1 Cerebellum
2 Corona radiata
3 Frontal lobe
4 Internal capsule
5 Lentiform nucleus
6 Occipital lobe
7 Temporal lobe

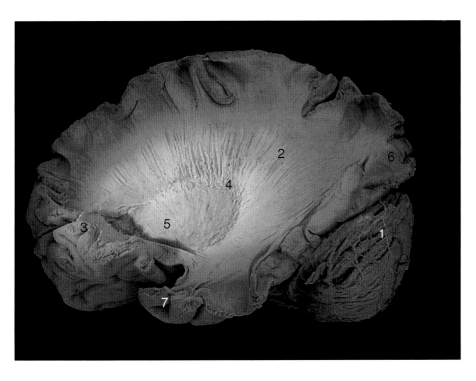

Fig. 10.51
Deeper dissection from the lateral side to show the lentiform nucleus. ×0.65

Fig. 10.52
The lentiform and caudate nuclei as viewed from the lateral surface. ×0.7

  1 Caudate nucleus
  2 Cerebellum
  3 Choroid plexus
  4 Corpus callosum
  5 Frontal lobe
  6 Lateral ventricle
  7 Lentiform nucleus
  8 Occipital lobe
  9 Parietal lobe
 10 Temporal lobe

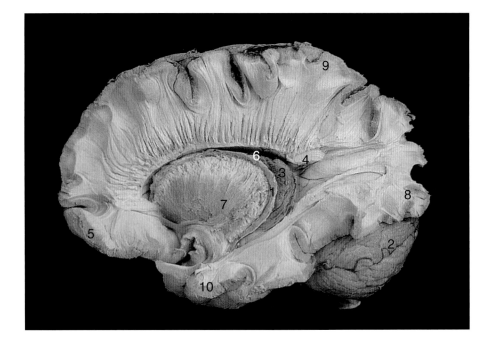

Fig. 10.53
Caudate nucleus and diencephalon in a dissection of the medial side of the brain. ×0.63

  1 Caudate nucleus
  2 Cerebellum
  3 Fornix
  4 Frontal lobe
  5 Internal capsule
  6 Mamillary body
  7 Mamillothalamic tract
  8 Midbrain
  9 Occipital lobe
 10 Optic chiasma
 11 Pons
 12 Stria terminalis
 13 Thalamic nuclei

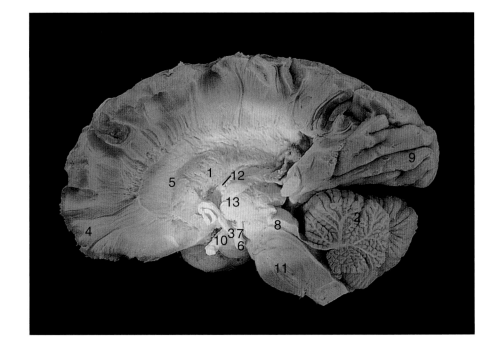

Figures 10.54–10.56 Sections to demonstrate connections between the rostral part (head) of the caudate nucleus and the lentiform nucleus across the internal capsule. The striped or striated appearance caused by these connections gives rise to the name "corpus striatum".

Fig. 10.54
Thick coronal section through both cerebral hemispheres. Mulligan stain. ×0.7

1 Caudate nucleus	**7** Frontal lobe
2 Claustrum	**8** Insula
3 Connections between the	**9** Internal capsule
caudate nucleus and	**10** Lateral ventricle
the lentiform nucleus	**11** Lentiform nucleus
4 Corpus callosum	**12** Longitudinal fissure
5 External capsule	**13** Septum pellucidum
6 Extreme capsule	**14** Temporal lobe

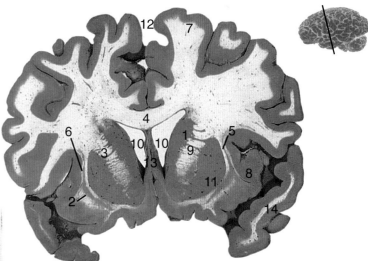

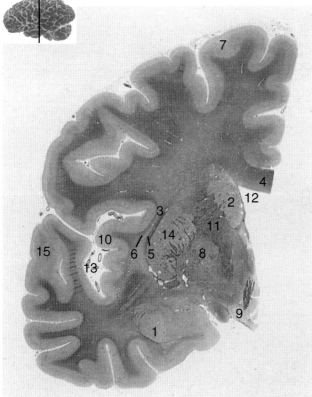

Fig. 10.55
An histological section through a cerebral hemisphere to show the structure of the corpus striatum. The relationship between the caudate, lentiform and amygdaloid nuclei is also illustrated. Phosphotungstic acid and hematoxylin stain. ×1.1

1 Amygdaloid nucleus	**9** Hypothalamus
2 Caudate nucleus	**10** Insula
3 Claustrum	**11** Internal capsule
4 Corpus callosum	**12** Lateral ventricle
5 External capsule	**13** Middle cerebral artery
6 Extreme capsule	**14** Putamen
7 Frontal lobe	**15** Temporal lobe
8 Globus pallidus	

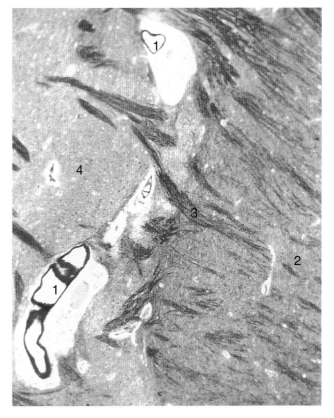

Fig. 10.56
Histological section showing nerve fibers passing between the putamen and the globus pallidus. A higher magnification of Fig. 10.55. Phosphotungstic acid and hematoxylin stain. ×29

1 Blood vessel	**3** Nerve fibers
2 Globus pallidus	**4** Putamen

● *The term "pallidus", i.e. pale, describes the appearance of this structure in unstained sections or in sections stained to demonstrate gray matter, for example with Mulligan stain.*

Figures 10.57–10.61 Dissections and histological preparations showing the relationships of the basal ganglia. The dissections in Figures 10.57, 10.59 and 10.60 are from the same specimen, to show the relationship between the corpus striatum and thalamus.

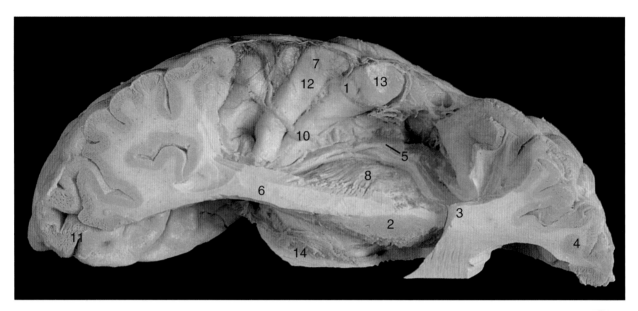

Fig. 10.57
A cerebral hemisphere dissected from above to show the medial to lateral relationships of the thalamus, caudate nucleus and lentiform nucleus. ×1

1 Auditory cortex	**6** Internal capsule	**11** Occipital lobe
2 Caudate nucleus	**7** Lateral aspect of brain	**12** Superior temporal gyrus
3 Corpus callosum	**8** Lentiform nucleus	**13** Temporal lobe
4 Frontal lobe	**9** Medial aspect of brain	**14** Thalamus
5 Insula	**10** Middle cerebral artery (branches)	

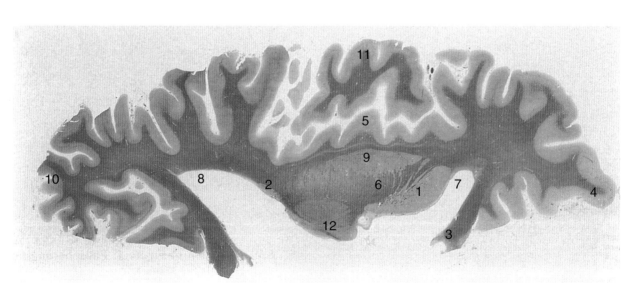

Fig. 10.58
Horizontal histological section through one cerebral hemisphere to illustrate the relationships of the caudate and lentiform nuclei to the thalamus. Solochrome cyanin and nuclear fast red stain. ×0.93

1 Caudate nucleus (head)	**4** Frontal lobe	**7** Lateral ventricle (anterior horn)	**10** Occipital lobe
2 Caudate nucleus (tail)	**5** Insula	**8** Lateral ventricle (posterior horn)	**11** Temporal lobe
3 Corpus callosum	**6** Internal capsule	**9** Lentiform nucleus	**12** Thalamus

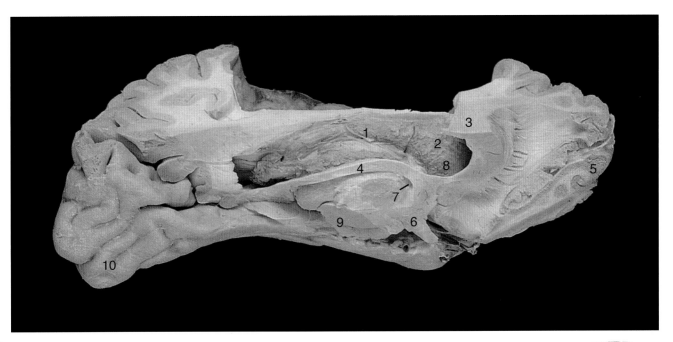

Fig. 10.59

A cerebral hemisphere dissected from the medial side to show the superior to inferior relationships of the thalamus and caudate nucleus. The septum pellucidum has been removed. ×0.95

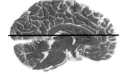

1 Caudate nucleus (body)	5 Frontal lobe	8 Lateral ventricle
2 Caudate nucleus (head)	6 Hypothalamus	9 Midbrain
3 Corpus callosum	7 Interventricular foramen	10 Occipital lobe
4 Fornix		

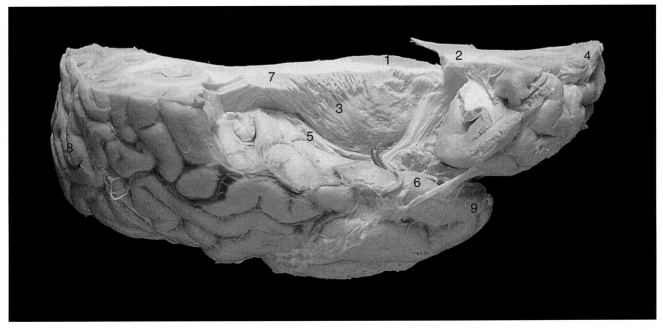

Fig. 10.60

A cerebral hemisphere dissected from the lateral surface to illustrate the relationships between the external capsule and lentiform nucleus. ×0.95

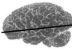

1 Caudate nucleus	4 Frontal lobe	7 Medial aspect of brain
2 Corpus callosum	5 Inferior longitudinal fasciculus	8 Occipital lobe
3 External capsule	6 Lateral aspect of brain	9 Temporal lobe

Fig. 10.61

Coronal histological section through part of one cerebral hemisphere showing the caudate and lentiform nuclei, thalamus and subthalamus. Solochrome cyanin and light green stain. ×2.5

1 Caudate nucleus (body)
2 Caudate nucleus (tail)
3 Corpus callosum
4 External capsule
5 Extreme capsule
6 Fornix
7 Insular cortex
8 Internal capsule
9 Lateral ventricle (body)
10 Lateral ventricle (inferior horn)

11 Lentiform nucleus
12 Subthalamus
13 Thalamus

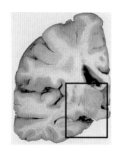

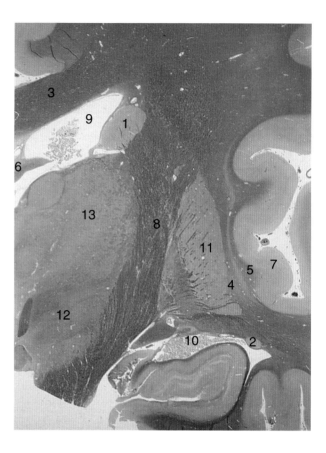

Figures 10.62–10.64 Sections illustrating the position and structure of the substantia nigra.

Fig. 10.62

Half a brain dissected from the medial side to demonstrate the position and relationships of the substantia nigra and red nucleus. ×0.65

1 Anterior commissure
2 Caudate nucleus
3 Cerebellum
4 Cerebral aqueduct
5 Cerebral hemisphere
6 Cerebral peduncle
7 Inferior colliculus
8 Fourth ventricle
9 Mamillary body

10 Mamillothalamic tract
11 Medulla
12 Midbrain
13 Pons
14 Red nucleus
15 Substantia nigra
16 Superior colliculus
17 Thalamus

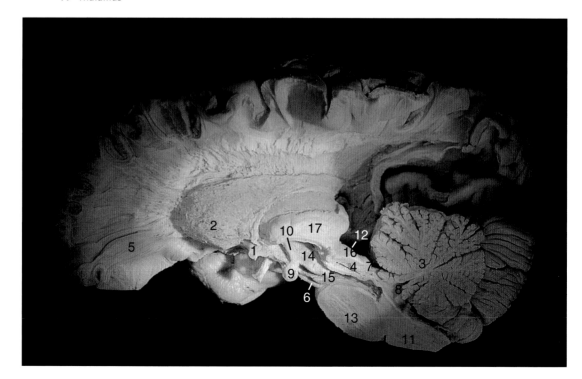

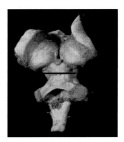

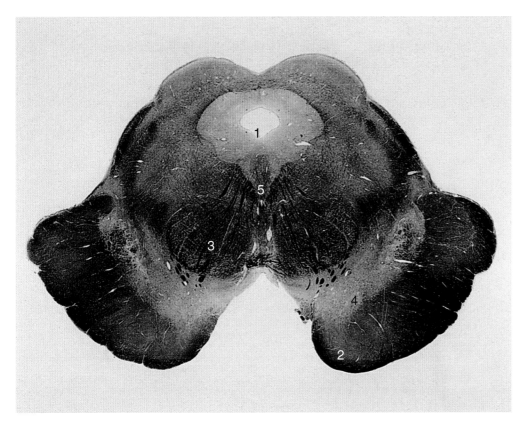

Fig. 10.63
A transverse histological section of the midbrain to show the position of the substantia nigra.
Weigert–Pal stain. ×5.6

1 Cerebral aqueduct
2 Cerebral peduncle
3 Red nucleus
4 Substantia nigra
5 Tegmentum

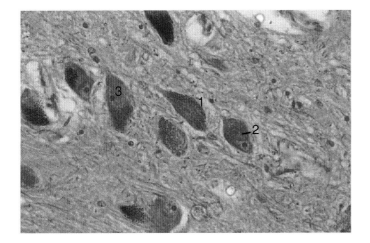

Fig. 10.64
Cells of the substantia nigra showing their brown neuromelanin
pigmentation. Solochrome cyanin and nuclear fast red stain. ×510

1 Cell body
2 Neuromelanin
3 Nucleus

11 Diencephalon

The name diencephalon means "between brain", and refers to the part lying between the brainstem and the cerebral hemispheres. The diencephalon surrounds the third ventricle and is subdivided into four parts: the thalamus, the subthalamus, the hypothalamus and the epithalamus.

The thalamus is a paired structure, with right and left thalami forming the upper part of the lateral walls of the third ventricle. Each is an oval mass of gray matter divided into medial, lateral and anterior parts by a Y-shaped band of white matter, the internal medullary lamina. Each of the three parts can be further subdivided into several nuclei. Their positions and connections are shown in the diagrams on pp. 142–143.

The thalamus is linked to the sensory systems, basal ganglia, cerebellum, brainstem and cerebral cortex. These connections enable the thalamus to act as an intermediary between subcortical structures and the cerebral cortex. Most cortical connections are grouped in bundles, the thalamic peduncles or radiations. Thalamic nuclei connected to localized areas of cerebral cortex are often called "specific nuclei" and those not so connected have "non-specific" connections. Some nuclei fall into both categories. The medial and lateral geniculate bodies lie slightly separated from the main mass of the thalamus. They are part of the auditory and visual pathways, respectively.

The subthalamus lies below and caudal to the thalamus. Its most prominent nucleus, the subthalamic nucleus, is functionally part of the basal ganglia, and involved in movement control.

The hypothalamus lies below the rostral end of the thalamus, forming the floor and lower part of the lateral walls of the third ventricle. It contains several nuclei and has a variety of important functions. By virtue of its connections with both the nervous and endocrine systems, it is central to the process of homeostasis. Homeostasis is the automatic maintenance of balance and stability in the internal functions of the body in spite of a changing external environment. Reactions may be physiological or behavioral. For example, if we are thirsty, antidiuretic hormone is secreted to promote water retention by the kidneys and we drink fluids. The hypothalamus monitors the state of the body both via the circulation and through afferent nervous pathways. Its responses are similarly mediated, either through circulating hormones or through efferent connections to other parts of the nervous system. The best defined hypothalamic nuclei are the supraoptic nucleus, the paraventricular nucleus and the suprachiasmatic nucleus. The supraoptic and paraventricular nuclei are connected to the posterior lobe of the pituitary gland by neural tracts. Their neurons are neurosecretory, producing the hormones vasopressin (antidiuretic hormone, ADH) and oxytocin. The hormones are transported down their axons to the posterior pituitary for storage. The suprachiasmatic nucleus is the "body clock". It is connected to the reticular formation and to the corpus striatum, and controls the daily rhythm of sleeping and waking, as well as our sense of the passage of time. Through its connections with the autonomic nervous system, the hypothalamus is involved in the regulation of body temperature and the circulation. It also controls food and water intake. Activation of nuclei in the posterior part of the hypothalamus stimulates the sympathetic nervous system. Anterior nuclei have parasympathetic effects. The lateral and ventromedial nuclei regulate food and water intake. The hypothalamus is also a component of the limbic system involved in emotional behavior. As a part of the endocrine system, it regulates the activity of the anterior lobe of the hypophysis by producing hormones known as releasing and inhibitory factors. These hormones are released into blood vessels in the median eminence and are carried by a system of portal vessels to the capillary plexus of the adenohypophysis.

The hypothalamus is anatomically and physiologically linked to the hypophysis or pituitary gland. The hypophysis consists of two parts, the adenohypophysis or anterior lobe and the neurohypophysis or posterior lobe. In the embryo the adenohypophysis develops from Rathke's pouch, an outgrowth of the roof of the mouth. It has no neural connections with the hypothalamus but is linked to it via its blood supply, the portal system. It is composed of endocrine cells of epithelial origin from the roof of the stomodeum. The neurohypophysis is in direct neural continuity with the hypothalamus. It develops as an outgrowth from the diencephalon in the embryo. The hypophyseal stalk contains tracts connecting it to the adult hypothalamus. Neurosecretory neurons in the hypothalamus secrete hormones, the releasing factors, into capillaries of the portal system in the hypothalamus. Production of releasing factors is controlled by a feedback mechanism according to the levels of hormones circulating in the blood, for example estrogen. They are transported via portal veins in the hypophyseal stalk to a second capillary bed in the adenohypophysis which supplies the endocrine cells. These cells respond to the releasing factors by producing hormones that regulate the activity of other endocrine glands throughout the body. A textbook of endocrinology should be consulted for further information on the structure and functions of the hypophysis.

The main tracts of the hypothalamus are the fornix, medial forebrain bundle, mamillothalamic tract and dorsal longitudinal fasciculus.

The epithalamus lies above the thalamus. It consists of the habenular nuclei and their associated tracts, and the pineal gland. The habenular nuclei and their tracts are part of the limbic system. The pineal gland is an endocrine gland and its cells, the pinealocytes, produce a hormone, melatonin, which is associated with reproductive behavior and the regulation of physiological and behavioral rhythms, for example the sleep/wake cycle. Melatonin secretion shows a diurnal rhythm related to light and darkness.

The pineal gland is believed to have evolved from a median third eye in extinct lower vertebrates. In modern vertebrates it is no longer photosensitive itself, but receives information about light levels indirectly via a complex neural pathway from the retina (see diagram).

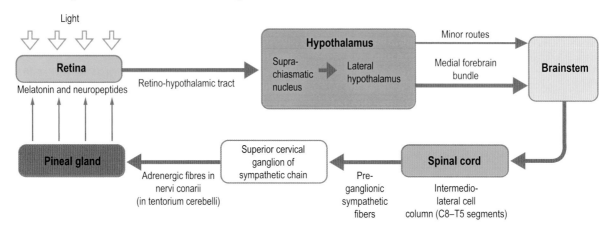

- *In the thalamic syndrome, pain perception is distorted or exaggerated on the side opposite the lesion.*

- *Rudimentary awareness of sensations, especially pain, exists at thalamic level.*

- *The rhythmic pattern of melatonin secretion is disturbed by "jet lag".*

A series of diagrams to illustrate the afferent and efferent connections of the thalamus.

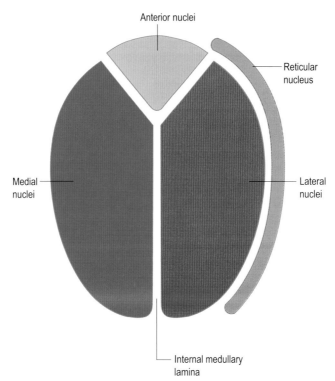

Diagrammatic view of the thalamus from above, as if sectioned into anterior, medial and lateral subdivisions by cutting along the internal medullary lamina.

The thalamus viewed from the lateral side as if cut into dorsal and ventral tiers of lateral thalamic nuclei. The medial and lateral geniculate bodies are anatomically separate from the rest of the thalamus, though functionally linked to it.

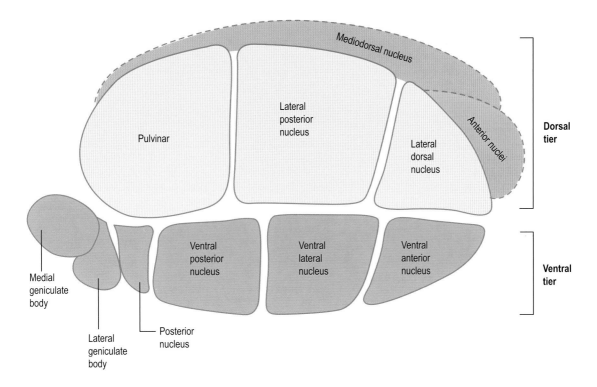

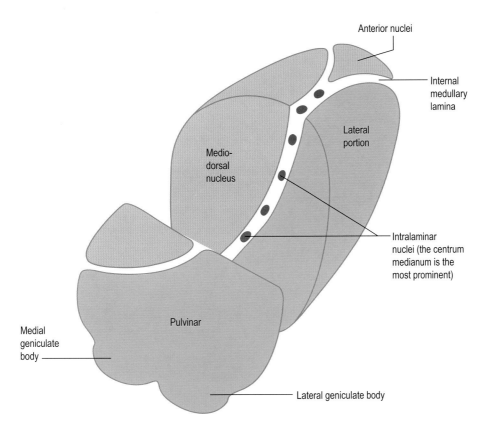

Diagrammatic view of the thalamus sectioned to show the mediodorsal nucleus and the intralaminar nuclei.

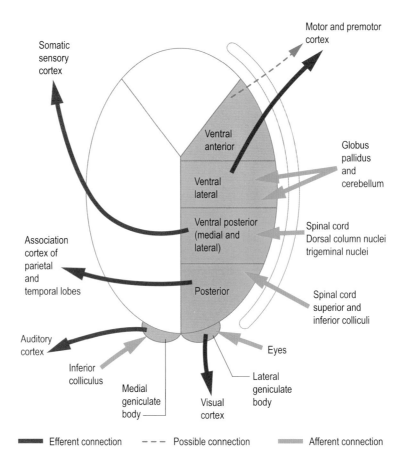

Somatic sensory cortex

Motor and premotor cortex

Ventral anterior

Globus pallidus and cerebellum

Ventral lateral

Ventral posterior (medial and lateral)

Spinal cord Dorsal column nuclei trigeminal nuclei

Association cortex of parietal and temporal lobes

Posterior

Spinal cord superior and inferior colliculi

Auditory cortex

Eyes

Inferior colliculus

Lateral geniculate body

Medial geniculate body

Visual cortex

Diagram showing the afferent and efferent connections of the ventral groups of specific thalamic nuclei in the lateral subdivision.

━━━ Efferent connection   - - - Possible connection   ▤▤▤ Afferent connection

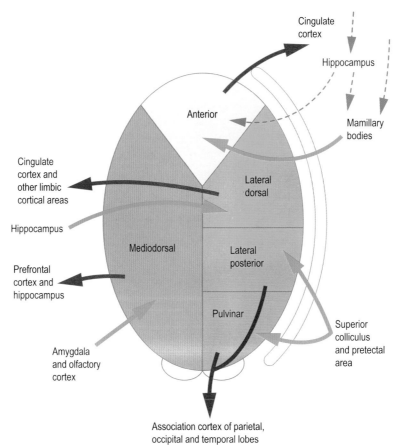

Cingulate cortex

Hippocampus

Anterior

Mamillary bodies

Cingulate cortex and other limbic cortical areas

Lateral dorsal

Hippocampus

Mediodorsal

Lateral posterior

Prefrontal cortex and hippocampus

Pulvinar

Superior colliculus and pretectal area

Amygdala and olfactory cortex

Association cortex of parietal, occipital and temporal lobes

Diagram showing the afferent and efferent connections of the dorsal groups of specific thalamic nuclei in the lateral subdivision.

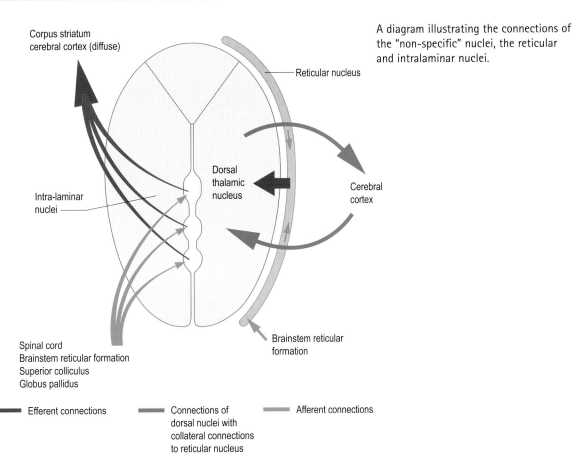

Corpus striatum
cerebral cortex (diffuse)

Reticular nucleus

A diagram illustrating the connections of
the "non-specific" nuclei, the reticular
and intralaminar nuclei.

Dorsal
thalamic
nucleus

Cerebral
cortex

Intra-laminar
nuclei

Spinal cord
Brainstem reticular formation
Superior colliculus
Globus pallidus

Brainstem reticular
formation

Efferent connections

Connections of
dorsal nuclei with
collateral connections
to reticular nucleus

Afferent connections

Superior thalamic peduncle
to the premotor and motor
cortex and the somatic
sensory cortex

Posterior thalamic peduncle
to the cortex of the parietal,
occipital and temporal lobes

Anterior thalamic peduncle
to the cortex of the frontal
lobe and cingulate gyrus

Parietal
lobe

Frontal
lobe

Thalamus

Occipital
lobe

Temporal
lobe

Inferior thalamic peduncle
to the orbital cortex of the
frontal lobe, the temporal pole
and the amygdaloid nucleus

Diagram to show the thalamic peduncles (radiations) projected onto the brain surface, lateral view.

Figures 11.1–11.5 Dissections and histological preparations showing the anatomy of the diencephalon as a whole.

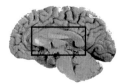

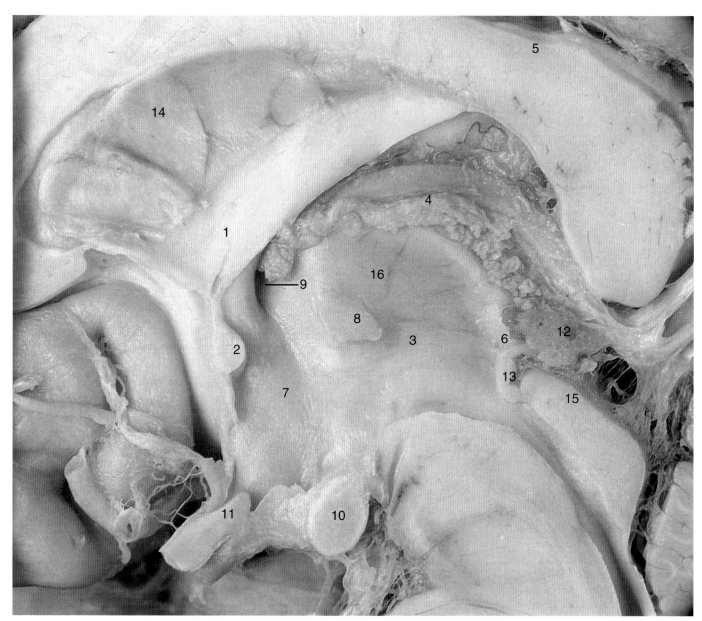

Fig. 11.1
Sagittal section of the brain to show the positions of the thalamus, hypothalamus and epithalamus. ×2.2

1 Anterior column of fornix	7 Hypothalamus	12 Pineal body (gland) (part of epithalamus)
2 Anterior commissure	8 Interthalamic connection or adhesion	13 Posterior commissure
3 Cavity of third ventricle	9 Interventricular foramen	14 Septum pellucidum
4 Choroid plexus of third ventricle	10 Mamillary body	15 Superior colliculus
5 Corpus callosum	11 Optic chiasma	16 Thalamus
6 Epithalamus		

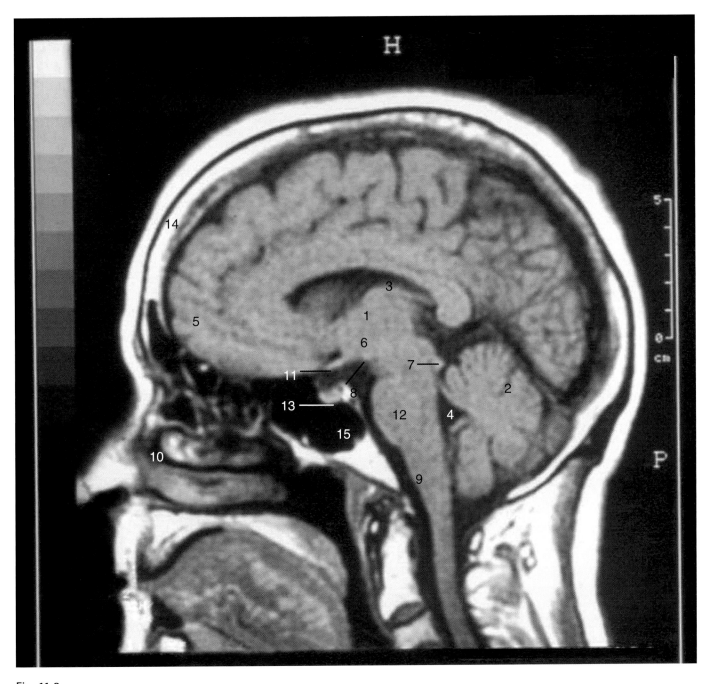

Fig. 11.2
A sagittal MRI scan showing the shapes and relationships of the thalamus and hypothalamus.

1 Anterior portion of thalamus
2 Cerebellum
3 Fornix
4 Fourth ventricle
5 Frontal lobe
6 Hypothalamus
7 Inferior colliculus
8 Mamillary body

9 Medulla oblongata
10 Nose
11 Optic chiasma
12 Pons
13 Sella turcica
14 Skull bone
15 Sphenoidal sinus

Dr. R. Abbott LRI

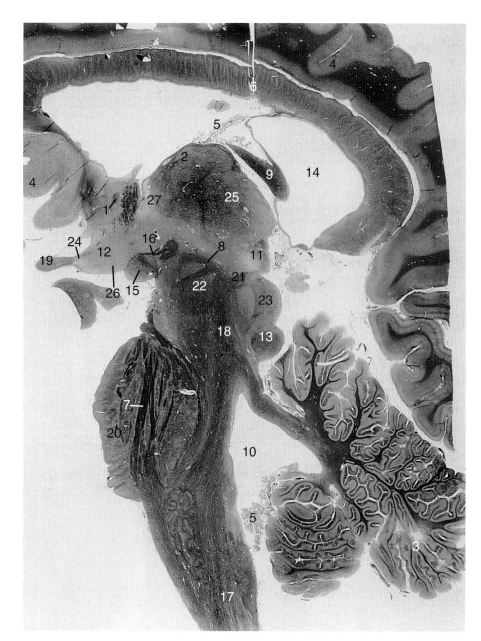

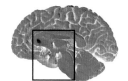

Fig. 11.3
A sagittal histological section of the brainstem and part of the forebrain to illustrate the nuclei and tracts of the diencephalon. Myelin stain. ×2.4

1 Anterior commissure
2 Anterior thalamic nuclei
3 Cerebellum
4 Cerebral cortex
5 Choroid plexus
6 Corpus callosum
7 Corticospinal tract
8 Fasciculus retroflexus (or habenulointer-
   peduncular tract)
9 Fornix
10 Fourth ventricle
11 Habenular area (trigone)
12 Hypothalamus
13 Inferior colliculus
14 Lateral ventricle
15 Mamillary body of hypothalamus
16 Mamillothalamic tract
17 Medulla oblongata
18 Midbrain
19 Optic chiasma
20 Pons
21 Pretectal area
22 Red nucleus
23 Superior colliculus
24 Supraoptic region of hypothalamus
25 Thalamus
26 Tuberal region of hypothalamus
27 Ventral thalamic nuclei

CAM

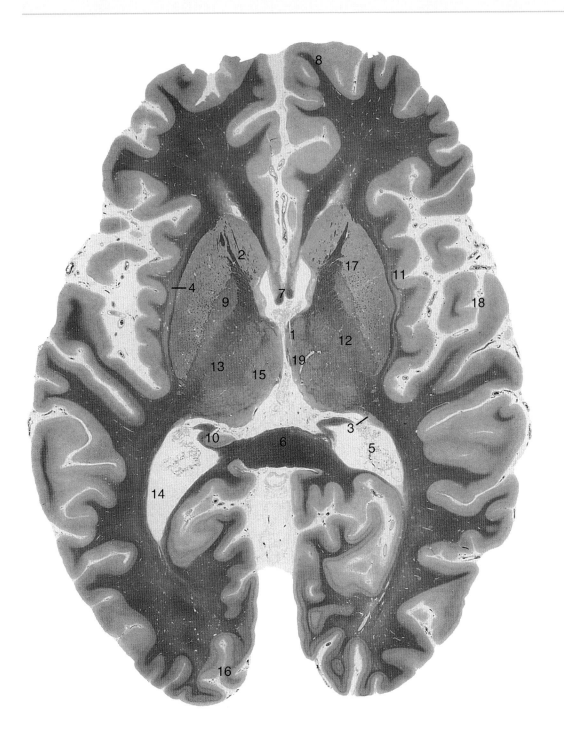

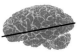

Fig. 11.4
Horizontal section through the brain showing the division of the thalamus into medial, lateral and anterior nuclear groups and the relationship between the thalamus and the basal ganglia. Solochrome cyanin and nuclear fast red stain. ×1.1

1 Anterior thalamic nuclei	**8** Frontal lobe of cerebral hemisphere	**14** Lateral ventricle
2 Caudate nucleus (head)	**9** Globus pallidus	**15** Medial thalamic nuclei
3 Caudate nucleus (tail)	**10** Hippocampus	**16** Occipital lobe
4 Claustrum	**11** Insula	**17** Putamen
5 Choroid plexus	**12** Internal capsule	**18** Temporal lobe
6 Corpus callosum	**13** Lateral thalamic nuclei	**19** Thalamus
7 Fornix		

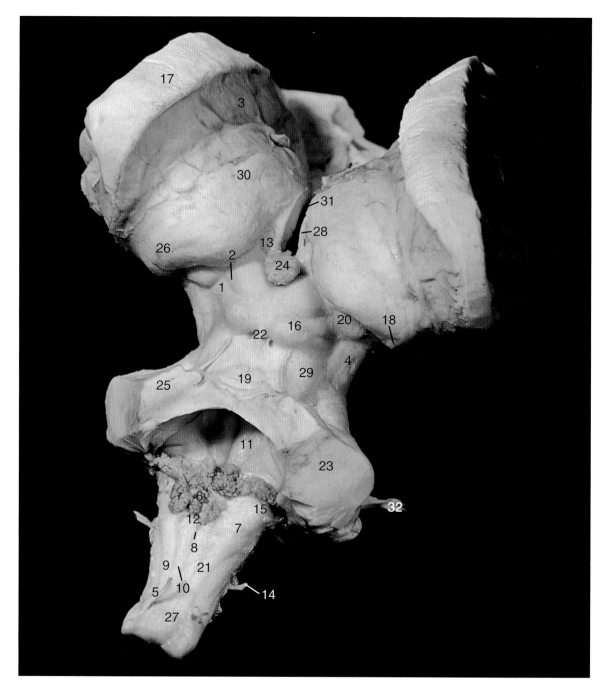

The diencephalon and brainstem superimposed on the base of the brain to illustrate their approximate relationship.

Fig. 11.5
A dissection of the diencephalon and brainstem viewed from the dorsal surface. ×1.65

1 Brachium of inferior colliculus	**12** Gracile tubercle	**23** Middle cerebellar peduncle
2 Brachium of superior colliculus	**13** Habenula	**24** Pineal gland
3 Caudate nucleus	**14** Hypoglossal nerve rootlets	**25** Pons
4 Cerebral peduncle	**15** Inferior cerebellar peduncle	**26** Pulvinar of thalamus
5 Cervical dorsal root	**16** Inferior colliculus	**27** Spinal cord
6 Choroid plexus	**17** Internal capsule	**28** Stria medullaris thalami
7 Cuneate tubercle	**18** Lateral geniculate body	**29** Superior cerebellar peduncle
8 Dorsal median sulcus	**19** Lingula of cerebellum	**30** Thalamus
9 Fasciculus cuneatus	**20** Medial geniculate body	**31** Third ventricle
10 Fasciculus gracilis	**21** Medulla oblongata	**32** Trigeminal nerve
11 Fourth ventricle	**22** Midbrain	

Figures 11.6–11.10 Sections through the diencephalon at various levels to demonstrate the nuclei of the thalamus, and the structure of the subthalamus and epithalamus.

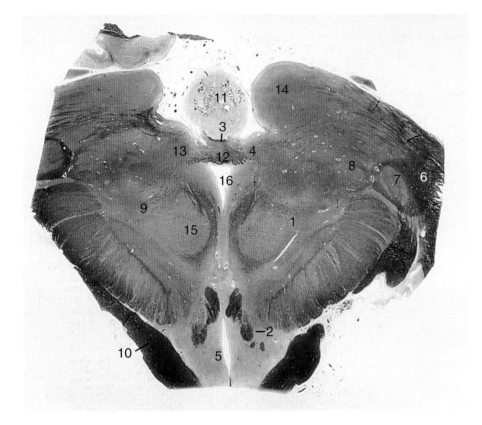

Fig. 11.6
A section passing through the transition between the midbrain and diencephalon. Myelin stain and counterstain. ×2

1 Dentatorubrothalamic fibers
2 Fornix
3 Habenular commissure
4 Habenular nucleus
5 Hypothalamus
6 Internal capsule
7 Lateral geniculate body
8 Medial geniculate body
9 Medial lemniscus, spinothalamic and trigeminothalamic tracts
10 Optic tract
11 Pineal gland
12 Posterior commissure
13 Pretectal nuclei
14 Pulvinar of thalamus
15 Red nucleus
16 Third ventricle becoming cerebral aqueduct

MHMS

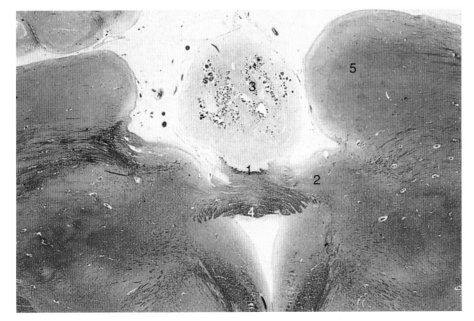

Fig. 11.7
A higher magnification view of the epithalamus demonstrating the habenular nuclei and the habenular commissure. Myelin stain and counterstain. ×4.2

1 Habenular commissure
2 Habenular nucleus
3 Pineal gland
4 Posterior commissure
5 Pulvinar of thalamus

MHMS

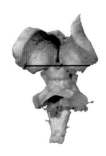

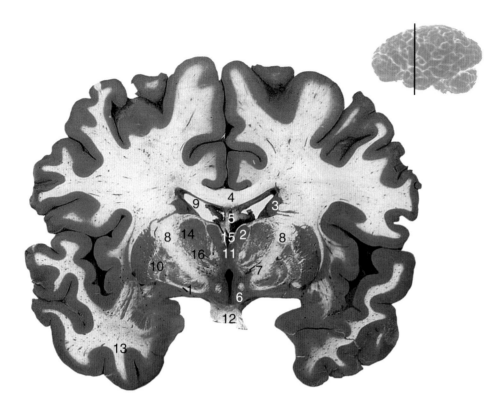

Fig. 11.8

A coronal thick slice through the forebrain at the rostral end of the diencephalon to show the anterior part of the thalamus, the hypothalamus and their relationships. Mulligan stain. ×0.86

1 Ansa lenticularis
2 Anterior thalamic nucleus
3 Caudate nucleus
4 Corpus callosum
5 Fornix
6 Hypothalamus
7 Inferior thalamic peduncle (radiation)
8 Internal capsule
9 Lateral ventricle
10 Lentiform nucleus
11 Midline thalamic nuclei
12 Optic chiasma
13 Temporal lobe
14 Thalamus
15 Third ventricle
16 Ventral anterior thalamic nucleus

Fig. 11.9

A histological section passing through the middle of the thalamus, with adjacent portions of the subthalamus and hypothalamus. Myelin stain. ×2.3

1 Caudate nucleus
2 External medullary lamina
3 Fornix
4 Globus pallidus
5 Hypothalamus
6 Internal capsule
7 Internal medullary lamina
8 Interthalamic adhesion and midline thalamic nuclei
9 Lateral dorsal thalamic nucleus
10 Lenticular fasciculus
11 Lentiform nucleus
12 Mamillothalamic tract
13 Medial (or mediodorsal) thalamic nucleus
14 Optic tract
15 Reticular thalamic nucleus
16 Stria medullaris thalami
17 Subthalamic nucleus
18 Thalamic fasciculus
19 Third ventricle
20 Ventral lateral thalamic nucleus
21 Zona incerta

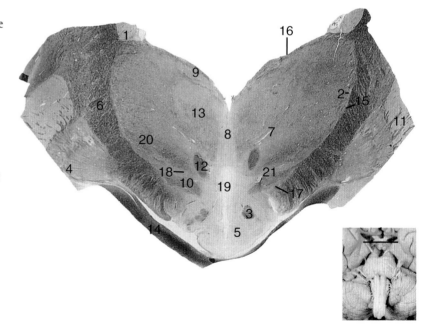

CXWMS

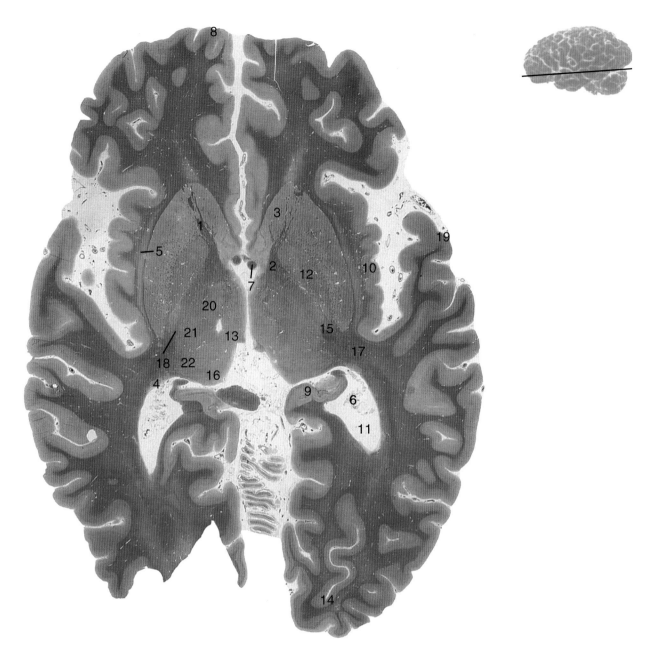

Fig. 11.10
A horizontal section through both cerebral hemispheres and diencephalon showing the medial and ventral thalamic nuclei and the anterior and somatic sensory thalamic radiations. Solochrome cyanin and nuclear fast red stain. ×1

1 Anterior limb of internal capsule	**9** Hippocampus	**16** Pulvinar of thalamus
2 Anterior thalamic peduncle (radiation)	**10** Insula	**17** Retrolentiform part of internal capsule
3 Caudate nucleus (head)	**11** Lateral ventricle	**18** Somatic sensory thalamic peduncle (radiation)
4 Caudate nucleus (tail)	**12** Lentiform nucleus	**19** Temporal lobe
5 Claustrum	**13** Medial thalamic nuclei	**20** Ventral anterior thalamic nucleus
6 Choroid plexus	**14** Occipital lobe	**21** Ventral lateral thalamic nucleus
7 Fornix	**15** Posterior limb of internal capsule	**22** Ventral posterior thalamic nucleus
8 Frontal lobe		

Figures 11.11–11.18 Dissections and histological preparations demonstrating the anatomy and relationships of the hypothalamus.

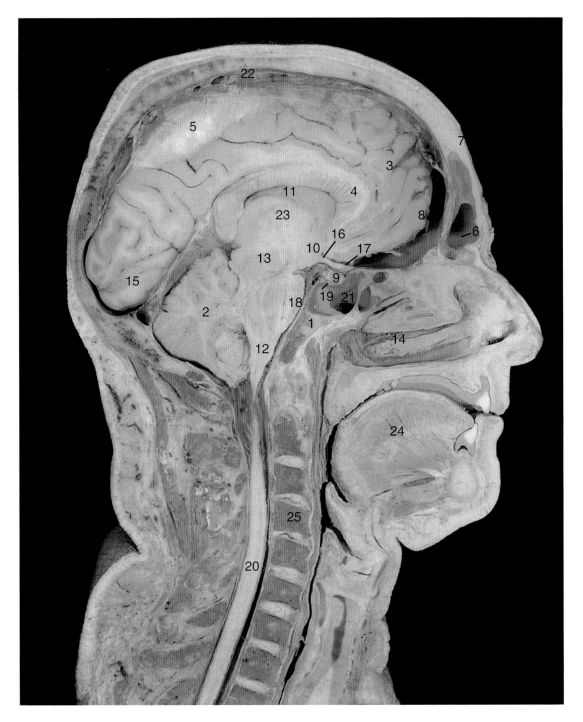

Fig. 11.11
A sagittal section of the head to show the relationships of the hypothalamus *in situ.* ×0.63

1 Body of sphenoid bone
2 Cerebellum
3 Cerebral hemisphere
4 Corpus callosum
5 Falx cerebri
6 Frontal air sinus
7 Frontal bone

8 Frontal lobe
9 Hypophysis
10 Hypothalamus
11 Lateral ventricle
12 Medulla oblongata
13 Midbrain

14 Nasal cavity
15 Occipital lobe
16 Optic chiasma
17 Optic nerve
18 Pons
19 Sella turcica (hypophyseal fossa)

20 Spinal cord
21 Sphenoidal air sinus
22 Superior sagittal sinus
23 Thalamus
24 Tongue
25 Vertebral column

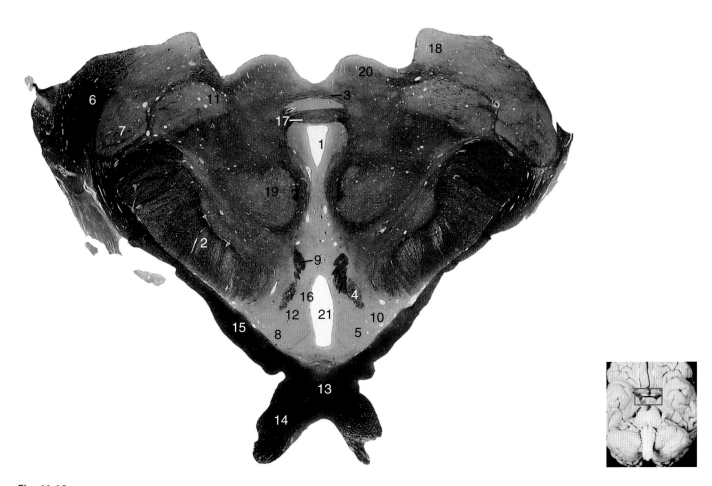

Fig. 11.12
A section through the transition between the midbrain and diencephalon orientated to pass through the optic chiasma. Weigert stain. ×3

1 Cerebral aqueduct	**8** Lateral area of hypothalamus	**15** Optic tract
2 Crus cerebri	**9** Mamillothalamic tract	**16** Periventricular hypothalamic area
3 Commissure of the superior colliculus	**10** Medial forebrain bundle	**17** Posterior commissure
4 Fornix	**11** Medial geniculate body	**18** Pulvinar of thalamus
5 Hypothalamus	**12** Medial hypothalamic area	**19** Red nucleus
6 Internal capsule	**13** Optic chiasma	**20** Superior colliculus
7 Lateral geniculate body	**14** Optic nerve	**21** Third ventricle

● *Tumors of the anterior pituitary can produce visual field defects by compressing the optic chiasma (see Vision, p. 241).*

Figures 11.13–11.16 Sections illustrating the structure of the neuroendocrine nuclei of the chiasmatic region of the hypothalamus.

Figures 11.13 and 11.14 Sections showing the position and structure of the supraoptic nucleus. Weigert stain.

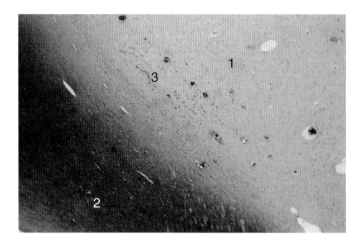

Fig. 11.13
A low power view showing the supraoptic nucleus and the optic tract. ×26

1 Gray matter of hypothalamus   3 Supraoptic nucleus
2 Optic tract

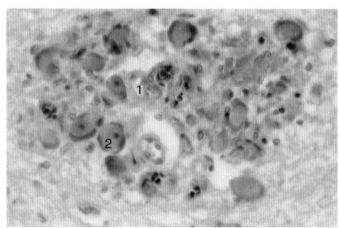

Fig. 11.14
A high magnification view of the specialized neurosecretory cells and profuse blood supply of the supraoptic nucleus. ×648

1 Capillary   2 Neurosecretory cell

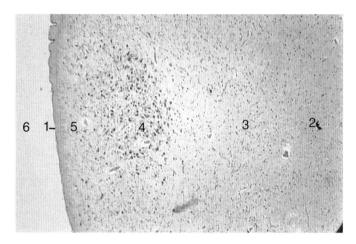

Fig. 11.15
A section to illustrate the position and structure of the paraventricular nucleus. Cresyl violet stain. ×40

1 Ependyma
2 Lateral hypothalamic area
3 Medial hypothalamic area
4 Paraventricular nucleus
5 Periventricular hypothalamic area
6 Third ventricle

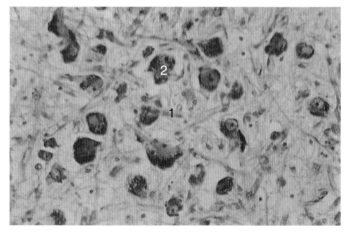

Fig. 11.16
High magnification view of the paraventricular nucleus showing its neurosecretory cells and profuse blood supply. Cresyl violet stain. ×520

1 Capillary
2 Neurosecretory cell

● *Hypothalamic tumors, like those of the pituitary, can cause under- or oversecretion of hormones. An example of this is acromegaly, in which a resumption of skeletal and muscular growth occurs in adults due to an overproduction of growth hormone. The hands, jaw and feet are particularly affected.*

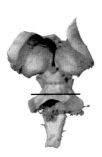

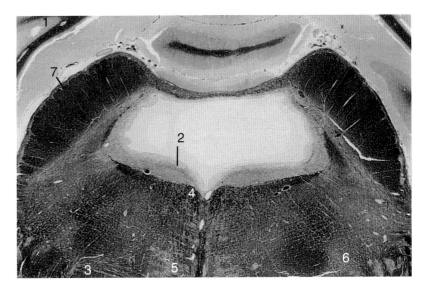

Fig. 11.17
A transverse paraffin wax section of the pons showing the dorsal longitudinal fasciculus, a connection between the hypothalamus and brainstem parasympathetic nuclei. Weigert stain. ×7.3

1 Cerebellum
2 Dorsal longitudinal fasciculus
3 Medial lemniscus
4 Medial longitudinal fasciculus

5 Pons
6 Reticular formation
7 Superior cerebellar peduncle

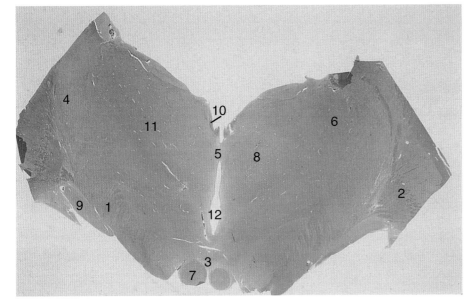

Fig. 11.18
A coronal section through the caudal end of the diencephalon demonstrating the position of the mamillary bodies in relation to other diencephalic structures. Luxol fast blue stain. ×2.3

1 Crus cerebri
2 Globus pallidus
3 Hypothalamus
4 Internal capsule
5 Interthalamic adhesion
6 Lateral thalamic nuclei
7 Mamillary body
8 Medial thalamic nuclei
9 Optic tract
10 Stria medullaris thalami
11 Thalamus
12 Third ventricle

CXWMS

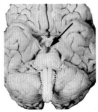

NEURAL AND CIRCULATORY CONNECTIONS OF THE HYPOTHALAMUS

NEURAL

AFFERENT	EFFERENT	EFFECT
Reticular formation	Reticular formation	Changes sleep/wake state
Limbic system	Limbic system	Emotional or behavioral response
Chemo- and baroreceptors and volume receptors via solitary nucleus		Monitors blood pressure, volume and O^2/CO^2
	Autonomic nervous system	Physiological response, e.g. heart rate, sweating

CIRCULATORY

AFFERENT	EFFERENT	EFFECT
Chemical, e.g. blood levels of metabolites		Monitors levels of substances, e.g. glucose, and helps regulate appetite
Physical changes in circulation, e.g. temperature, osmolarity		Monitors and adjusts physical states, e.g. helps regulate water intake, urine output
Endocrine		Monitors levels of hormones in circulation, e.g. sex hormones in control of reproductive cycles
	Endocrine	Secretes hormones, e.g. oxytocin, ADH, hormones to control the anterior pituitary*

* For the effects of the hormones produced by the hypophysis see a textbook of endocrinology.

Summary

1. The diencephalon consists of the thalamus, subthalamus, hypothalamus and epithalamus.
2. The thalamus is a structural and functional intermediary in pathways linking the cerebral cortex with subcortical structures.
3. The thalamus is the major sensory relay center for the somatic senses of touch, pain, temperature and conscious proprioception.
4. Some conscious perception of pain can occur in the thalamus.
5. The thalamus is subdivided into groups of nuclei, each with different functions and connections.
6. The subthalamus participates in movement control by the basal ganglia.
7. The hypothalamus is an endocrine organ, producing oxytocin and antidiuretic hormone. It also secretes hormones that regulate the secretory activity of the anterior lobe of the pituitary gland.
8. The hypothalamus is an important component of the autonomic and limbic systems.
9. The epithalamus is an important component of the endocrine system. It includes the pineal gland, which secretes melatonin.
10. The epithalamus is an important component of the limbic system. It includes the habenular nuclei.

12 Commissural Fibers

Commissures pass from one side of the brain to the other carrying impulses in both directions. There are several bundles of commissural fibers: the corpus callosum, anterior commissure, posterior commissure, hippocampal commissure (commissure of the fornix) and habenular commissure.

The corpus callosum connects broad regions of the cortex in all the lobes with the corresponding regions in the other hemisphere. It is divided into four regions: the rostrum, genu, body and splenium. The rostrum and genu connect anterior parts of the frontal lobe, and their radiating fibers form the forceps minor (frontal forceps). The body connects the remainder of the frontal lobe and the parietal lobe. The splenium connects regions of the temporal and occipital lobes, and their radiating fibers form the forceps major. A group of fibers in the splenium (tapetum) sweeps inferiorly over the ventricle and optic radiation, and connects with the temporal lobe.

The anterior commissure is a small bundle of fibers shaped like bicycle handlebars straddling the midline. It is divided into two parts: fibers lying rostrally in the commissure connecting the olfactory structures, and fibers lying caudally connecting the middle and inferior temporal gyri.

The posterior commissure lies in the lower part of the pineal stalk. Its composition is poorly understood but one important component consists of fibers crossing the midline from the pretectal area to the contralateral Edinger-Westphal nucleus from which the constrictor muscle of the pupil is supplied (see Brainstem cranial nerve nuclei, p. 185). These are part of the pathway for the pupillary light reflex. Both pupils constrict when a light is shone into one because of this commissural connection. This is known as the consensual light reflex.

The fornix is the main tract of the limbic system connecting the hippocampus with the hypothalamus. Most of its fibers are ipsilateral but some cross, forming the hippocampal commissure.

Small commissures also link the colliculi of the midbrain. The habenular commissure lies in the upper part of the pineal stalk and connects the two habenular nuclei to the contralateral olfactory areas. The habenular nuclei are part of the limbic system.

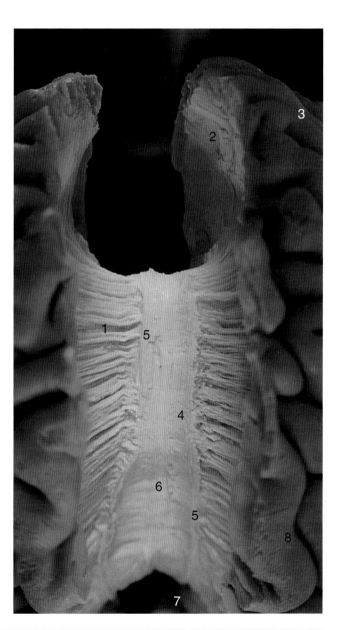

Fig. 12.1
The corpus callosum connecting the two hemispheres as viewed from above. ×1.6

1 Corpus callosum (commissural fibers)
2 Frontal forceps
3 Frontal lobe
4 Indusium griseum (position of)
5 Lateral longitudinal stria
6 Medial longitudinal stria
7 Occipital lobe
8 Parietal lobe

Fig. 12.2
Thick coronal slice of the cerebral hemispheres showing the corpus callosum. Mulligan stain. ×0.76

1 Caudate nucleus
2 Cerebral cortex (gray matter)
3 Cerebral white matter
4 Claustrum
5 Corpus callosum
6 Insula
7 Hypothalamus
8 Lateral sulcus
9 Lateral ventricle
10 Lentiform nucleus
11 Optic tract
12 Septum pellucidum
13 Superior longitudinal fissure
14 Temporal lobe

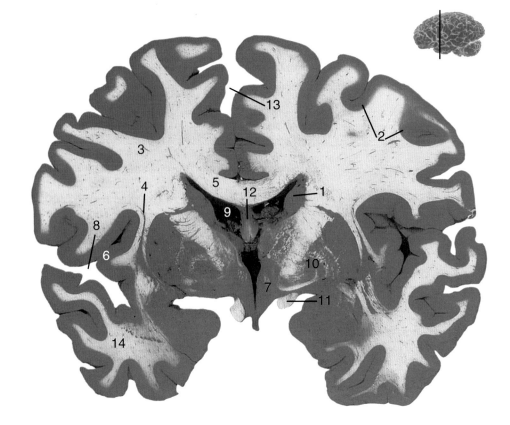

Fig. 12.3
Paraffin wax histological section of the corpus callosum showing the indusium griseum. Cresyl violet stain. ×193

1 Corpus callosum
2 Indusium griseum

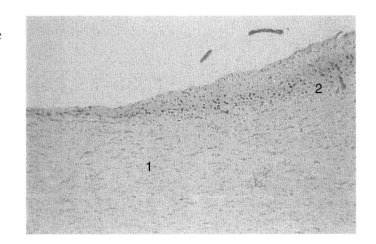

Fig. 12.4
Horizontal section through the brain showing the
anterior commissure. Note its "bicycle handlebar" shape.
×0.7

1 Anterior commissure
2 Caudate nucleus
3 Cerebellum
4 Frontal lobe
5 Insula
6 Lateral ventricle
7 Lentiform nucleus
8 Occipital lobe
9 Pineal gland
10 Temporal lobe
11 Thalamus

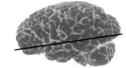

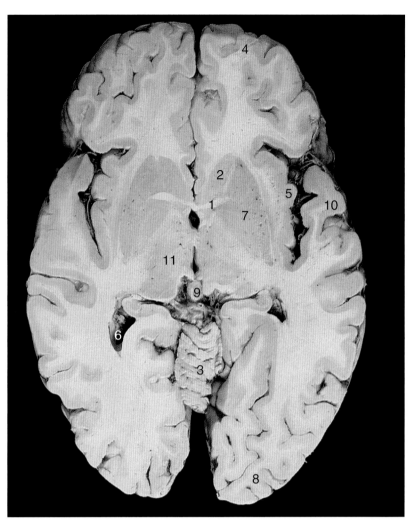

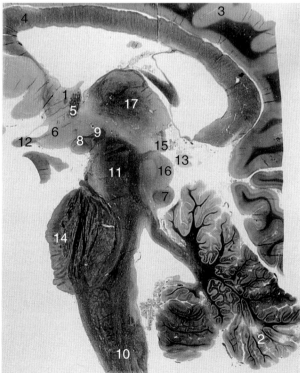

Fig. 12.5
Sagittal section passing through brainstem, cerebellum, diencephalon and
part of cerebral hemisphere showing the anterior and posterior
commissures and the corpus callosum. Myelin stain. ×1.6

1 Anterior commissure
2 Cerebellum
3 Cerebral hemisphere
4 Corpus callosum
5 Fornix
6 Hypothalamus
7 Inferior colliculus
8 Mamillary body
9 Mamillothalamic tract
10 Medulla oblongata
11 Midbrain
12 Optic chiasma
13 Pineal gland
14 Pons
15 Posterior commissure
16 Superior colliculus
17 Thalamus

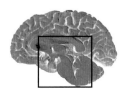

CAM

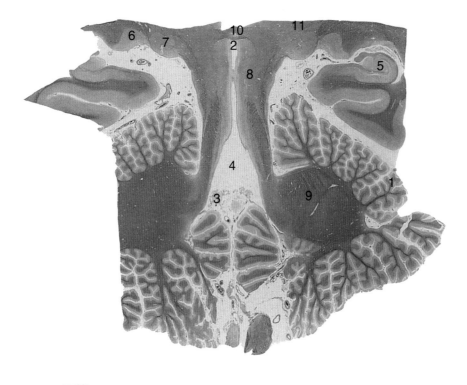

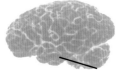

Fig. 12.6
Longitudinal section of brainstem showing the posterior commissure. Solochrome cyanin and nuclear fast red stain. ×1.2

1 Cerebellum
2 Cerebral aqueduct
3 Choroid plexus
4 Fourth ventricle
5 Hippocampus
6 Lateral geniculate body
7 Medial geniculate body
8 Midbrain
9 Middle cerebellar peduncle
10 Posterior commissure
11 Thalamus

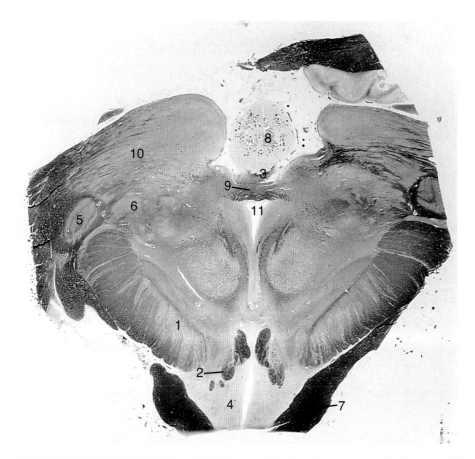

Fig. 12.7
Histological section through the transition between the midbrain and diencephalon orientated to pass through the posterior and habenular commissures. Weigert-Pal stain. ×2.6

1 Cerebral peduncle
2 Fornix
3 Habenular commissure
4 Hypothalamus
5 Lateral geniculate body
6 Medial geniculate body
7 Optic tract
8 Pineal gland
9 Posterior commissure
10 Thalamus
11 Third ventricle

MHMS

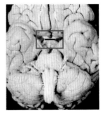

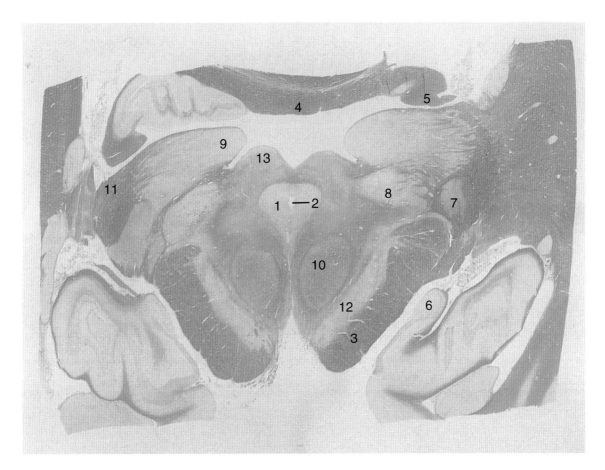

Fig. 12.8
Paraffin wax histological section through the brainstem at the junction of midbrain and diencephalon, to demonstrate the hippocampal commissure (commissure of the fornix). Luxol fast blue stain. ×2.3

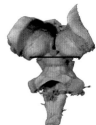

1 Central (periaqueductal) gray matter of midbrain	8 Medial geniculate body
2 Cerebral aqueduct	9 Pulvinar of thalamus
3 Cerebral peduncle	10 Red nucleus
4 Commissure of fornix	11 Retrolentiform part of internal capsule
5 Crus of fornix	12 Substantia nigra
6 Hippocampal formation	13 Superior colliculus
7 Lateral geniculate body	CAM

Summary

1. Commissural fibers pass from one side of the brain to the other, across the neuraxis.
2. The corpus callosum is the largest commissural pathway.
3. The corpus callosum connects broad regions of cortex in each cerebral hemisphere with equivalent areas on the other side.
4. The anterior commissure links olfactory regions of the frontal lobes and parts of the temporal lobes.
5. The hippocampal commissure is part of the fornix.
6. Other commissural pathways associated with the diencephalon and midbrain are the posterior commissure, the habenular commissure and the commissures of the superior and inferior colliculi.

13 Brainstem

The brainstem consists of the midbrain, the pons and the medulla. All of these are midline structures that are overgrown by the cerebral hemispheres during development. Therefore, most parts of the brainstem can be seen only when the brain is viewed from below or in section.

Rostrally, the brainstem is continuous with the diencephalon. Caudally, it blends with the first cervical segment of the spinal cord. Dorsally, it is connected to the cerebellum by the superior, middle and inferior cerebellar peduncles.

The brainstem lies on the floor of the cranial cavity. The medulla rests on the basi-occiput, the pons on the sphenoid bone as far forward as the dorsum sellae. The midbrain passes through the tentorial notch of the tentorium cerebelli.

All of the cranial nerves except the first and second arise from the brainstem; the first (olfactory) nerve is composed of processes of bipolar neurons in the olfactory epithelium and the second (optic) nerve is a drawn-out brain pathway rather than a true peripheral nerve. Cranial nerves III to XII, which originate from the brainstem, arise from or terminate in aggregations of gray matter (i.e. nerve cells) that form nuclei. These will be described in more detail in the next chapter (Brainstem Cranial Nerve Nuclei). Certain other brainstem nuclei, for example nucleus gracilis and nucleus cuneatus, are not associated with cranial nerves, but form part of sensory or motor functional systems. The most important of these will be covered in the section on somatic sensory pathways (see p. 223).

The white matter of the brainstem is arranged in bundles or tracts. These may be local connections within the brainstem itself or projection fibers linking brainstem structures to other parts of the central nervous system, often as parts of functional systems.

The most important tracts clearly visible in brainstem sections are listed in the table below.

The reticular formation forms the central core of the brainstem. Although it appears anatomically ill-defined, it is functionally complex and important. Some areas have distinctive neurotransmitters. The reticular formation is involved in four aspects of brain function: maintaining arousal of the cerebral cortex, e.g. in the sleep/wake cycle; controlling visceral functions such as respiration and the cardiovascular system; modulating pain perception; and movement control. Afferent connections come from all the sensory systems of the brain to the reticular formation, and efferent pathways go to the cerebral cortex as well as other parts of the brainstem, diencephalon and spinal cord. Many of these connections pass through the central tegmental tract. Two groups of cells in the reticular formation can be distinguished by size. The larger cells are 50–70 µm in diameter. They give rise to long sensory and motor pathways between the reticular formation and the spinal cord. The smaller group of cells, 20–25 µm in diameter, are those responsible for modulating cortical function.

The reticular formation in the pons and medulla can be divided anatomically into three zones: the raphe nuclei, the medial zone and the lateral zone.

1. The raphe nuclei lie close to the midline. They contain serotonin and 5-hydroxytryptamine (5HT). Their neurons have ascending connections to the whole cerebral cortex,

MAJOR TRACTS VISIBLE IN BRAINSTEM SECTIONS AND THEIR FUNCTIONS	
Function	Tracts
Sensory pathways (ascending tracts) for the somatic senses and hearing	Spinothalamic tracts (touch, pain, temperature) Medial lemniscus (touch, pressure, conscious proprioception) Spinocerebellar tracts (unconscious proprioception) Lateral lemniscus (auditory) Spinal tract and nucleus of the trigeminal nerve (touch, pain and temperature from the head)
Motor pathways for movement control (descending tracts)	Pyramidal tracts (corticospinal and corticobulbar tracts) Extrapyramidal tracts (rubrospinal tract, reticulospinal tract, tectospinal tract, vestibulospinal tract)
Connections with the cerebellum Connecting brainstem nuclei to each other	Inferior, middle and superior cerebellar peduncles Medial longitudinal fasciculus

especially sensory and limbic areas. This pathway is part of the reticular activating system important in maintaining the level of arousal of the cerebral cortex. Descending pathways from the raphe nuclei to the spinal cord form part of a pain control mechanism blocking transmission in pain pathways (see p. 224).

2. The medial zone gives rise to the reticulospinal tracts, which are part of the extrapyramidal system of descending tracts for movement control (see Descending tracts, p. 285).

3. The lateral zone is concerned with visceral functions. It contains the cardiovascular and respiratory centers. Norepinephrine (noradrenaline) is its most important neurotransmitter. The locus ceruleus is a well-defined nucleus, containing neuromelanin pigment which gives it a dark blue-gray color. It sends noradrenergic nerve fibers via the central tegmental tract. These go to the thalamus, hypothalamus and the entire cerebral cortex, especially sensory and limbic areas. It is an important component of the reticular activating system, which functions during changes in alertness level. The locus ceruleus, together with the raphe nuclei, vary their level of activity in rapid eye movement (REM) sleep.

In the midbrain, there are areas linked to the reticular formation, both structurally and functionally. These are the periaqueductal gray and the ventral tegmental areas.

The periaqueductal gray contains the endogenous opiates dynorphin and enkephalin. Through their connection to the raphe nuclei and the spinal cord, they are part of the pain control mechanism (see p. 224).

The ventral tegmental area gives off connections to the limbic cortex, basal ganglia and the amygdaloid nucleus. These form the mesolimbic pathways (see Limbic system, p. 319).

● *An alternative definition of the brainstem includes the diencephalon.*

● *Brainstem injuries may be fatal by directly damaging reticular formation centers for control of vital functions.*

● *Uncal tumors of the temporal lobe may cause the temporal lobe to herniate into the tentorial notch, compressing the midbrain. Herniation (coning) can also occur in a patient with a raised intracranial pressure if a lumbar puncture is performed, due to sudden decompression when CSF is withdrawn. (See ventricles, p. 93)*

Fig. 13.1
Anterior view of a computer-reconstructed image of the brain from MRI scans. The brainstem and spinal cord appear white.

1 Brainstem
  a Midbrain
  b Pons
  c Medulla oblongata
2 Cerebellum
3 Frontal lobe
4 Longitudinal fissure
5 Spinal cord
6 Temporal lobe

Prof. F. W. Zonneveld UUH

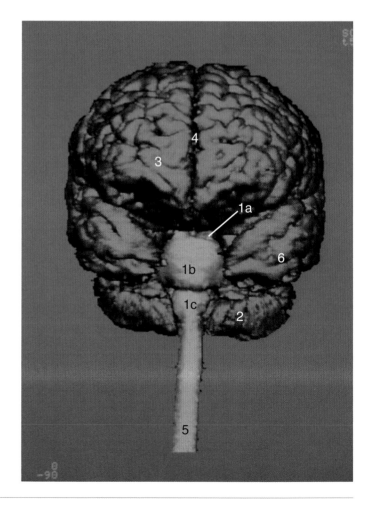

● *Some antidepressant drugs act by enhancing transmission at synapses that utilize norepinephrine (noradrenaline) or serotonin.*

● *Antipsychotic drugs such as thorazine block dopaminergic transmission in the mesolimbic pathways.*

● *Serotonin specific re-uptake inhibitors (SSRIs) are a class of antidepressant drugs that act by preventing serotonin released at synapses from being taken back into the neuron terminals. In this way the neurotransmitter action of serotonin is prolonged.*

Figures 13.2–13.4 Anatomy and relationships of the brainstem *in situ*.

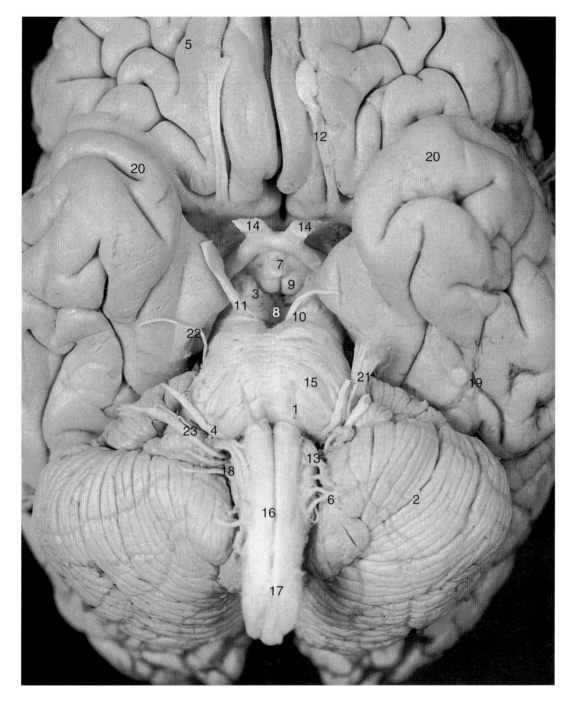

Fig. 13.2
The brain viewed from the basal aspect showing the brainstem and associated structures including the blood vessels and cranial nerves. The meninges have been removed. ×1.3

1 Abducens nerve (VI)
2 Cerebellum
3 Cerebral peduncle
4 Facial nerve and nervus intermedius (VII)
5 Frontal lobe
6 Hypoglossal nerve (XII) roots
7 Hypothalamus
8 Interpeduncular fossa

9 Mamillary body
10 Midbrain (cerebral peduncle)
11 Oculomotor nerve (III)
12 Olfactory tract
13 Olive
14 Optic nerve (II)
15 Pons
16 Pyramid

17 Pyramidal decussation
18 Roots of glossopharyngeal (IX), vagus (X) and accessory (XI) nerves
19 Surface blood vessels
20 Temporal lobe
21 Trigeminal nerve (V)
22 Trochlear nerve (IV)
23 Vestibulocochlear nerve (VIII)

Figures 13.3 and 13.4 A dissection and an NMR (nuclear magnetic resonance) image to demonstrate the relationships of the brainstem in the cranial cavity.

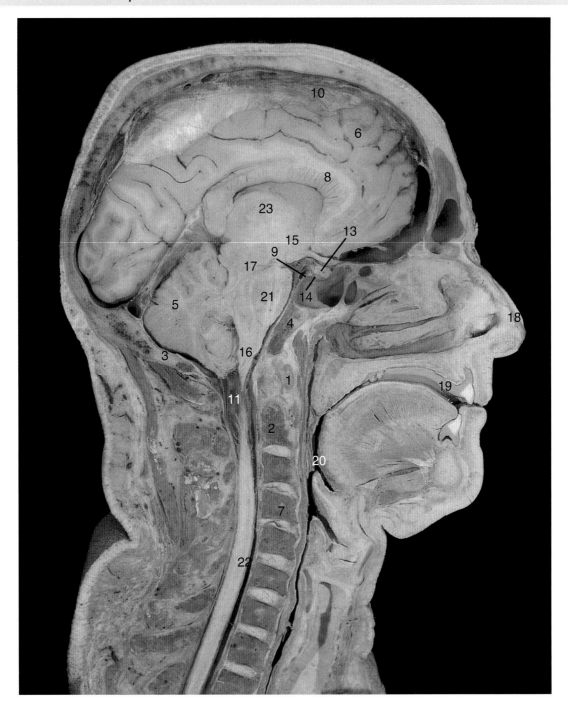

Fig. 13.3
A sagittal section of the head. ×0.62

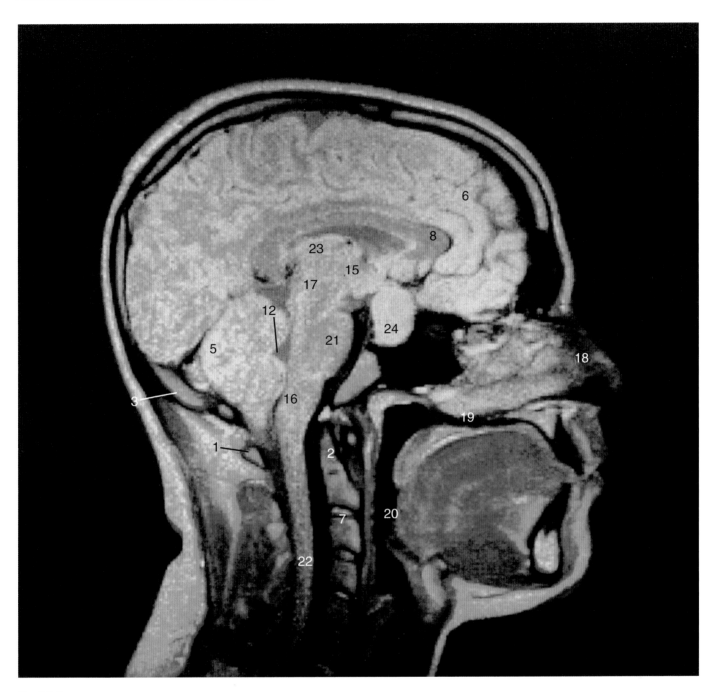

Fig. 13.4
A sagittal nuclear magnetic resonance (NMR) image of the head in a patient with a tumor of the hypophysis. Three different black-and-white images were superimposed to form this color composite by displaying the first as red, second as green, and third as shades of blue. This allows simultaneous viewing of all three original images and can simplify their interpretation.

1	Atlas	**9**	Dorsum sellae	**17**	Midbrain
2	Axis	**10**	Falx cerebri	**18**	Nose
3	Basi-occiput	**11**	Foramen magnum	**19**	Oral cavity
4	Body of sphenoid	**12**	Fourth ventricle	**20**	Pharynx
5	Cerebellum	**13**	Hypophysis	**21**	Pons
6	Cerebral hemisphere	**14**	Hypophyseal fossa	**22**	Spinal cord
7	Cervical vertebra	**15**	Hypothalamus	**23**	Thalamus
8	Corpus callosum	**16**	Medulla oblongata	**24**	Tumor

Elscint Ltd

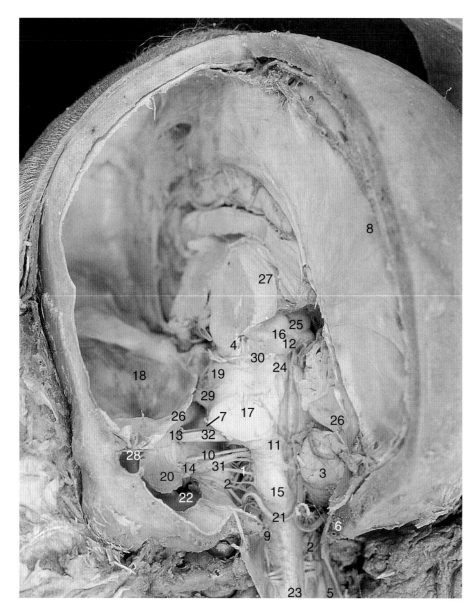

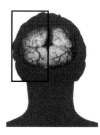

Fig. 13.5
Oblique posterior view of a dissection to display some cranial nerves leaving the brainstem through their foramina in the skull. Almost all of the cerebellum, the right cerebral hemisphere and the right side of the tentorium cerebelli have been removed. ×0.6

 1 Accessory nerve (cranial root) (XI)
 2 Accessory nerve (spinal root) (XI)
 3 Cerebellum
 4 Cerebral peduncle
 5 Dura mater
 6 Edge of foramen magnum
 7 Facial nerve (VII)
 8 Falx cerebri
 9 First cervical nerve root (CI)
10 Glossopharyngeal nerve (IX)
11 Inferior cerebellar peduncle
12 Inferior colliculus
13 Internal auditory meatus
14 Jugular foramen
15 Medulla
16 Midbrain (tectum)
17 Middle cerebellar peduncle
18 Middle cranial fossa
19 Pons
20 Posterior cranial fossa
21 Posterior inferior cerebellar artery
22 Sigmoid sinus
23 Spinal cord
24 Superior cerebellar peduncle
25 Superior colliculus
26 Tentorium cerebelli
27 Thalamus
28 Transverse sinus
29 Trigeminal nerve (V)
30 Trochlear nerve (IV)
31 Vagus nerve (X)
32 Vestibulocochlear nerve (VIII)

OXF

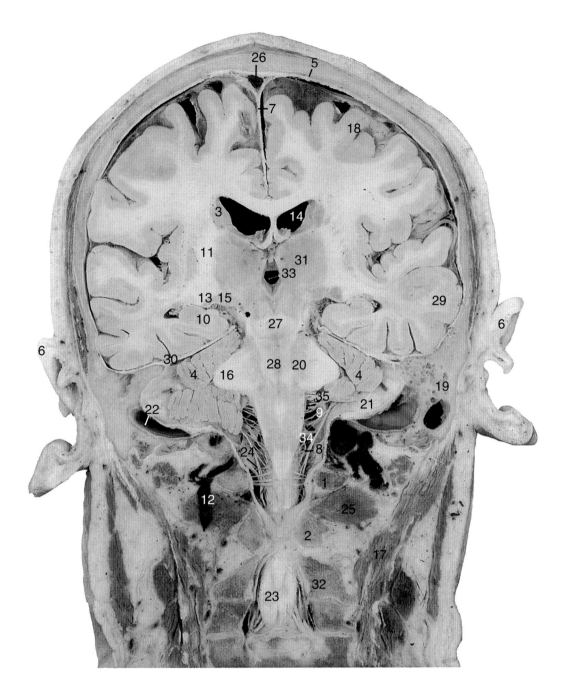

Fig. 13.6
A coronal section of the head and neck viewed from behind. The specimen shows the relationships of the brainstem *in situ* and its continuity with the spinal cord and diencephalon (thalamus). ×0.73

1 Atlas	**13** Lateral geniculate body	**25** Subcapital muscles
2 Axis	**14** Lateral ventricle	**26** Superior sagittal sinus
3 Caudate nucleus	**15** Medial geniculate body	**27** Tegmentum of midbrain
4 Cerebellum	**16** Middle cerebellar peduncle	**28** Tegmentum of pons
5 Dura mater	**17** Muscles of posterior triangle of the neck	**29** Temporal lobe
6 Ear	**18** Parietal lobe	**30** Tentorium cerebelli
7 Falx cerebri	**19** Petrous temporal bone	**31** Thalamus
8 First cervical nerve root (C1)	**20** Pons	**32** Third cervical vertebra
9 Glossopharyngeal and vagus nerve roots	**21** Posterior cranial fossa	**33** Third ventricle
10 Hippocampus	**22** Sigmoid sinus	**34** Vertebral artery
11 Internal capsule	**23** Spinal cord	**35** Vestibulocochlear nerve (VIII)
12 Internal jugular vein	**24** Spinal root of accessory nerve (XI)	UN

Figures 13.7–13.9 Dissections and histological preparations to demonstrate the anatomy of the isolated brainstem.

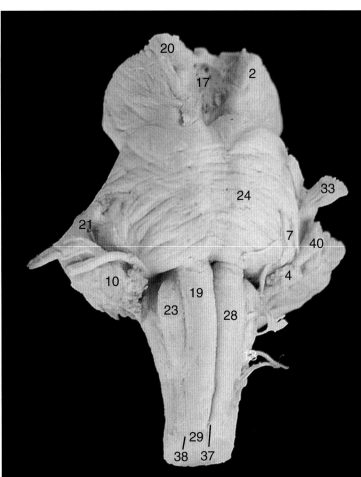

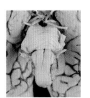

Fig. 13.7
The brainstem viewed from the ventral aspect. ×1.5

Fig. 13.8
The same brainstem viewed from the left side. ×1.5

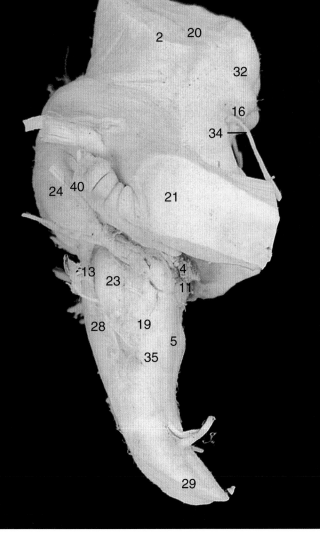

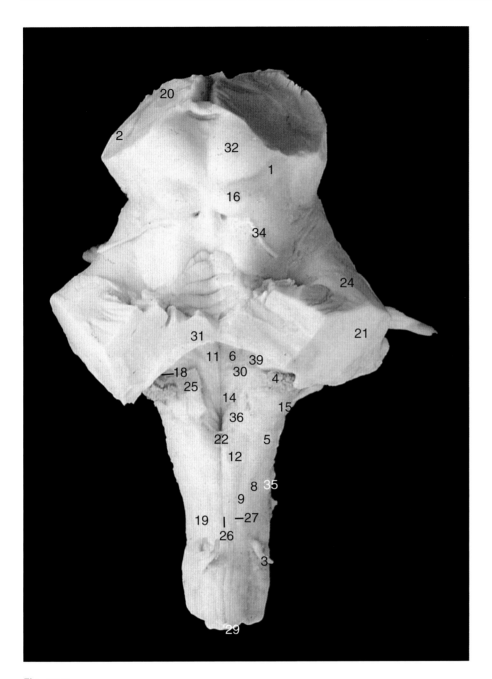

A diagram representing the floor of the fourth ventricle, labeled as in Figure 13.9. The dashed lines indicate the position of the sulcus limitans (see Embryology, p. 23).

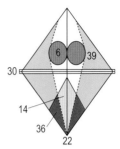

Fig. 13.9
A dorsal view of the brainstem in Figure 13.7. ×1.8

1 Brachium of inferior colliculus	**15** Inferior cerebellar peduncle	**28** Pyramid
2 Cerebral peduncle	**16** Inferior colliculus	**29** Spinal cord
3 Cervical (C1) dorsal roots	**17** Interpeduncular fossa	**30** Stria medullaris
4 Choroid plexus of fourth ventricle	**18** Lateral recess of fourth ventricle	**31** Superior cerebellar peduncle
5 Cuneate tubercle	**19** Medulla oblongata	**32** Superior colliculus
6 Facial colliculus	**20** Midbrain	**33** Trigeminal nerve (V)
7 Facial nerve (VII)	**21** Middle cerebellar peduncle	**34** Trochlear nerve (IV)
8 Fasciculus cuneatus	**22** Obex	**35** Tuberculum cinereum
9 Fasciculus gracilis	**23** Olive	**36** Vagal trigone
10 Flocculus of cerebellum	**24** Pons	**37** Ventral (anterior) median fissure
11 Fourth ventricle	**25** Posterior inferior cerebellar artery	**38** Ventrolateral (anterolateral) sulcus
12 Gracile tubercle	**26** Posterior (dorsal) median sulcus	**39** Vestibular area
13 Hypoglossal nerve (XII)	**27** Posterolateral (dorsolateral) sulcus	**40** Vestibulocochlear nerve
14 Hypoglossal trigone		

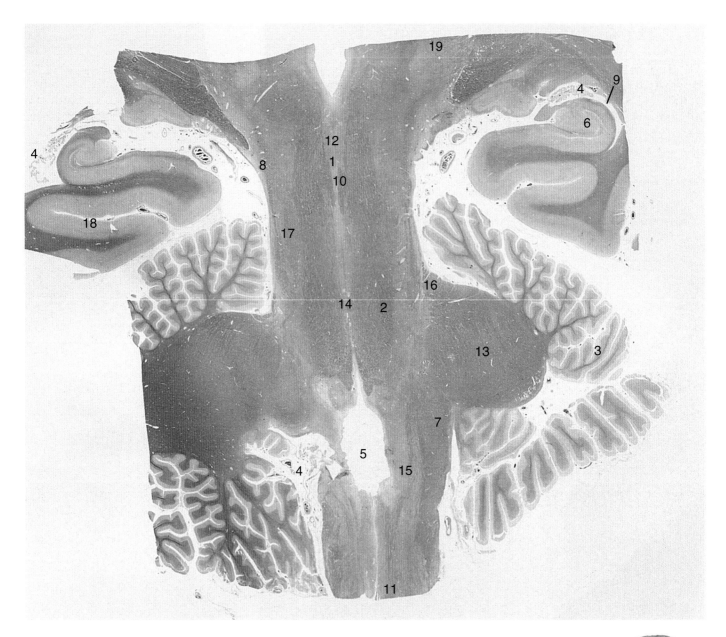

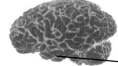

Fig. 13.10
A longitudinal histological section through the brainstem with part of the cerebellum and thalamus. This section shows tracts passing through the brainstem and connecting it to adjacent structures. Solochrome cyanin and nuclear fast red stain. ×2.4

1 Aqueduct (of Sylvius)	**8** Lateral lemniscus	**14** Pons
2 Central tegmental tract	**9** Lateral ventricle	**15** Solitary tract
3 Cerebellum	**10** Medial longitudinal fasciculus	**16** Superior spinocerebellar tract
4 Choroid plexus	**11** Medulla oblongata	**17** Superior cerebellar peduncle
5 Fourth ventricle	**12** Midbrain	**18** Temporal lobe cortex
6 Hippocampal formation	**13** Middle cerebellar peduncle	**19** Thalamus
7 Inferior cerebellar peduncle		

Midbrain

The midbrain can be divided into three zones visible in transverse sections. The roof or tectum consists of the superior and inferior colliculi (see Fig. 13.9) and lies dorsal to the cerebral aqueduct (of Sylvius). Below this is the tegmentum which contains a variety of nuclei and tracts.

The base of the midbrain consists of the two crura cerebri. These are made up of descending motor pathways, the corticospinal, corticobulbar and corticopontine tracts. One crus cerebri plus one half of the tegmentum constitutes a cerebral peduncle.

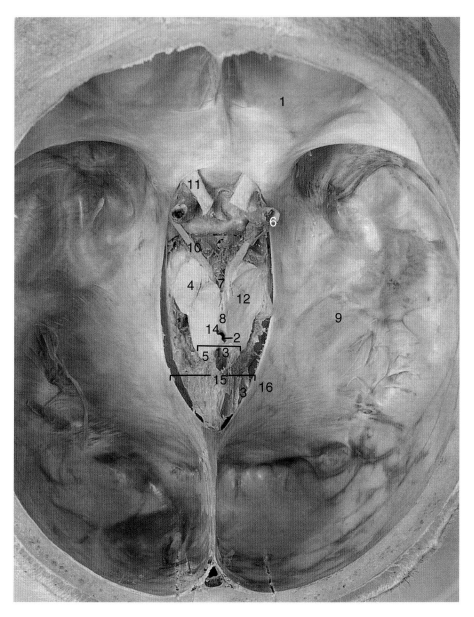

Fig. 13.11
A dissection of the midbrain *in situ* demonstrating its anatomy and relationships. The midbrain is sectioned at the level of the inferior colliculi. ×0.9

 1 Anterior cranial fossa
 2 Cerebral aqueduct
 3 Cerebellum
 4 Crus cerebri
 5 Inferior colliculus
 6 Internal carotid artery
 7 Interpeduncular fossa
 8 Midbrain
 9 Middle cranial fossa
10 Oculomotor nerve
11 Optic nerve
12 Substantia nigra
13 Tectum (bracketed)
14 Tegmentum
15 Tentorial notch (bracketed)
16 Tentorium cerebelli

Pons

The pons consists of a large basal or basilar portion and a small dorsal or tegmental portion in the floor of the fourth ventricle. Corticospinal and corticobulbar fibers run longitudinally through the basilar portion. Transverse pontine fibers, which are axons of the neurons comprising the pontine nuclei, cross it to enter the cerebellum in the middle cerebellar peduncle. The tegmental portion contains cranial nerve nuclei and a variety of ascending and descending tracts.

Figures 13.12–13.16 Dissections and histological preparations demonstrating the anatomy of the pons.

Fig. 13.12
The pons viewed from the ventral aspect to show its general anatomy and relationships. The cerebellum has been removed. ×1.8

  1 Basilar portion of pons
  2 Crus cerebri of midbrain
  3 Facial nerve (VII)
  4 Hypoglossal nerve (XII)
  5 Interpeduncular fossa
  6 Occipital lobe
  7 Oculomotor nerve (III)
  8 Olive
  9 Posterior cerebral artery
 10 Posterior communicating artery
 11 Pyramid of medulla oblongata
 12 Temporal lobe
 13 Transverse pontine fibers
 14 Trigeminal nerve (V)
 15 Vestibulocochlear nerve (VIII)

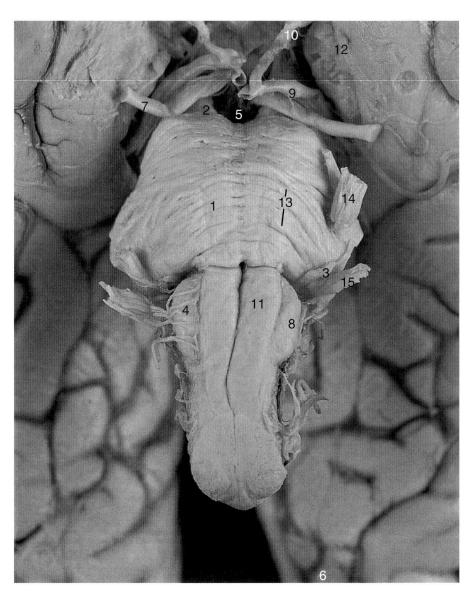

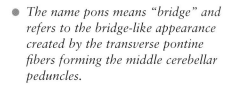

● *The name pons means "bridge" and refers to the bridge-like appearance created by the transverse pontine fibers forming the middle cerebellar peduncles.*

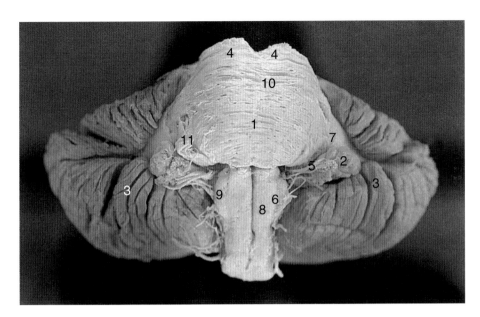

Fig. 13.13
A superficial dissection of the brainstem and cerebellum showing transverse pontine fibers crossing the basilar portion of the pons and entering the middle cerebellar peduncle. ×1

1 Basilar portion of pons
2 Cerebellar flocculus
3 Cerebellar hemisphere
4 Crus cerebri
5 Facial nerve (VII)
6 Hypoglossal nerve (XII)
7 Middle cerebellar peduncle
8 Pyramid of medulla oblongata
9 Olive
10 Transverse pontine fibers
11 Vestibulocochlear nerve (VIII)

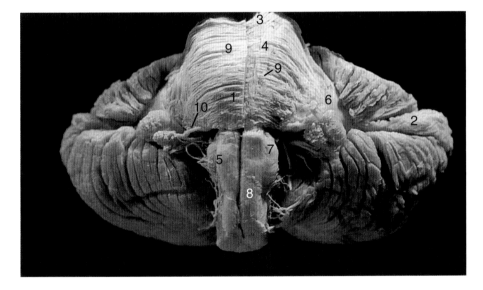

Fig. 13.14
A deep dissection of the left-hand side of the pons. This demonstrates the corticospinal fibers coursing longitudinally through the basilar portion of the pons, interweaving with the transverse pontine fibers. ×1.3

1 Basilar portion of pons
2 Cerebellum
3 Crus cerebri of midbrain
4 Corticospinal fibers
5 Medulla oblongata
6 Middle cerebellar peduncle
7 Olive
8 Pyramid
9 Transverse pontine fibers
10 Vestibulocochlear and facial nerves (VIII and VII)

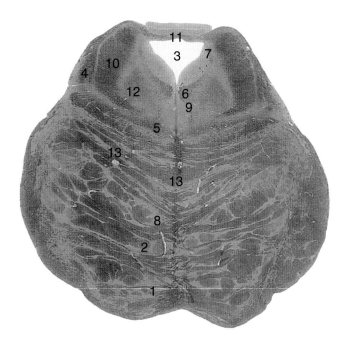

Fig. 13.15
A transverse section of the pons rostral to the middle cerebellar peduncle. Weigert stain. ×4.2

1 Basilar portion of pons
2 Corticospinal/corticobulbar fibers
3 Fourth ventricle
4 Lateral lemniscus
5 Medial lemniscus
6 Medial longitudinal fasciculus
7 Mesencephalic nucleus and tract of trigeminal nerve
8 Pontine nuclei
9 Reticular formation
10 Superior cerebellar peduncle
11 Superior medullary velum
12 Tegmental portion of pons
13 Transverse pontine fibers

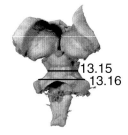

Fig. 13.16
A transverse section through the pons and the middle cerebellar peduncle. Luxol fast blue stain. ×3.6

1 Basilar portion of pons
2 Corticospinal tract
3 Facial nerve (VII)
4 Fourth ventricle
5 Medial lemniscus
6 Middle cerebellar peduncle
7 Reticular formation
8 Spinothalamic tracts
9 Tegmental portion of pons
10 Trapezoid body
11 Trigeminal nerve fibers
12 Vestibular nuclei

CAM

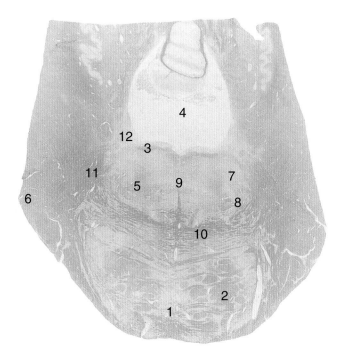

Medulla Oblongata

The medulla oblongata is the hindmost portion of the brainstem. At its caudal end its structure shows a gradual transition to that of the first cervical segment of the spinal cord. Rostrally, it is continuous with the pons. Tracts ascending and descending between the spinal cord and higher brain centers all pass through the medulla. It also contains several cranial nerve nuclei and other nuclei associated with functional systems.

Figures 13.17–13.19 Sections showing the structure and relationships of the medulla oblongata.

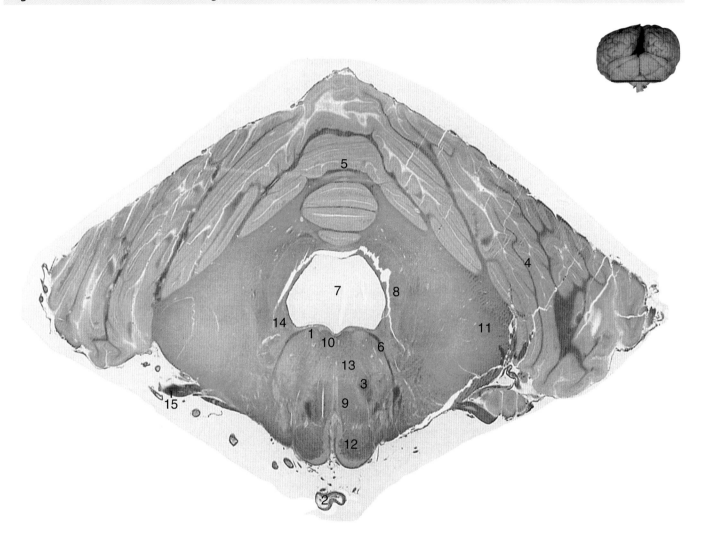

Fig. 13.17
A coronal section through the brainstem at the junction between the pons and the medulla oblongata, with the cerebellum attached. Weigert-Pal stain, celloidin-embedded section cut by Mr. P. A. Runnicles. ×1.8

1 Abducens nucleus	**6** Facial nerve (VII)	**11** Middle cerebellar peduncle
2 Basilar artery	**7** Fourth ventricle	**12** Pyramid
3 Central tegmental tract	**8** Inferior cerebellar peduncle	**13** Reticular formation
4 Cerebellar hemisphere	**9** Medial lemniscus	**14** Vestibular nuclei
5 Cerebellar vermis	**10** Medial longitudinal fasciculus	**15** Vestibulocochlear nerve (VIII)

MHMS

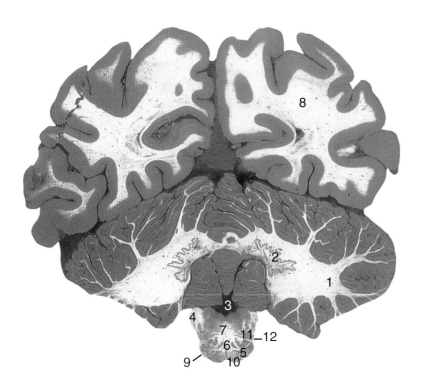

Fig. 13.18
Thick coronal slice through the brain showing the anatomy and relationships of the medulla oblongata at the level of the olive. Mulligan stain. ×0.95

1 Cerebellum
2 Dentate nucleus
3 Fourth ventricle
4 Inferior cerebellar peduncle
5 Inferior olivary nucleus
6 Medial lemniscus
7 Medulla oblongata
8 Occipital lobe
9 Olive
10 Pyramid
11 Spinal trigeminal nucleus and tract
12 Tuberculum cinereum

● *Enlarged views of sections through the medulla oblongata at this level can be found on p. 183.*

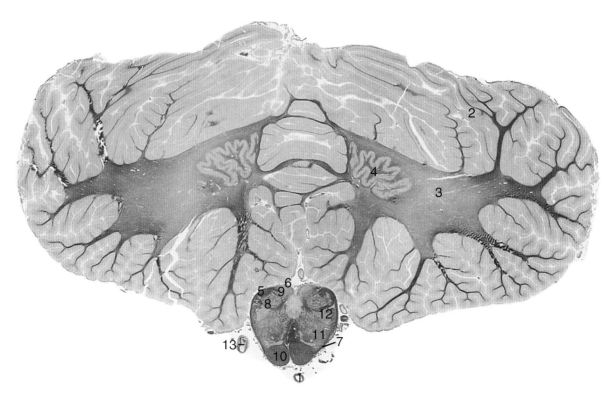

Fig. 13.19
Coronal section through the brainstem and cerebellum showing the anatomy and relationships of the medulla oblongata caudal to the olive. Weigert-Pal stain and celloidin-embedded section cut by Mr. P. A. Runnicles. ×1.6

1 Anterior spinal artery	6 Fasciculus gracilis	11 Reticular formation
2 Cerebellar cortex	7 Medulla oblongata	12 Spinal trigeminal nucleus and tract
3 Cerebellar white matter	8 Nucleus cuneatus	13 Vertebral artery
4 Dentate nucleus	9 Nucleus gracilis	
5 Fasciculus cuneatus	10 Pyramid	

MHMS

Figures 13.20 and 13.21 are transverse sections through the junction between the lower medulla oblongata and the first cervical segment of the spinal cord. In this transitional zone the arrangement of gray matter changes from the discrete nuclei typical of the brainstem to the central butterfly-shaped mass of spinal cord gray matter. The most prominent feature of the white matter is the pyramidal decussation. The pyramidal or corticospinal tract is the major nervous pathway for the control of voluntary movement. It connects the motor cortex of the cerebral hemisphere with the contralateral side of the spinal cord. Approximately 80% of its fibers decussate at the transition from brainstem to spinal cord. The resulting concentration of decussating fibers is known as the pyramidal decussation.

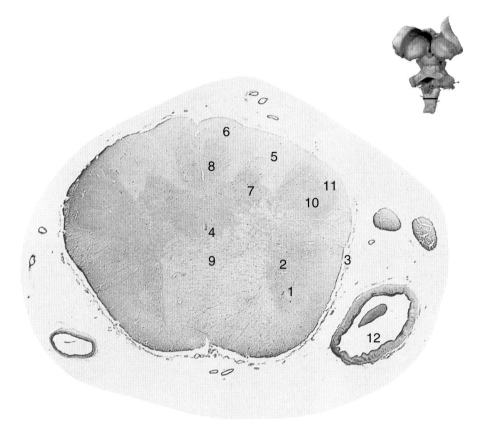

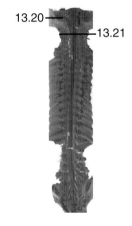

Fig. 13.20
A section of medulla oblongata passing through the pyramidal decussation. Thionin stain. ×7.3

1 Accessory nerve nucleus
2 Anterior horn
3 Arachnoid mater
4 Central gray matter
5 Fasciculus cuneatus
6 Fasciculus gracilis
7 Nucleus cuneatus
8 Nucleus gracilis
9 Pyramidal decussation
10 Spinal trigeminal nucleus
11 Spinal trigeminal tract
12 Vertebral artery

Fig. 13.21
A section through the first cervical segment (C1) of the spinal cord. Myelin stain. ×4.9

1 Anterior (ventral) horn
2 Anterior (ventral) median sulcus
3 Cervical nerve roots
4 Fasciculus cuneatus
5 Fasciculus gracilis
6 Lateral corticospinal tract
7 Posterior (dorsal) horn
8 Spinal trigeminal nucleus
9 Spinal trigeminal tract
10 Vertebral artery

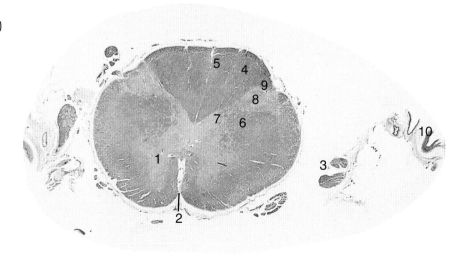

Figures 13.22–13.26 The position and histology of the reticular formation.

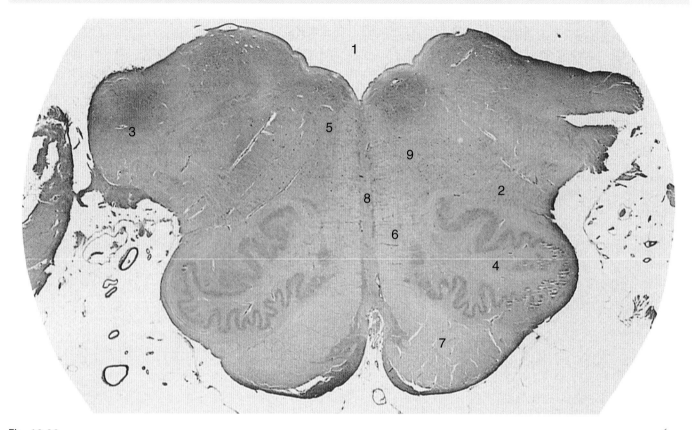

Fig. 13.22
A transverse section of the upper medulla oblongata showing the most important reticular nuclei. Thionin stain. ×9.2

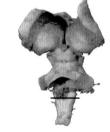

1 Fourth ventricle
2 Lateral reticular nucleus
3 Inferior cerebellar peduncle
4 Inferior olivary nucleus
5 Magnocellular nucleus

6 Medial lemniscus
7 Pyramid
8 Raphe nucleus
9 Reticular formation

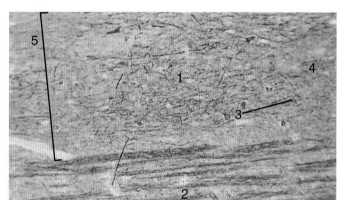

Fig. 13.23
Section to contrast the histology of the reticular formation in the medulla with that of a myelinated tract, the medial lemniscus. Palmgren stain. ×62

1 Loosely arranged nerve fibers
2 Medial lemniscus
3 Nerve cell bodies
4 Nerve fiber bundles
5 Reticular formation

● *The term "brainstem death" refers to a situation in which damage to the brainstem is irreversible and so severe that recovery of its vital functions such as the maintenance of breathing and heartbeat is impossible. A list of tests designed to assess brainstem function must be carried out before deciding to turn off life support equipment or remove organs for donation. Such tests are a legal requirement to prevent misdiagnosis. Consult a textbook for details.*

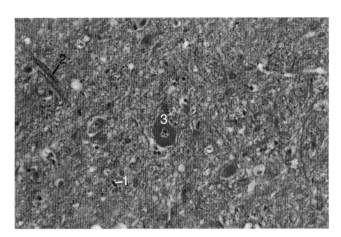

Fig. 13.24
High power view of the reticular formation in the pons to show widely scattered cells and fibers. Luxol fast blue and acid fuchsin stain. ×390

1 Glial cell nucleus
2 Nerve fibers
3 Neuron

CXWMS

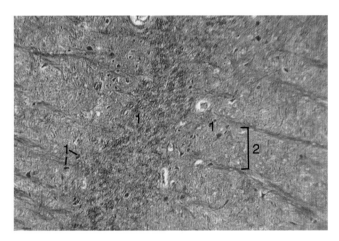

Fig. 13.25
A section of the medulla oblongata at the same level as Figure 13.22 to demonstrate the relationship between the raphe nucleus and the medial lemniscus. Palmgren stain. ×183

1 Cells of raphe nucleus
2 Fibers of medial lemniscus

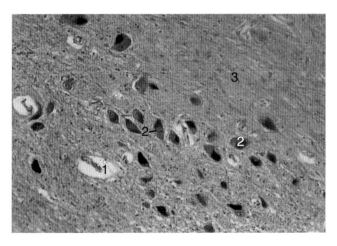

Fig. 13.26
A section showing the pigmented cells of the locus ceruleus. Hematoxylin and eosin stain. ×154

1 Blood vessel
2 Pigmented neurons
3 Unpigmented nervous tissue

- *The reticular activating system (see p. 166) is the component of the reticular formation responsible for maintaining awareness. General anesthetics abolish consciousness by suppressing transmission of impulses through the reticular activating system.*

- *The reticular formation contains some pathways that inhibit the transmission of impulses from pain receptors to the brain. The production of analgesia by acupuncture may involve stimulation of these pathways.*

- *Serotonin is a widespread inhibitory transmitter in the reticular formation. Tryptophan is a precursor of serotonin synthesis. It is present in milk. This may account for the effectiveness of milk-based drinks in relieving insomnia in many individuals.*

- *Some groups of cells in the reticular formation are pigmented. The largest of these is the locus ceruleus in the floor of the fourth ventricle. The noradrenergic neurons of this nucleus have widespread connections throughout the brain.*

- *No blood–brain barrier exists in the locus ceruleus.*

Summary

1. The brainstem consists of the midbrain, pons and medulla oblongata.
2. The brainstem contains ascending and descending tracts, cranial nerve nuclei III–XII and the reticular formation.
3. The brainstem is responsible for the control of vital body functions such as breathing and the circulation.
4. Severe brainstem damage causes deep, irreversible coma and death.

14 Brainstem Cranial Nerve Nuclei

Cranial nerves III–XII arise from the brainstem and appear in order from rostral to caudal. The oculomotor (III) and trochlear (IV) nerves emerge from the midbrain; the trigeminal (V), abducens (VI), facial (VII) and vestibulocochlear (VIII) nerves emerge from the pons and the junction between the pons and medulla oblongata; and the glossopharyngeal (IX), vagus (X), accessory (XI) and hypoglossal (XII) nerves emerge from the medulla oblongata.

● *Cranial nerves III–XII beyond their exit from the skull are considered as part of the peripheral nervous system and are not covered in this book.*

Figures 14.1–14.13 Dissections and histological preparations to demonstrate cranial nerves and their nuclei in the brainstem.

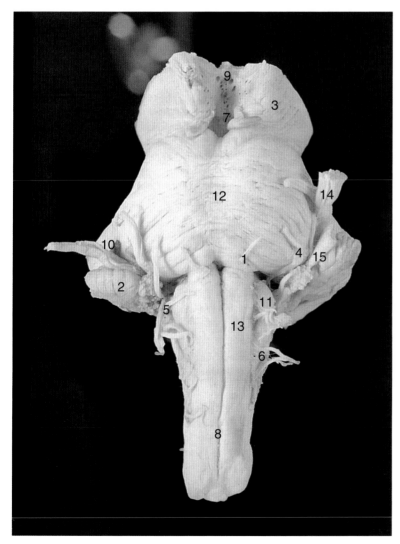

Fig. 14.1
The brainstem viewed from below (anteriorly) to demonstrate the emergence of cranial nerves. ×1.46

1 Abducens nerve (VI)
2 Cerebellar flocculus
3 Crus cerebri
4 Facial nerve (VII)
5 Glossopharyngeal (IX), vagus (X) and accessory (XI) nerve rootlets
6 Hypoglossal nerve rootlets (XII)
7 Interpeduncular fossa
8 Medulla oblongata
9 Midbrain
10 Middle cerebellar peduncle
11 Olive
12 Pons
13 Pyramid
14 Trigeminal nerve (V)
15 Vestibulocochlear nerve (VIII)

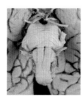

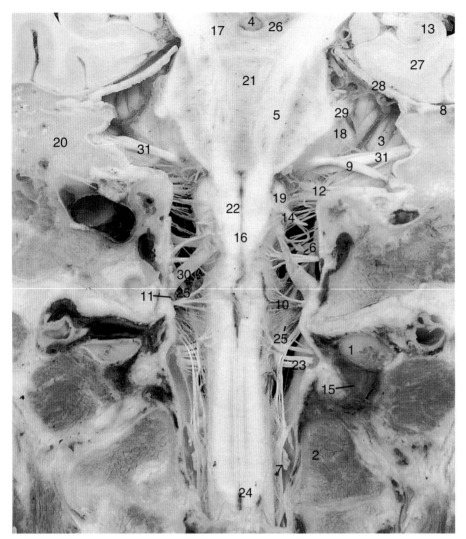

Fig. 14.2
An anterior view of a coronal section through the brainstem *in situ* showing cranial nerve roots and upper cervical spinal nerve roots in relation to the skull and vertebral column. ×1.5

1 Atlas
2 Axis
3 Cerebellum
4 Cerebral aqueduct
5 Corticospinal tract
6 Cranial root of accessory nerve (XI)
7 Denticulate ligament
8 Dura mater
9 Facial nerve (VII)
10 First cervical nerve (CI) roots
11 Foramen magnum
12 Glossopharyngeal nerve (IX)
13 Hippocampal formation
14 Hypoglossal nerve (XII)
15 Internal jugular vein
16 Medulla oblongata
17 Midbrain
18 Middle cerebellar peduncle
19 Olive
20 Petrous temporal bone
21 Pons
22 Pyramid
23 Second cervical nerve (C2) roots
24 Spinal cord
25 Spinal root of accessory nerve (XI)
26 Tegmentum of midbrain
27 Temporal lobe
28 Tentorium cerebelli
29 Trigeminal nerve (V)
30 Vertebral artery
31 Vestibulocochlear nerve (VIII)

UN

● *For the optic and olfactory nerves see Vison and Smell p. 241 and p. 275.*

● *Unlike spinal nerves, which all contain both sensory and motor fibers, cranial nerves may be either mixed or purely motor or sensory. The mixed cranial nerves contain fibers associated with both motor and sensory brainstem nuclei.*

● *Motor cranial nerve nuclei supplying extraocular and tongue muscles lie closer to the midline of the brainstem than autonomic or sensory nuclei. This pattern derives from their embryonic origin from the alar plate (sensory)*

or basal plate (motor). See Embryology p. 23 for discussion.

● *In a clinical examination of the cranial nerves, motor, sensory and autonomic functions are all utilized to assess function. Loss of cranial nerve function may be due to a lesion of the nerve itself (infranuclear) or its nuclei in the brainstem (intranuclear), or to loss of ascending or descending connections between the brainstem and higher centers (supranuclear) (see Somatic Sensory and Motor Pathways, p. 223).*

Nuclei of the Oculomotor and Trochlear Nerves

The oculomotor nucleus contains an autonomic (parasympathetic) component, the Edinger-Westphal nucleus, that supplies the pupillary sphincter and ciliary muscle. Groups of somatic motor cells within the main nucleus supply the superior, medial and inferior rectus and the inferior oblique muscles of the eye, and the levator palpebrae superioris muscle of the upper eyelid.

Figures 14.3–14.5 Histological preparations illustrating the anatomy of the oculomotor and trochlear nuclei and nerves.

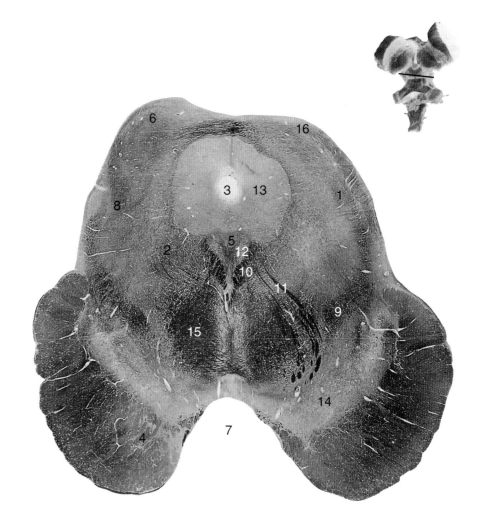

Fig. 14.3
An oblique section through the midbrain, passing through the rostral end of one inferior colliculus and the caudal end of the contralateral superior colliculus, demonstrating the nucleus and fibers of the oculomotor nerve. Weigert stain. ×4.5

1 Anterolateral system
2 Central tegmental tract
3 Cerebral aqueduct
4 Crus cerebri
5 Edinger-Westphal nucleus
6 Inferior colliculus
7 Interpeduncular fossa
8 Lateral lemniscus
9 Medial lemniscus
10 Medial longitudinal fasciculus
11 Oculomotor nerve fibers (III)
12 Oculomotor nucleus
13 Periaqueductal gray matter
14 Substantia nigra
15 Superior cerebellar peduncle
16 Superior colliculus

● *A person with a lesion of the oculomotor nerve will show some or all of the following features:*
   An inability to adduct the eye on the affected side, due to paralysis of the medial rectus muscle on the affected side.
   A lateral strabismus (squint) due to unopposed action of the lateral rectus muscle, which is supplied by the abducens (VI) nerve.

Ptosis, a drooping of the upper eyelid, due to paralysis of the levator palpebrae superioris muscle on the affected side.
Dilatation of the pupil and failure of the light reflex if the parasympathetic supply to the sphincter pupillae muscle of the iris is lost. The dilator pupillae muscle is unaffected because it is supplied by sympathetic nerves.

The trochlear nerve (IV) supplies only the superior oblique muscle of the eye. It is the only nerve that emerges from the dorsum of the brainstem. From the nucleus, the nerve fibers pass caudally and decussate in the superior medullary velum over the fourth ventricle before leaving the brain.

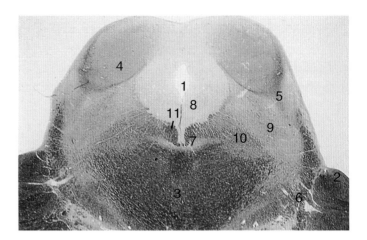

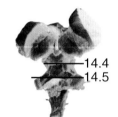

Fig. 14.4
A transverse section of the tectum and tegmentum of the midbrain to show the position of the nucleus of the trochlear nerve. Weigert stain. ×2.5

1	Cerebral aqueduct	6	Medial lemniscus
2	Crus cerebri	7	Medial longitudinal fasciculus
3	Decussation of superior cerebellar peduncle	8	Periaqueductal gray matter
4	Inferior colliculus (tectum)	9	Reticular formation
5	Lateral lemniscus	10	Tegmentum
		11	Trochlear nucleus

MHMS

Fig. 14.5
A transverse section of the rostral end of the pons immediately behind the inferior colliculus, demonstrating the decussation and emergence of the fibers of the trochlear nerve. Weigert stain. ×3.7

1 Basilar portion of pons
2 Central tegmental tract
3 Corticospinal tract
4 Decussating fibers of trochlear nerve (IV)
5 Emerging fibers of trochlear nerve (IV)
6 Fourth ventricle
7 Lateral lemniscus
8 Medial lemniscus
9 Medial longitudinal fasciculus
10 Superior cerebellar peduncle
11 Superior medullary velum
12 Transverse pontine fibers

* The red bracket indicates the depth of the basilar portion of the pons.

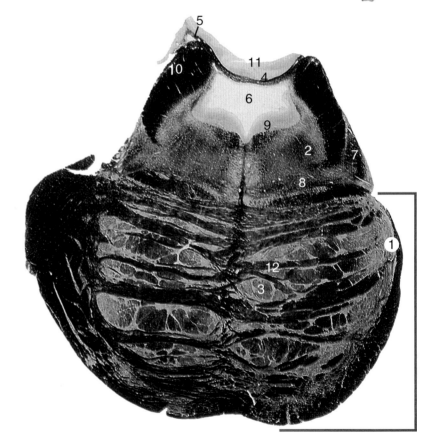

● *Function of the trochlear nerve is tested by asking the patient to look obliquely downwards. With a lesion of the trochlear nerve, the function of the superior oblique muscle is lost. When looking down, if this muscle acts normally, the eyes tilt inferiorly and converge towards the midline (intorsion). Damage to the trochlear nerve causes these movements to fail on the affected side and the patient looks downward and outward (extorsion). The patient, on looking down (e.g. during reading), will also tilt their head to the side opposite the lesion to avoid diplopia (double vision).*

Nuclei of the Trigeminal Nerve

Four nuclei are associated with each trigeminal nerve. A chain of nuclei receiving sensory fibers from the nerve extends through the brainstem and down into the spinal cord as far as the third cervical segment. Of these, the spinal nucleus (or nucleus of the descending tract of V) is concerned with touch, pain and temperature, the principal (or main) sensory nucleus with touch, and the mesencephalic nucleus with proprioception. The motor nucleus lies in the pons. Its fibers enter only the mandibular division of the trigeminal nerve and innervate muscles of mastication. Maxillary and ophthalmic divisions of the nerve are sensory.

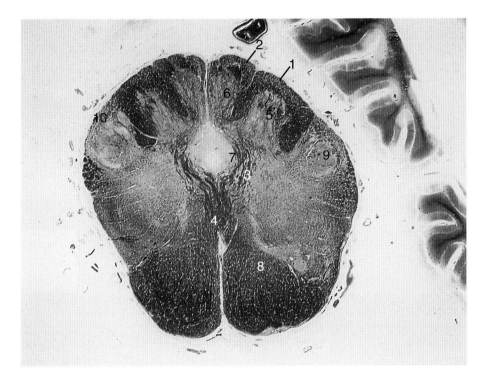

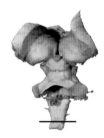

Fig. 14.6
A transverse section of the caudal end of the medulla oblongata showing the spinal nucleus and spinal tract of the trigeminal nerve. Weigert-Pal stain. ×6.1

1 Fasciculus cuneatus
2 Fasciculus gracilis
3 Internal arcuate fibers
4 Medial lemniscus
5 Nucleus cuneatus
6 Nucleus gracilis
7 Position of X and XII nuclei
8 Pyramid
9 Spinal nucleus of the trigeminal nerve
10 Spinal tract of the trigeminal nerve

MHMS

- *The spinal nucleus of the trigeminal nerve receives afferent fibers from all three divisions of the trigeminal nerve. It also receives fibers from the facial, glossopharyngeal and vagus nerves, and upper cervical segments of the spinal cord. It, therefore, receives a complete "map" of sensory information from the head, beyond the territory of the trigeminal nerve itself.*

- *To test sensory function in the trigeminal nerve, it is important to test each division of the nerve separately. Tactile sensation is tested by touching the skin with a piece of cotton. Temperature is tested with a cold object, e.g. the side of a tuning fork. Pain is not normally assessed to avoid distressing the patient.*

- *The corneal reflex is an important protective reflex for the eye involving both the trigeminal nerve (sensory,*

ophthalmic division) and the facial nerve (motor). If the reflex is normal, the patient will blink when the cornea is touched gently with a piece of cotton.

- *Motor trigeminal function is tested by examining the function of the jaw muscles. Function of the masseter muscle can be detected by feeling it contract as the patient clenches their jaws together. If motor function is impaired, when the patient opens their mouth, the jaw will deviate to the affected side due to paralysis of the lateral pterygoid muscle.*

- *In trigeminal neuralgia, there is intense pain in the area supplied by one of the divisions of the trigeminal nerve.*

Fig. 14.7
A transverse section through the pons demonstrating the nuclei of the trigeminal nerve and some features of the abducens and facial nerves. Weigert stain. ×3.1

1 Abducens nerve (VI)
2 Abducens nucleus
3 Corticospinal tract
4 Facial nerve (VII)
5 Fourth ventricle
6 Lateral lemniscus
7 Mesencephalic tract and nucleus of trigeminal nerve
8 Middle cerebellar peduncle
9 Motor nucleus of trigeminal nerve
10 Pontine genu of facial nerve
11 Principal sensory nucleus of trigeminal nerve
12 Spinal tract and nucleus of trigeminal nerve
13 Trigeminal nerve fibers (V)

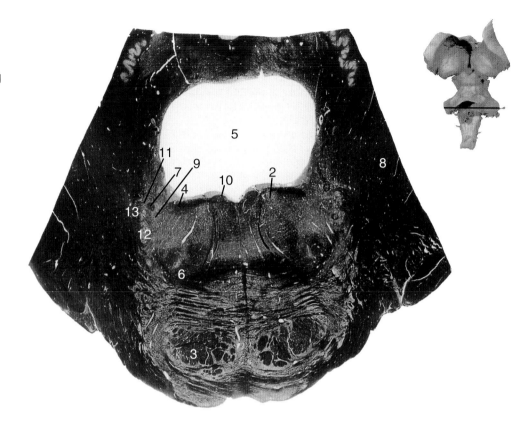

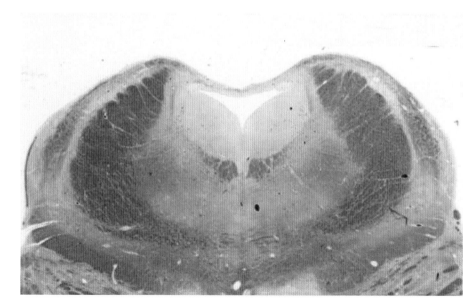

Fig. 14.8
A section of part of the floor of the fourth ventricle in the rostral third of the pons to show the mesencephalic tract and nucleus of the trigeminal nerve. Solochrome cyanin stain. ×7.5

1 Fourth ventricle
2 Medial lemniscus
3 Medial longitudinal fasciculus
4 Mesencephalic tract and nucleus of trigeminal nerve
5 Superior cerebellar peduncle
6 Superior medullary velum

Dr. A. Fletcher LRI

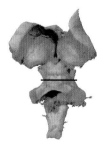

Nuclei of the Abducens, Facial and Vestibulocochlear Nerves

The abducens nerve (VI) supplies the lateral rectus muscle of the eye. As they leave their nucleus, the fibers of the facial nerve (VII) arch around the abducens nucleus forming a bulge, the facial colliculus, in the floor of the fourth ventricle.

The facial nerve arises from three nuclei: the motor nucleus controls the muscles of facial expression, the superior salivatory nucleus supplies parasympathetic innervation for salivatory and lachrymal glands, and the solitary nucleus is a sensory nucleus for the sense of taste. In addition, the spinal nucleus of the trigeminal nerve receives a few facial nerve sensory fibers from the ear.

Six nuclei receive incoming sensory fibers in the vestibulocochlear nerve. These are the dorsal and ventral cochlear nuclei, associated with the cochlear division of the nerve, i.e. the sense of hearing, and the superior, inferior, medial and lateral vestibular nuclei associated with the vestibular division of the nerve, i.e. with the sense of equilibrium.

Figures 14.9 and 14.10 Histological sections demonstrating the nuclei of the abducens and facial nerves.

Fig. 14.9
A section through the tegmental portion of the pons to show the nuclei and fibers of the abducens and facial nerves. Weigert stain. ×7.5

1 Abducens nucleus
2 Abducens nerve (VI) fibers
3 Basilar portion of pons
4 Corticospinal tract
5 Facial colliculus
6 Facial motor nucleus
7 Facial nerve (VII) fibers
8 Fourth ventricle
9 Medial lemniscus
10 Medial longitudinal fasciculus
11 Pontine genu of facial nerve
12 Spinal nucleus of trigeminal nerve (V)
13 Spinal tract of trigeminal nerve
14 Superior salivatory nucleus
15 Tectospinal tract
16 Tegmental portion of pons
17 Transverse pontine fibers

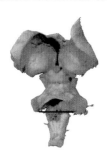
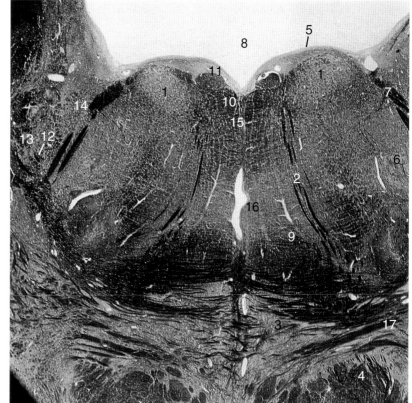

- Testing of the vestibulocochlear nerve is considered under Hearing (p. 259) and Equilibrium (p. 271).

- The medial longitudinal fasciculus links the oculomotor, trochlear and abducens nuclei with the vestibular nuclei. It enables eye movements to be coordinated with head position and movements.

- A patient with damage to the abducens nerve will lose the ability to abduct the eye on the affected side due to paralysis of the lateral rectus muscle.

- Facial movements are important in emotional expression, and the facial motor nucleus probably has connections with the limbic areas of the cerebral cortex.

- Motor function in the facial nerve is tested by observing movements of facial expression. In a lower motor neuron lesion, such as Bell's palsy, where the nerve itself is affected, the entire face will be paralyzed ipsilateral to the lesion. In an upper motor neuron lesion involving higher movement control centers, e.g. cerebral cortex, the muscles of the upper face will be spared and the patient will be able to wrinkle their forehead (see p. 285 for an explanation). Autonomic fibers in the facial nerve supply the salivary and lachrymal glands. These functions are not normally tested directly in a general neurological examination but the patient may report dryness of the eyes or mouth. Taste may also be affected if the lesion occurs proximal to the point where the chorda tympani nerve leaves the main trunk of the facial nerve.

Fig. 14.10

A section of the floor of the fourth ventricle demonstrating connections from the medial longitudinal fasciculus to the abducens nucleus. Luxol fast blue and acid fuchsin stain. ×10.3

1 Abducens nucleus
2 Facial nerve (VII)
3 Fibers from medial longitudinal fasciculus to abducens nucleus (arrow)
4 Fourth ventricle
5 Medial longitudinal fasciculus
6 Median sulcus
7 Pontine genu of facial nerve
8 Sulcus limitans
9 Tectospinal tract   CXWMS

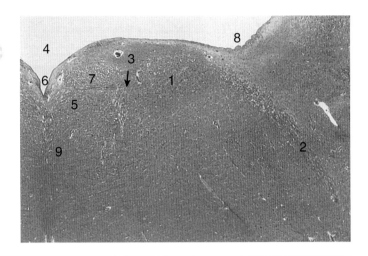

Figures 14.11 and 14.12 Histological sections to illustrate the nuclei of the vestibulocochlear nerve.

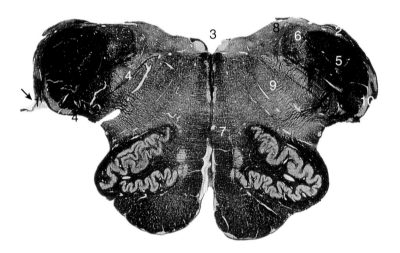

Fig. 14.11

A transverse section of the medulla oblongata showing the dorsal and ventral cochlear nuclei and the medial and inferior vestibular nuclei. Weigert stain. ×3.95

1 Cochlear nerve (VIII) (arrow)
2 Dorsal cochlear nucleus
3 Fourth ventricle
4 Glossopharyngeal nerve (IX)
5 Inferior cerebellar peduncle
6 Inferior vestibular nucleus
7 Medial lemniscus
8 Medial vestibular nucleus
9 Reticular formation
10 Ventral cochlear nucleus

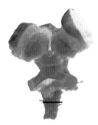

Fig. 14.12

A transverse section of the pons demonstrating the superior, medial and lateral vestibular nuclei. Luxol fast blue and acid fuchsin stain. ×3.3

1 Abducens nucleus
2 Basilar portion of pons
3 Corticospinal tract
4 Dentate nucleus
5 Facial nerve (VII)
6 Fourth ventricle
7 Lateral vestibular nucleus
8 Medial lemniscus
9 Medial vestibular nucleus
10 Middle cerebellar peduncle
11 Spinal nucleus of the trigeminal nerve
12 Superior vestibular nucleus

CXWMS

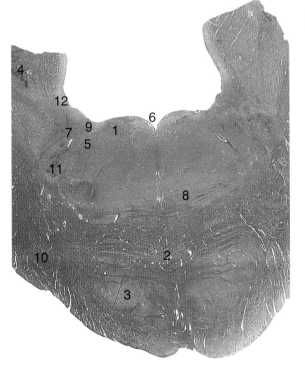

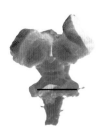

The Glossopharyngeal, Vagus, Accessory and Hypoglossal Nerves and their Nuclei

The glossopharyngeal (IX), vagus (X) and accessory (XI) nerves emerge in sequence from the medulla oblongata, in the longitudinal groove between the olive and the inferior cerebellar peduncle.

The glossopharyngeal is a mixed nerve. It contains motor fibers from the nucleus ambiguus to supply the stylopharyngeus muscle, and parasympathetic fibers from the inferior salivatory nucleus for the parotid gland. Sensory fibers from taste buds on the posterior third of the tongue, from the oropharynx, from the carotid sinus (baroreceptor for the control of blood pressure) and the carotid body (chemoreceptor for the control of respiration) all terminate in the solitary nucleus. Sensory fibers from the middle ear terminate in the spinal trigeminal nucleus (see pp. 225-226).

The vagus is also a mixed nerve. Sensory fibers from the aortic arch, baro- and chemoreceptors, and the respiratory and gastrointestinal tracts terminate in the solitary nucleus, forming part of the reflex mechanisms for cardiovascular function, respiration and gastrointestinal tract mobility. Taste fibers enter the solitary nucleus from taste buds on the epiglottis, and somatic sensory fibers from the external ear go to the spinal trigeminal nucleus.

Visceral efferent (parasympathetic) fibers in the vagus nerve from the nucleus ambiguus supply the heart. Their action is to slow the heart rate. The dorsal motor nucleus supplies parasympathetic innervation to the respiratory and digestive tracts. The nucleus ambiguus supplies muscles of the larynx and pharynx.

The accessory nerve is a purely motor nerve. Its nucleus is an elongated column of cells extending in the anterior horn of the first five or six cervical segments of the spinal cord. These cells give rise to its spinal root. It also has a cranial root arising from the nucleus ambiguus (sometimes viewed as part of the vagus). The spinal root ascends through the foramen magnum to join the cranial root. The fibers in the accessory nerve arising from the accessory nucleus supply the trapezius and sternocleidomastoid muscles in the neck. Fibers from the nucleus ambiguus supply the muscles of the pharynx.

The hypoglossal nerve emerges from the medulla by multiple rootlets between the pyramid and the olive. It is a purely motor nerve that innervates the intrinsic and extrinsic muscles of the tongue.

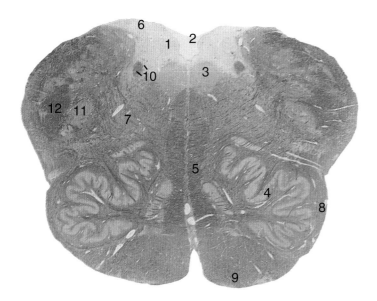

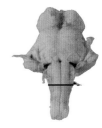

Fig. 14.13
A transverse section of the medulla oblongata showing the solitary nucleus, nucleus ambiguus, dorsal motor nucleus of the vagus and hypoglossal nucleus. Myelin stain. ×6

 1 Dorsal motor nucleus of vagus nerve
 2 Fourth ventricle
 3 Hypoglossal nucleus
 4 Inferior olivary nucleus
 5 Medial lemniscus
 6 Medial vestibular nucleus
 7 Nucleus ambiguus
 8 Olive
 9 Pyramid
10 Solitary nucleus and tract
11 Spinal nucleus of trigeminal nerve
12 Spinal tract of trigeminal nerve

- *Testing of function in the glossopharyngeal and vagus nerves is based on their providing sensory and motor supplies to the pharynx. If the back of the pharynx is touched, e.g. with a tongue depressor, there should be a gag reflex if the sensory pathway through the glossopharyngeal nerve is intact. The soft palate should rise symmetrically if the patient is asked to make a sound, e.g. "Ah", when the motor innervation is normal. The tone of the voice can also indicate function of the vagus nerve, since it supplies the intrinsic muscles of the larynx. Paralysis of a vocal cord will cause hoarseness and inability to cough because the vocal cords cannot be apposed.*

- *The accessory nerve is tested by assessing the power of the trapezius and/or sternocleidomastoid muscles in the neck. The former can be tested by asking the patient to shrug their shoulders, the latter by asking him/her to turn the head, in each case against resistance provided by pressure of the examiner's hand. Rotation of the head in the direction opposite to the affected side will be weakened if the nerve is damaged.*

- *Examination of the hypoglossal nerve relies on its motor supply to the intrinsic and extrinsic muscles of the tongue. In a hypoglossal nerve lesion, the tongue on the affected side undergoes atrophy and may show fine involuntary movements (fasciculation). If the tongue is protruded, it will deviate to the affected side due to weakness of the genioglossus muscle.*

Summary

1. Cranial nerves I and II are atypical because they do not develop from the brainstem.
2. Cranial nerve I (olfactory) is connected to the forebrain; cranial nerve II (optic) is connected to the diencephalon, also part of the forebrain.
3. Cranial nerves III to XII arise in sequence from the brainstem.
4. Unlike spinal nerves, which contain motor, sensory and autonomic fibers, cranial nerves may be functionally specialized, i.e. purely sensory or purely motor.
5. Each cranial nerve arises from one or more nuclei in the brainstem. Mixed nerves possess multiple nuclei.
6. Competent examination of the cranial nerves depends on an understanding of their functional components.
7. Abnormal cranial nerve function may be the result of a lesion in the nerve itself (infranuclear), its nucleus/nuclei (intranuclear) or the connections between the nucleus and higher levels in the brain (supranuclear).

15 Cerebellum

The cerebellum is the largest part of the hindbrain. It consists of two cerebellar hemispheres united by a central, median vermis. The surface of the cerebellum is deeply folded. Major folds, the fissures, subdivide the cerebellum into superior and inferior halves, and demarcate subdivisions, the anterior, posterior and flocculonodular lobes within each hemisphere. The fissures and the lobes that they demarcate form early in the development of the cerebellum; they also have functional significance. The flocculonodular lobe forms first, is mainly concerned with equilibrium and is separated from the rest of the cerebellum by the posterior lateral fissure. The anterior lobe, lying rostral to the next fissure to form, the primary fissure, is mainly associated with proprioception (the sense of position) while the remainder of the cerebellum is concerned with complex processes of automatic motor control.

The cerebellum is similar in structure to the cerebral hemisphere: the cerebellar cortex (gray matter) forms folds (folia) on the surface and surrounds the white matter, within which are embedded the intracerebral or deep nuclei, i.e. the dentate, emboliform, globose and fastigial nuclei.

The cerebellar cortex has three cellular layers: the outermost molecular layer is mainly synaptic, containing sparse, small stellate and basket cells; the middle layer is composed of the giant Purkinje cells whose dendrites branch in the molecular layer and whose axons pass into the granular layer and enter the white matter; and the granular layer is innermost and is densely populated by small granule and larger but much sparser Golgi cells.

The white matter of the cerebellum resembles a tree with repeated branching. The trunk of the tree is the medullary center, while the branches are the arbor vitae. There are three types of fiber in the white matter: intrinsic, afferent and efferent. Intrinsic fibers connect different areas in the same hemisphere or the same area in both hemispheres.

The afferent and efferent fibers connect the cerebellum with other parts of the central nervous system. Their fibers are aggregated into three bundles in each hemisphere called the superior, middle and inferior peduncles. Afferent fibers make up the bulk of the white matter. They enter via the middle and inferior cerebellar peduncles and terminate in the cerebellar cortex, and many have collateral connections to the deep nuclei. A large proportion of the afferent fibers terminate as "mossy fibers" in the granular layer. "Climbing fibers" from the inferior olivary complex end on Purkinje cell dendrites. Each Purkinje cell is connected to only one climbing fiber, but receives several thousand connections via the mossy fibers and granule cells. The Purkinje cells are the output cells of the cerebellar cortex. With the exception of a minority, located in the flocculonodular lobe, their axons do not leave the cerebellum but project to the deep cerebellar nuclei. It is from these deep nuclei that most cerebellar efferents arise. The axons of the minority group of Purkinje cells project directly to the brainstem, especially to the inferior olivary nucleus.

The cerebellum coordinates muscular activity and controls the force, direction and extent of voluntary movements. It is also important as a center for body equilibrium (flocculonodular lobe) and in the maintenance of posture. Its sensory input via its afferent pathways is from the eyes, ears, cutaneous sensory receptors and proprioceptors. In turn, the efferent connections pass to motor control centers in the brainstem, some of which in turn are linked to the cerebral cortex. There is no direct output to the cerebral cortex, or to the spinal cord.

Functionally, the cerebellum can be considered as three parts: the archicerebellum, paleocerebellum and neocerebellum. The first consists of the flocculonodular lobe, the second includes the anterior lobe, pyramid and uvula, and the third is the remainder of the hemisphere. The fastigial nucleus is the deep nucleus associated with the archicerebellum, the globose and emboliform nuclei are linked to the paleocerebellum, and the dentate nucleus is the deep nucleus of the neocerebellum.

- *Each cerebellar hemisphere assists in the control of movement on its own side of the body.*

- *In spite of its large sensory input, no conscious sensations are perceived in the cerebellum.*

- *The inhibitory neurotransmitter for basket, stellate, Purkinje and Golgi cells is gamma-aminobutyric acid (GABA). The excitatory transmitter of the granule cells is glutamate.*

- *The sensory role of the cerebellum is important when proprioception is used to assess features such as the size or weight of objects held in the hand. Functional MRI scans show activation of the dentate nucleus.*

- *In locomotion, proprioception from the neck muscles assists vision in monitoring and controlling the direction of movement.*

For cerebellar connections see pp. 301–309.

Figures 15.1–15.4 The cerebellum *in situ*.

Fig. 15.1
Mid-sagittal section of the brainstem and cerebellum. ×0.6

1 Choroid plexus of fourth ventricle
2 Fourth ventricle
3 Hemisphere of cerebellum
4 Medulla oblongata
5 Midbrain
6 Pons
7 Vermis of cerebellum

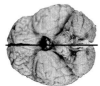

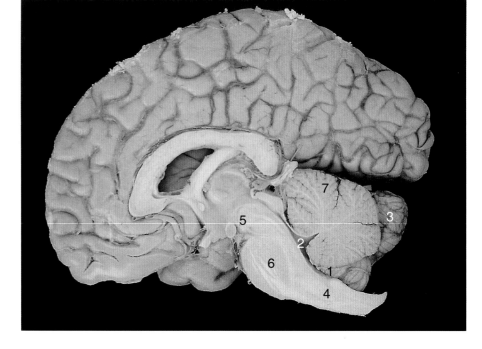

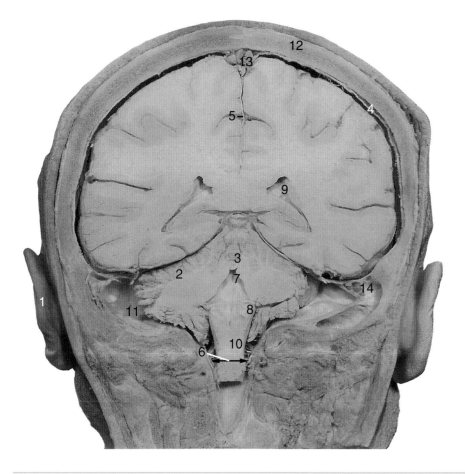

Fig. 15.2
Coronal section passing through the posterior cranial fossa. ×0.68

1 Auricle
2 Cerebellar hemisphere
3 Cerebellar vermis
4 Dura mater
5 Falx cerebri
6 Foramen magnum (arrows)
7 Fourth ventricle
8 Inferior cerebellar peduncle (restiform body)
9 Lateral ventricle
10 Medulla oblongata
11 Posterior cranial fossa
12 Skull vault
13 Superior sagittal sinus
14 Transverse sinus

RCS

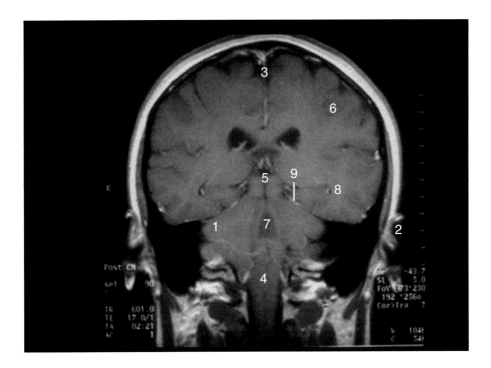

Fig. 15.3
A coronal MRI scan showing the relationship of the cerebellum to the cerebral hemisphere and brainstem.

1 Cerebellum
2 Ear
3 Falx cerebri
4 Medulla oblongata
5 Midbrain
6 Parietal lobe
7 Pons
8 Temporal lobe
9 Tentorium cerebelli

Mr. J. Wasserberg QEH

Fig. 15.4
Sagittal image of the normal adult brain as visualized by nuclear magnetic resonance technique (NMR).

 1 Brainstem
 2 Cerebellum
 3 Corpus callosum
 4 Cranial vault
 5 Fourth ventricle
 6 Frontal lobe
 7 Nose
 8 Occipital lobe
 9 Parietal lobe
10 Pharynx
11 Spinal cord
12 Vertebral column

Dr. R. Abbot LRI

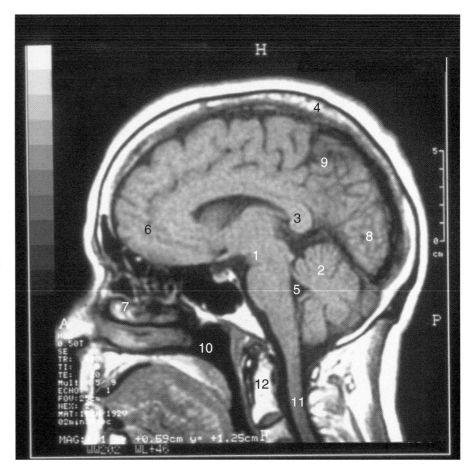

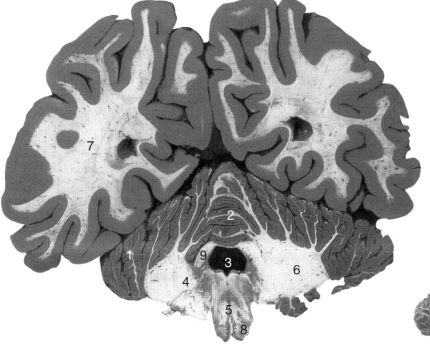
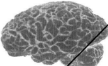

Fig. 15.5
Thick transverse slice through the brainstem, cerebellum and both cerebral hemispheres to show the relationship of the cerebellum to the fourth ventricle. Mulligan stain. ×1

1 Cerebellar hemisphere
2 Cerebellar vermis
3 Fourth ventricle
4 Inferior cerebellar peduncle
5 Medulla oblongata
6 Middle cerebellar peduncle
7 Occipital lobe
8 Pyramid of medulla
9 Superior cerebellar peduncle

Figures 15.6 and 15.7 The cerebellum and brainstem.

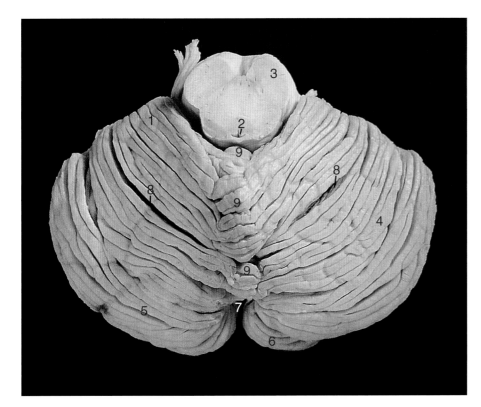

Fig. 15.6
Superior surface of cerebellum attached to the brainstem. The blood vessels have been removed. ×1.05

1 Anterior lobe
2 Cerebral aqueduct
3 Crus cerebri
4 Hemisphere of cerebellum
5 Horizontal fissure
6 Posterior lobe
7 Posterior notch
8 Primary fissure
9 Superior vermis

Fig. 15.7
Cerebellum and brainstem from below. The blood vessels have been removed. ×1.1

1 Flocculus
2 Hemisphere
3 Inferior cerebellar peduncle (restiform body)
4 Medulla oblongata
5 Middle cerebellar peduncle (brachium pontis)
6 Pons
7 Posterolateral fissure (arrow)
8 Posterior notch
9 Pyramid of medulla
10 Tonsil
11 Transverse pontine fibers
12 Trigeminal nerve (V)
13 Vallecula
14 Vermis

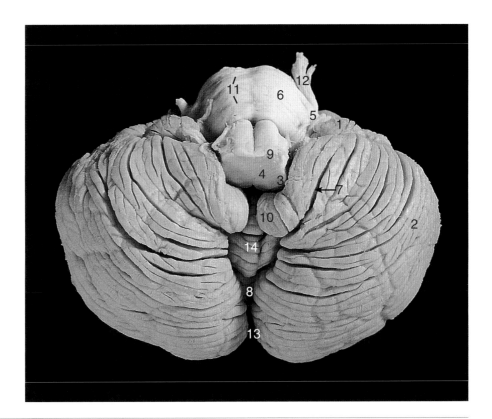

Figures 15.8–15.14 The white matter of the cerebellum. Fibers form the medullary center and the branching arbor vitae.

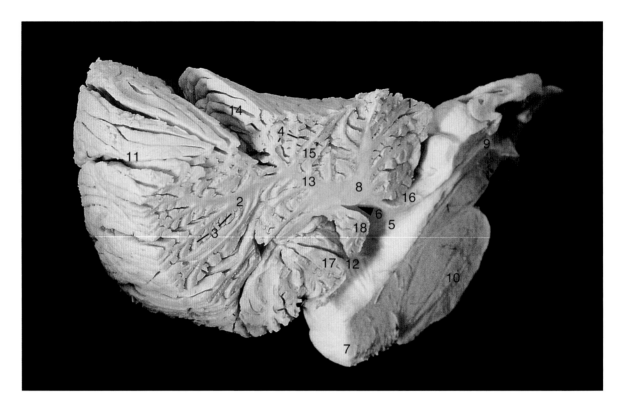

Fig. 15.8
Sagitally sectioned cerebellum viewed obliquely to show the arbor vitae. ×1.65

1 Anterior lobe
2 Arbor vitae
3 Cortex
4 Folia
5 Fourth ventricle
6 Lateral recess of fourth ventricle (arrowhead)

7 Medulla oblongata
8 Medullary center of cerebellum
9 Midbrain
10 Pons
11 Posterior lobe
12 Posterolateral fissure

13 Primary lamina of arbor vitae
14 Primary fissure
15 Secondary lamina of arbor vitae
16 Lingula ⎫
17 Uvula ⎬ of vermis
18 Nodule ⎭

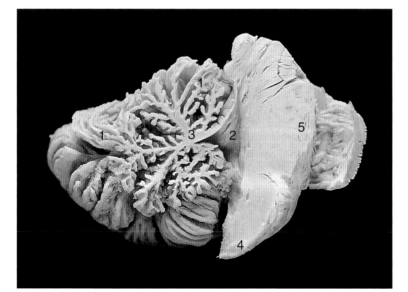

Fig. 15.9
The fibrous skeleton of the cerebellum. (The cellular structure has been removed on the sectioned face of the cerebellum.) ×1.1

1 Arbor vitae
2 Fourth ventricle
3 Medullary center
4 Medulla oblongata
5 Pons

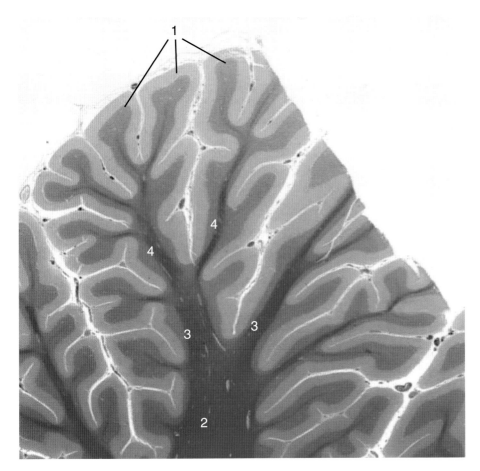

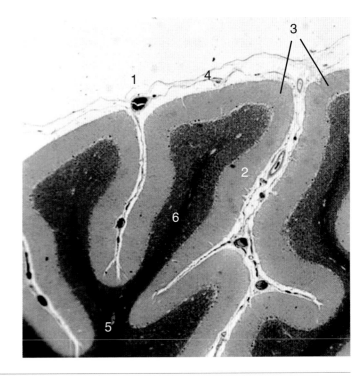

Fig. 15.10
Histological section of the arbor vitae. Luxol fast blue and cresyl violet stain. ×8.9

1 Folia
2 Medullary center
3 Primary lamina of arbor vitae
4 Secondary lamina of arbor vitae

Fig. 15.11
Three folia from an adjacent histological section to Figure 15.10, showing the arbor vitae in relation to the cerebellar cortex. Silver stain. ×20

1 Blood vessel
2 Cortex
3 Folia
4 Pia mater
5 Secondary lamina of arbor vitae
6 Tertiary lamina of arbor vitae

Figures 15.12–15.14 Afferent, efferent and intracortical fibers of arbor vitae and the cerebellar cortex. All three figures share the following labels:

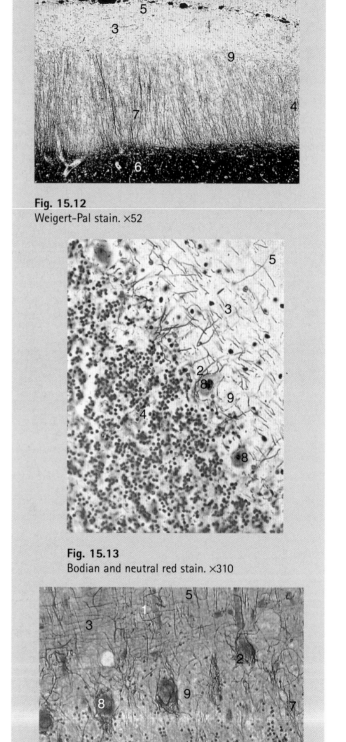

Fig. 15.12
Weigert-Pal stain. ×52

Fig. 15.13
Bodian and neutral red stain. ×310

Fig. 15.14
Palmgren stain. ×340

1 Climbing fibers (afferent) around Purkinje cells
2 Basket cell processes
3 Fibers (intracortical) parallel to cortical surface
4 Granular layer
5 Molecular layer
6 Myelinated fibers of arbor vitae
7 Myelinated fibers in granular layer
8 Purkinje cell bodies
9 Purkinje cell layer

Figures 15.15–15.17 The cellular structure of the cerebellar cortex. The cortex consists of three cellular layers: granular, Purkinje and molecular.

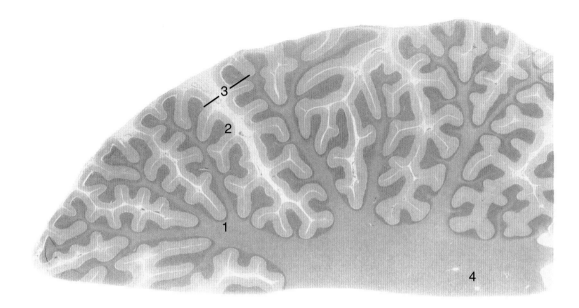

Fig. 15.15
Paraffin wax section showing the cerebellar cortex. Hematoxylin and eosin stain. ×3.9

1 Arbor vitae
2 Cerebellar cortex
3 Folia
4 Medullary center

CXWMS

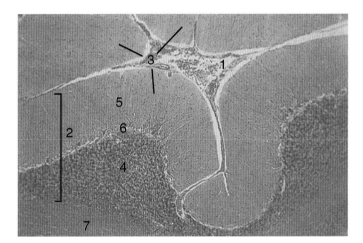

Fig. 15.16
Higher magnification of folia showing full thickness of cortex. Hematoxylin and eosin stain. ×88

1 Blood vessels in arachnoid mater
2 Cortex
3 Folia
4 Granular layer
5 Molecular layer
6 Purkinje layer
7 White matter of arbor vitae

CXWMS

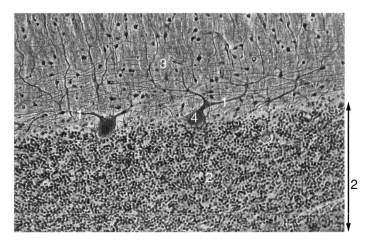

Fig. 15.17
Purkinje cells and their processes between the granular and molecular layers of the cerebellar cortex. Silver stain. ×253

1 Dendrites
2 Granular layer
3 Molecular layer
4 Purkinje cell body

CAM

The major nuclei are the dentate, emboliform, globose and fastigial nuclei. Axons from the dentate, emboliform and globose nuclei leave the cerebellum via the superior cerebellar peduncle. Axons from the fastigial nucleus leave via the inferior cerebellar peduncle.

Fibers from the dentate nucleus run to the red nucleus and thalamus.

The emboliform and globose nuclei send fibers to the red nucleus.

The fastigial nucleus is connected to the lateral vestibular nucleus and reticular formation.

Figures 15.18–15.21 The intracerebellar or deep nuclei.

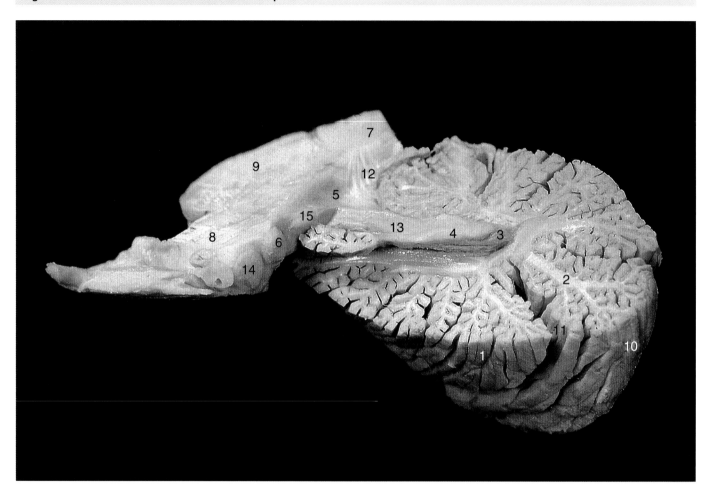

Fig. 15.18
Sagittally sectioned cerebellum and brainstem showing the dentate nucleus and superior cerebellar peduncle. ×1.6

1 Anterior lobe
2 Arbor vitae
3 Dentate nucleus
4 Fibers joining superior peduncle
5 Fourth ventricle
6 Inferior colliculus
7 Medulla oblongata
8 Midbrain
9 Pons
10 Posterior lobe
11 Primary fissure
12 Striae medullares
13 Superior cerebellar peduncle
14 Superior colliculus
15 Superior medullary velum

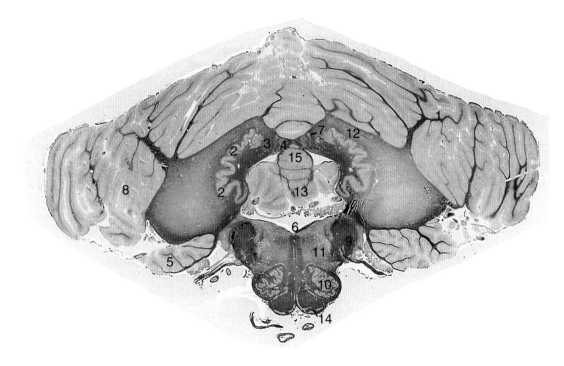

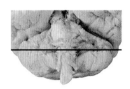

Fig. 15.19
Celloidin section through cerebellum and medulla oblongata showing the deep cerebellar nuclei. Weigert-Pal stain and celloidin-embedded section cut by Mr. P. A. Runnicles. ×1.4

1 Arbor vitae	**6** Fourth ventricle	**11** Medulla oblongata
2 Dentate nucleus	**7** Globose nucleus	**12** Medullary center
3 Emboliform nucleus	**8** Hemisphere	**13** Nodule
4 Fastigial nucleus	**9** Inferior cerebellar peduncle	**14** Pyramid of medulla
5 Flocculus	**10** Inferior olivary nucleus	**15** Uvula of vermis MHMS

Figures 15.20 and 15.21 High magnification views of the dentate nucleus. They share the following labels:

1 Cell bodies
2 Dentate nucleus
3 Folia
4 Hilus of dentate nucleus
5 Medullary center

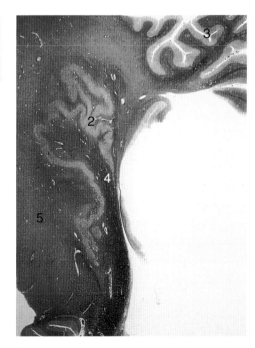

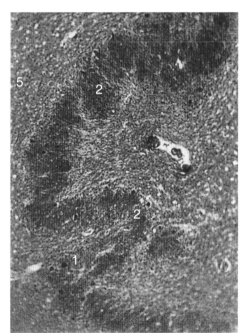

Fig. 15.20
Paraffin wax section of the dentate nucleus. Myelin stain and counterstain. ×2.8

MHMS

Fig. 15.21
Higher magnification of part of the dentate nucleus. Luxol fast blue and cresyl violet stain. ×65

CXWMS

Summary

1. The cerebellum lies dorsal to the brainstem and the fourth ventricle.

2. It consists of two hemispheres united by the vermis.

3. Its surface is covered by a cortex of gray matter deeply folded into folia.

4. The interior of the cerebellum is formed of white matter. It contains nerve fibers passing to and from the cerebellar cortex.

5. Deep inside the white matter lie the deep nuclei: the dentate, globose, fastigial and emboliform nuclei.

6. The cerebellum is connected to the brainstem by the superior, middle and inferior cerebellar peduncles, containing afferent and efferent connections between the cerebellum and other brain regions.

7. Afferent pathways to the cerebellum go to the cerebellar cortex and efferent pathways leave the cerebellum via the deep nuclei.

8. Sensory input to the cerebellum comes from all the general and special senses, and is utilized in the control of smooth coordinated movements.

9. Cerebellar function takes place at a subconscious level.

16 Spinal Cord

The spinal cord lies in the vertebral canal and is continuous with the medulla oblongata. Distally it tapers into the conus medullaris which in the adult ends at a variable level between the twelfth thoracic vertebra (T12) and the disk between the first and second lumbar vertebrae (L1–L2). Thirty-one pairs of spinal nerves arise from the cord and leave the vertebral column through the intervertebral foramina. Due to differential growth between the spinal cord and the vertebral column, the lower lumbar and sacral segments of the spinal cord lie opposite the lower thoracic and upper lumbar vertebrae in the adult. Their roots run obliquely downwards to the foramina. Those lying beyond the conus medullaris form a leash of nerves called the cauda equina or "horse's tail". Every nerve has an anterior or ventral (motor) and a posterior or dorsal (sensory) root, except that some individuals lack the dorsal root of the first cervical nerve (C1). The cord is surrounded and protected by all three layers of the meninges and by the cerebrospinal fluid, all of which are continuous with those around the brain. A longitudinal groove, the anterior (or ventral) median fissure, runs the entire length of the cord. Although there is no fissure posteriorly, a posterior (dorsal) median septum is seen in cross-section.

The spinal cord can be divided into cervical, thoracic, lumbar, sacral and coccygeal regions according to the parts of the body its nerves supply. Each of these can be further subdivided into segments, each giving rise to a pair of spinal nerves, i.e. eight cervical (C1–C8), twelve thoracic (T1–T12), five lumbar (L1–L5), five sacral (S1–S5) and one coccygeal. The gray matter of the cord is enlarged where the nerves of the brachial and lumbosacral plexuses arise; these swellings are called the cervical (C5–T1) and lumbar (L2–S3) enlargements.

In cross-section the spinal cord consists of an external layer of white matter and an inner core of gray matter, within which there is a minute central canal continuous with the fourth ventricle of the brain. The gray matter is shaped like a butterfly with the wings on each side being the anterior (ventral) and posterior (dorsal) horns. From T1 or T2 to L2 a lateral horn is discernible. The anterior horn is motor in function, the posterior horn is sensory and the lateral horn is sympathetic. Different levels of the cord can easily be distinguished in transverse sections because there is a preponderance of gray matter at lower (lumbar and sacral)

levels and of white matter at thoracic or cervical levels. Sections through the first cervical segment (C1) show a transitional arrangement between the spinal cord and the lower levels of the medulla oblongata.

The white matter is arranged around the gray matter into anterior, posterior and lateral white columns (or funiculi) and anterior and posterior white commissures. The columns contain nerve fibers grouped in tracts. Cell groupings within the gray matter may be described as nuclei or, in the dorsal horn, as layers, the laminae of Rexed. These have indistinct borders and much intermingling, and are difficult to demarcate in human material. The long ascending and descending tracts link the spinal cord with the brain. The fasciculi proprii are short tracts for local connections within the cord. The white commissures contain some fibers that remain on their own side and others that cross (decussate) from one side of the cord to the other.

Very simple nervous activity, for example the reflex arc, is possible in the spinal cord without involving the brain. More complex activity, voluntary movement and conscious sensations involve communication with the brain. Ascending tracts carry impulses up to the brain and are sensory in function. Descending tracts carry impulses down from the brain to the spinal cord and are motor.

Ascending tracts in the spinal cord are part of the ascending, sensory, nervous pathways that convey information about the general or somatic senses from the trunk and limbs to the brain. The somatic senses are touch, pain, temperature, itch, pressure and vibration, and proprioception, the sense of position. All are consciously perceived except for proprioception, which exists in two forms: unconscious from muscles, and conscious from joints and tendons. Pathways concerned with conscious sensations ultimately terminate in the primary sensory cortex, that is, the post-central gyrus, Brodmann's areas 1, 2 and 3. They do so on the opposite side to that on which the sensation is received by a peripheral sensory receptor, for example a nerve ending in the skin. This is because the ascending pathways concerned with these sensations decussate en route to the sensory cortex. They are also interrupted at one or more points along their course. A pathway consists of a chain of neurons and their processes linked together by synapses. The impulse passes from one neuron to the next along the course of the pathway, the successive neurons in the sequence being known as first-, second- and third-order neurons. The tracts in the spinal cord concerned with conscious sensations are the anterior spinothalamic tract, for crude, non-discriminating touch, the lateral spinothalamic tract for pain and temperature, and the fasciculus gracilis and fasciculus cuneatus, jointly known as the posterior columns, for fine touch, pressure, vibration and conscious proprioception. Unconscious proprioception is exceptional in that the tracts conveying this sensory information, the spinocerebellar tracts, terminate in the cerebellum, are predominantly uncrossed, and consist of only two neurons.

A number of structures in the brain are motor in function. These include the primary motor cortex (Brodmann's areas 4 and 6), the red nucleus, substantia nigra, corpus striatum, cerebellum, vestibular nuclei, inferior olivary nucleus, midbrain tectum and reticular formation. They give origin to descending tracts, which form motor pathways between some of the motor centers in the brain and the motor neurons in the anterior horn of the spinal cord. The former are known as upper motor neurons and the latter as lower motor neurons. Most motor pathways are therefore two-neuron chains. Lower motor neuron stimulation alone will cause a muscle to contract, but purposeful voluntary movements and the coordination of the actions of different muscles require the participation of upper motor neurons via the descending motor pathways. Like a sensory pathway, a motor pathway may decussate along its course and be interrupted by one or more synaptic relays. The major pathway for the control of voluntary movement of the trunk and limbs is the lateral corticospinal tract, which decussates in the brainstem, so bringing movements on each side of the body under the control of the opposite (contralateral) side of

the brain. It has a companion tract, the corticobulbar tract, which controls voluntary movement in the head through its connections with motor cranial nerve nuclei. Together they form the pyramidal tract. The name refers to its passage through the pyramid of the medulla oblongata during its descent. The remaining pathways do not pass through the medullary pyramid and are referred to as "extrapyramidal". They control postural and automatic movements of the neck, trunk and limbs.

The main ascending and descending tracts are summarized in the table below; for details see the appropriate chapters in the second section of the book.

- *The names of tracts indicate the origin and termination of the tract and the direction in which impulses flow, for example:* **spinocerebellar** – *from* **spinal** *cord to* **cerebellum** *(ascending);* **corticospinal** – *from motor* **cortex** *to* **spinal** *cord (descending).*

- *The most medially placed cells in the anterior horn supply axial muscles; more laterally placed cells supply the limbs.*

- *Due to intermingling of adjacent tracts, disease processes rarely affect one tract exclusively.*

- *Due to their different rates of embryonic development, vertebral level and spinal cord, segments do not coincide below cervical levels of the cord. This fact is important in assessing the effects of spinal injuries.*

- *The bladder is controlled by spinal cord segment S1, which lies opposite vertebrae T12 and L1. Spinal injuries at this level may paralyze the bladder.*

ASCENDING AND DESCENDING TRACTS

	ASCENDING TRACTS	DESCENDING TRACTS
ANTERIOR COLUMN	Anterior (ventral) spinothalamic	Anterior (ventral) corticospinal (pyramidal) Vestibulospinal Tectospinal Reticulospinal
LATERAL COLUMN	Spinocerebellar Lateral spinothalamic Spinotectal	Lateral corticospinal Rubrospinal Olivospinal
POSTERIOR COLUMN	Fasciculus gracilis Fasciculus cuneatus	Fasciculus interfascicularis Septomarginal fasciculus
DIFFUSE IN ANTERIOR AND LATERAL COLUMNS	Spinoreticular	

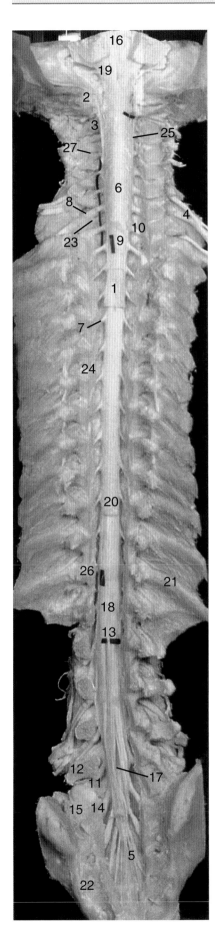

Fig. 16.1
A dissection of the adult spinal cord *in situ* to demonstrate its anatomy and relationships. ×0.3

1 Arachnoid mater	**15** First sacral vertebra (S1)
2 Atlas	**16** Fourth ventricle
3 Axis	**17** Lumbar cistern
4 Brachial plexus	**18** Lumbar enlargement
5 Cauda equina	**19** Medulla oblongata
6 Cervical enlargement	**20** Pia mater
7 Dorsal (posterior) root	**21** Ribs
8 Dorsal (posterior) root ganglion	**22** Sacrum
9 Dura mater	**23** Seventh cervical vertebra (C7)
10 Eighth cervical nerve root (C8)	**24** Sixth thoracic vertebra (T6)
11 Fifth lumbar nerve root (L5)	**25** Spinal root of accessory nerve
12 Fifth lumbar vertebra	**26** Twelfth thoracic vertebra (T12)
13 Filum terminale	**27** Ventral (anterior) root
14 First sacral nerve root (S1)	

OXF

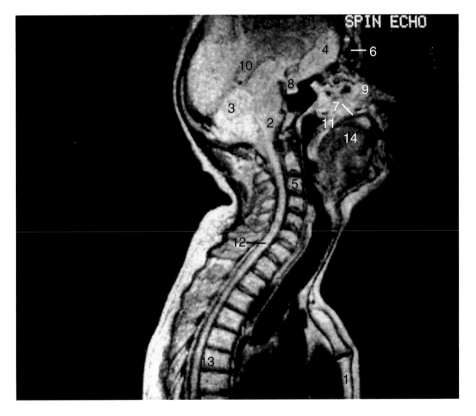

Fig. 16.2
An NMR image to illustrate the brain and spinal cord *in situ* and to demonstrate the pliability of the spinal cord.

1 Body of sternum	**8** Hypophysis
2 Brainstem	**9** Nose
3 Cerebellum	**10** Position of lateral ventricle
4 Cerebral hemisphere	**11** Soft palate
5 Cervical vertebrae	**12** Spinal cord
6 Frontal sinus	**13** Thoracic vertebrae
7 Hard palate	**14** Tongue

Elscint Ltd

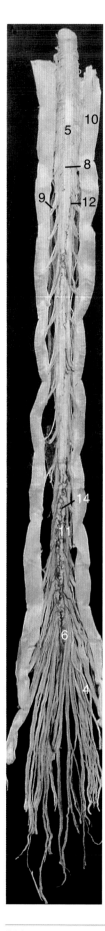

Fig. 16.3
Isolated spinal cord and meninges viewed from the dorsal (posterior) aspect. ×0.38

UN

Figures 16.3–16.7 Dissections and histological preparations to demonstrate the spinal cord in its meningeal coverings.

Spinal meninges differ from those around the brain in two important respects. First, the pia mater is more robust and sometimes is described as having two layers. There is a thick outer layer, the epi-pia, and a thin inner layer, the pia intima. Second, an epidural space containing fatty areolar tissue and a venous plexus lies between the dura mater and the bone of the vertebral canal. Figures 16.3–16.5 share the following labels:

1 Anterior (ventral) nerve roots
2 Anterior radicular artery
3 Anterior spinal artery
4 Cauda equina
5 Cervical enlargement
6 Conus medullaris
7 Denticulate ligament of the pia mater
8 Dorsal (posterior) columns
9 Dorsal (posterior) nerve roots
10 Dura and arachnoid mater, opened
11 Lumbar enlargement
12 Posterior spinal artery
13 Posterior radicular artery
14 Venous plexus

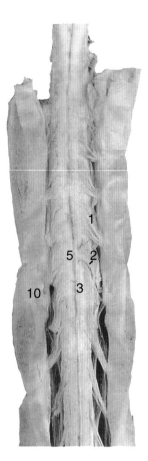

Fig. 16.4
The cervical enlargement viewed from the ventral (anterior) aspect. ×0.8

UN

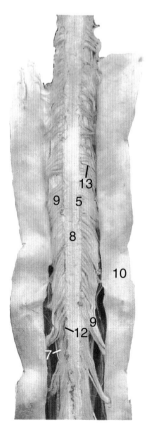

Fig. 16.5
The cervical enlargement viewed from the dorsal (posterior) aspect. ×0.78

UN

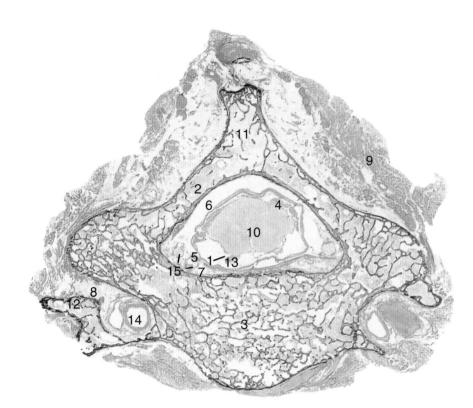

Fig. 16.6
Histological section through a cervical vertebra and the spinal cord *in situ*, to show the relationship between the spinal cord, bone and meninges. Block stained with silver nitrate, section stained with light green and Orange G. ×2

 1 Arachnoid and pia mater
 2 Arch or lamina of vertebra
 3 Body of vertebra
 4 Dorsal (posterior) nerve root
 5 Dura mater
 6 Epidural space
 7 Fat within epidural space
 8 Foramen transversarium
 9 Neck muscles
10 Spinal cord
11 Spine of vertebra
12 Transverse process
13 Ventral (anterior) nerve roots
14 Vertebral artery
15 Vessels in epidural space

Mr. D. Adams

Fig. 16.7
A section showing the structure of pia mater covering the spinal cord. Weigert-Pal stain. ×35

1 Arachnoid mater
2 Blood vessels
3 Dorsal (posterior) horn
4 Dorsal (posterior) nerve root
5 Dorsal (posterior) white columns
6 Gray matter
7 Lateral white column
8 Pia mater

CAM

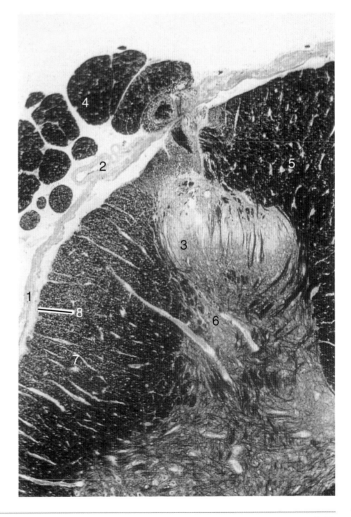

● *In spinal anesthesia, anesthetic solution may be introduced into either the epidural space or the subarachnoid space, where it mixes with the CSF.*

Figures 16.8–16.11 A sequence of paraffin wax sections showing regional variations in the arrangement of gray and white matter in the spinal cord. They share the following labels:

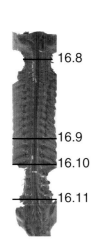

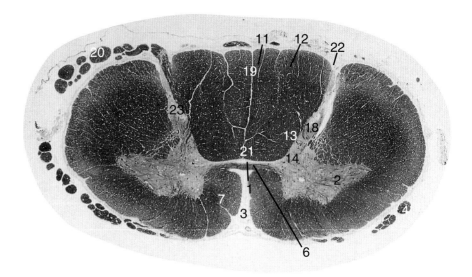

Fig. 16.8
Cervical region. Weigert stain. ×5.5

MHMS

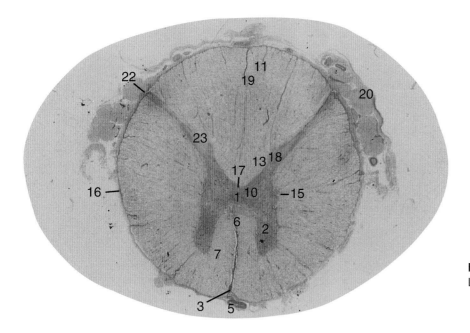

Fig. 16.9
Lower thoracic region. Van Gieson stain. ×12.5

Mr. D. Adams

 1 Anterior (ventral) gray commissure (part of Rexed's lamina X)
 2 Anterior (ventral) horn (Rexed's laminae VIII and IX)
 3 Anterior (ventral) median sulcus
 4 Anterior (ventral) nerve roots
 5 Anterior (ventral) spinal vessels
 6 Anterior (ventral) white commissure
 7 Anterior (ventral) white funiculus (or column)
 8 Cauda equina
 9 Central canal
10 Nucleus dorsalis; Clarke's nucleus (Rexed's lamina VI)
11 Fasciculus gracilis
12 Fasciculus cuneatus

13 Fasciculi proprii
14 Intermediate zone (Rexed's laminae VI and VII)
15 Lateral (intermediolateral) horn
16 Pia mater
17 Posterior (dorsal) gray commissure
18 Posterior (dorsal) horn (Rexed's laminae I to V)
19 Posterior median septum
20 Posterior (dorsal) nerve roots
21 Posterior (dorsal) white commissure
22 Posterolateral (dorsolateral) sulcus
23 Substantia gelatinosa (Rolandi) (Rexed's laminae II and III)

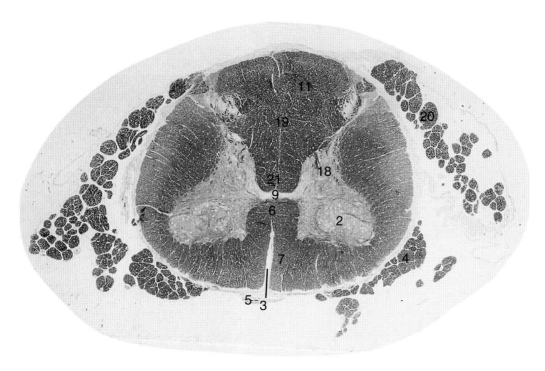

Fig. 16.10
Lumbar region. Weigert stain. ×7.9

MHMS

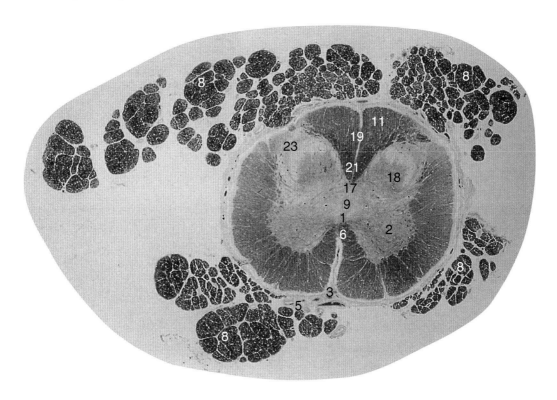

Fig. 16.11
Sacral region. Weigert stain. ×12.3

MHMS

● *Enkephalins and substance P are found in the substantia gelatinosa. Pain fibers in dorsal roots terminate there and throughout laminae I to III.*

Figures 16.12 and 16.13 Histological sections showing the cells and fibers of the spinal cord.

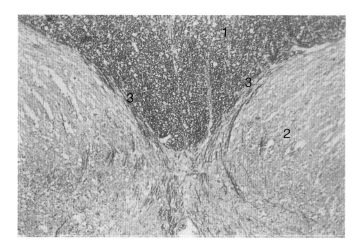

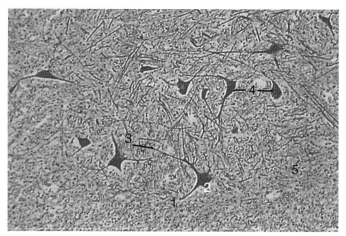

Fig. 16.12
A histological section showing fibers leaving the dorsal (posterior) horn to enter fasciculi proprii in the sacral spinal cord. Myelin stain. ×63

   1 Dorsal (posterior) column
   2 Dorsal (posterior) horn
   3 Fasciculi proprii

CAM

Fig. 16.13
Motor neurons in the anterior horn of the cervical spinal cord. Silver stain. ×100

   1 Axon
   2 Cell body
   3 Dendrite
   4 Motor neuron
   5 Neuropil

CAM

● *The large α motor neurons that supply skeletal muscle are cholinergic.*

● *If spinal cord disease or injury involves gray matter alone, it will affect sensory and/or motor functions only in the damaged segments. If white matter is damaged, ascending and descending tracts will be interrupted. The spinal cord, and the areas it supplies below the lesion, will be isolated. This can produce widespread sensory and motor impairment. Muscles innervated from spinal cord segments below the lesion may show hyperreflexia; spinal reflexes are exaggerated.*

Cauda Equina

The cauda equina (horse's tail) consists of the filum terminale, a pial and neuroglial strand, and the dorsal and ventral roots of the lumbar and sacral nerves. It lies in the lumbar cistern of the subarachnoid space.

● *Lumbar punctures below the level of L3–L4 will not encounter spinal cord. The needle passes between the spinal nerves, which are displaced. A sample of cerebrospinal fluid can be removed for analysis or solutions such as anesthetics introduced.*

Figures 16.14 and 16.15 Dissections showing the structure of the cauda equina.

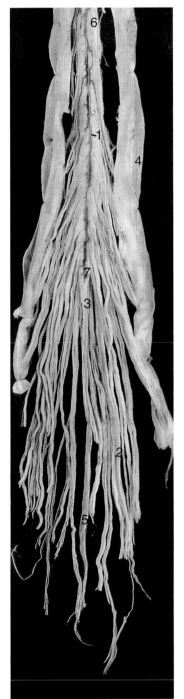

Fig. 16.14
The lumbar and sacral regions of the spinal cord and the cauda equina, in their meningeal coverings. The cauda equina has been spread to demonstrate individual nerve roots. The filum terminale has been severed in removing the spinal cord from the vertebral canal. ×0.72

   1 Anterior spinal artery
   2 Cauda equina
   3 Conus medullaris
   4 Dura and arachnoid mater
   5 Filum terminale
   6 Lumbar region of spinal cord
   7 Sacral region of spinal cord

UN

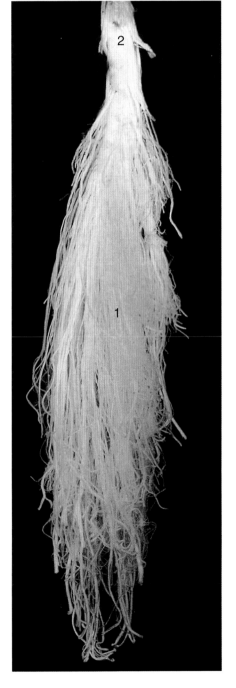

Fig. 16.15
An 18th century dissection of the cauda equina prepared by John Hunter, from the Hunterian Museum of the Royal College of Surgeons of England. ×0.75

   1 Frayed nerves of cauda equina
   2 Spinal cord

Fig. 16.16
MRI scan showing cauda equina *in situ*.

1 Abdominal cavity
2 Cauda equina
3 Ilium
4 Sacrum

● *Prolapse of an intervertebral disk may compress spinal nerve roots. This may cause pain in the dermatomes supplied by the affected nerves. Cervical and lumbar regions are particularly vulnerable because they are the most mobile parts of the spine.*

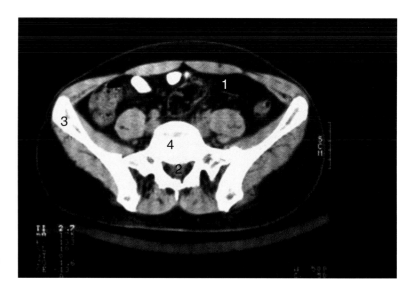

REGION OF SPINAL CORD	SEGMENTS OF SPINAL CORD	FUNCTIONS OF SEGMENTS		
CERVICAL	C1			Head/neck movements
	C2			
	C3		Breathing movements	
	C4			
	C5	Heart rate	Shoulder movements	
	C6			Wrist/elbow movements
	C7		Hand movements	
	C8			
THORACIC	T1			
	T2			
	T3			
	T4			
	T5			
	T6	Stability of the trunk		Sympathetic system
	T7			
	T8			
	T9			
	T10			
	T11		Ejaculation of semen	
	T12			
LUMBAR	L1			
	L2		Hip movements	
	L3		Extension of knee	
	L4		Movements of the foot	
	L5	Flexion of knee		
SACRAL	S1			
	S2		Hind gut/bladder control	Clitoral and penile erection
	S3			
	S4			
	S5			

This figure illustrates some of the most important body functions controlled by the spinal cord. Regions of the cord and individual segments within each region are given a common color code. The same color is used to indicate functions controlled by a segment or region. For example, the whole cervical region, and segments of the spinal cord C3 and C4, and "breathing movements" are all colored pale blue.

Sometimes activities are controlled by spinal cord segments in more than one region. For example, hand movements are controlled by C7, C8 and T1. Where this happens, the overlap in function is indicated on the chart by a wavy line between the regional colors, pale blue and dark blue.

Sometimes, a segment participates in more than one function. For example, L5 controls knee flexion and is also involved with L4 and S1 in foot movements. Where this occurs, the functions are displayed in adjacent columns. This is to emphasize the dual functional role of the segment while avoiding overlaps in the figure.

Summary

1. The spinal cord is continuous cranially with the medulla oblongata.
2. The spinal cord lies in the vertebral canal, extending from C1 to a variable level between T12 and L2.
3. The spinal cord can be divided into segments, each of which gives rise to a pair of spinal nerves.
4. A butterfly-shaped area of gray matter lies in the center of the spinal cord, where it forms dorsal horns which are sensory and ventral horns which are motor.
5. White matter lies externally in the spinal cord, where it contains tracts of nerve fibers linking the cord with the brain.
6. Ascending tracts are sensory; descending tracts are principally motor.
7. Disease or injury to the spinal cord may impair function locally (in affected segments only) or have more widespread effects due to interruption of ascending or descending tracts.

Section 2
FUNCTIONAL SYSTEMS OF THE CENTRAL NERVOUS SYSTEM

17 Reflex Arc

The nervous system is able to make involuntary motor responses to sensory stimuli which are either painful or potentially damaging. This type of response is termed a reflex and it is dependent upon the integrity of a nervous pathway known as a reflex arc. The simplest type of arc, termed a monosynaptic reflex arc, consists of a receptor organ, an afferent neuron, an efferent neuron and an effector organ. The sensory receptor organs are located in skin, mucous membranes, connective tissue or muscles. They are innervated by primary sensory neurons whose cell bodies lie in the dorsal (posterior) root ganglia. These cells are unipolar, but their axons divide into two processes, a central process connecting the cell to the spinal cord and a peripheral one connecting it to the receptor. The peripheral processes of the axons form the sensory (afferent) fibers in peripheral nerves and the central processes form the nerve roots. When the receptor is stimulated, an impulse travels along the two processes of the axon to the dorsal (posterior) horn of the spinal cord.

In a polysynaptic reflex arc, the afferent fibers entering the cord synapse with one or more internuncial neurons which act as intermediate or messenger neurons. These in turn synapse with motor (efferent) neurons. The axons of the motor neurons pass out through the ventral root and to the effector organ (muscle or gland). Fibers from the internuncial neurons may ascend or descend in the cord to stimulate motor neurons at different segmental levels of the spinal cord. They may also cross to the opposite side of the cord and stimulate motor neurons.

Although such reflex arcs are at the spinal cord level, they may be influenced by the brain via the olivospinal, rubrospinal, reticulospinal, corticospinal, tectospinal and vestibulospinal tracts. These are all motor pathways or descending tracts. The effect of these motor connections is to suppress the activity of many reflex arcs in the spinal cord. As a result, we do not respond to harmless or even useful stimuli. For example, we do not withdraw our feet when they make contact with the ground while walking. These reflexes, many of which are primitive defense responses, are present in babies before the descending tracts are mature. They may reappear in adults if the descending pathways are interrupted by injury or disease. An example of this release from inhibition is Babinski's sign. In a normal adult the toes flex when the sole of the foot is stimulated. In babies, or in adults with lesions of the corticospinal tract, the toes extend.

A "stretch reflex" is the contraction of a muscle in response to stretching. Sensory receptors in the muscle itself (muscle spindles) or its tendon (Golgi tendon organs) are stimulated. Many such reflexes are monosynaptic, that is, there is no interneuron between the sensory and motor nerves. This arrangement maximizes the speed of the response by minimizing delays in transmission of the impulse at synapses.

Testing of spinal reflexes is an important stage in any neurological examination. In disease, the intensity, duration or speed of stretch reflexes may change. An example of this is seen in spasticity. When stretch reflexes are tested in these patients, there is an abnormal increase of muscle tone, and sometimes rapid oscillating limb movements known as clonus, due to the loss of inhibitory influences coming from the brain through descending tracts.

Deep tendon reflexes are involuntary contractions made by a muscle in response to a sudden stretching of its tendon. They are elicited clinically by tapping the tendon with a reflex hammer. The sensory and motor connections necessary for these reflexes lie within one or two segments of the spinal cord, so it is possible to test for damage in the spinal cord by assessing appropriate reflexes. For example, the knee-jerk reflex is served by segments L3 and L4, the biceps jerk by C5 and C6, the ankle jerk by S1 and S2. If a segment of the cord is damaged, the reflexes it controls are absent.

As well as the spinal reflexes, there are also reflexes involving the brainstem, which are mediated by the cranial nerves. For example, in the corneal reflex, if the cornea is touched, the eyelids close to protect the eye. The sensory fibers for this reflex run in the ophthalmic division of the trigeminal nerve, but the orbicularis oculi muscle which shuts the eye receives its motor innervation from the facial nerve.

- *Reflex arcs in the spinal cord play an important role in maintaining muscle tone and posture.*

- *Flexor and extensor muscles of the same limb do not contract simultaneously in a reflex. There are connections between the afferent flexor nerve fibers which synapse with extensor motor neurons of the same limb and inhibit them. This effect is called the law of reciprocal innervation.*

- *In a normal individual, stimulation of one lower limb may result in extension of the contralateral limb. This response is known as the crossed extensor reflex. Its anatomical basis is the connection of incoming sensory fibers to contralateral motor neurons in the spinal cord, via internuncial neurons whose axons cross the midline.*

- *The muscle spindles which act as stretch receptors in striated muscles are modified muscle fibers. They have their own motor innervation by γ-motor neurons in the ventral horn of the spinal cord. This nerve supply sets the sensitivity level of the muscle spindle by regulating the tension of the modified muscle fibers.*

A diagram of the reflex arc

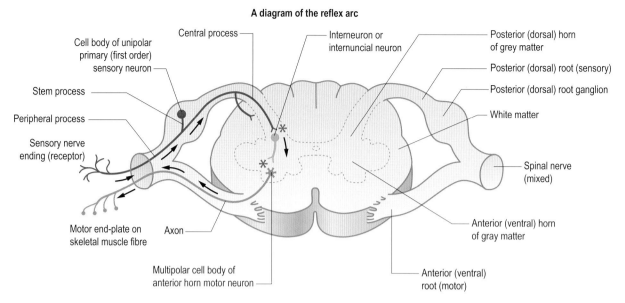

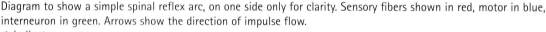

Cell body of unipolar primary (first order) sensory neuron

Central process

Interneuron or internuncial neuron

Posterior (dorsal) horn of grey matter

Posterior (dorsal) root (sensory)

Posterior (dorsal) root ganglion

Stem process

White matter

Peripheral process

Sensory nerve ending (receptor)

Spinal nerve (mixed)

Motor end-plate on skeletal muscle fibre

Axon

Anterior (ventral) horn of gray matter

Multipolar cell body of anterior horn motor neuron

Anterior (ventral) root (motor)

Diagram to show a simple spinal reflex arc, on one side only for clarity. Sensory fibers shown in red, motor in blue, interneuron in green. Arrows show the direction of impulse flow.
✳ Indicates synapses.

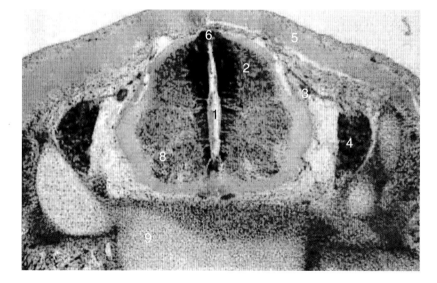

Fig. 17.1
A transverse paraffin wax section of the spinal cord and vertebral canal of a 25-mm CR embryo to show the components of a reflex arc. Hematoxylin and eosin stain. ×60
1 Central canal
2 Dorsal horn (gray matter)
3 Dorsal root
4 Dorsal root ganglion
5 Skin
6 Spinal cord
7 Spinal nerve (position of)
8 Ventral horn (gray matter)
9 Vertebral body

Summary

1. The reflex arc represents the simplest form of organization and activity in the central nervous system.
2. Reflexes are involuntary movements made in response to sensory stimuli.
3. Reflexes are important in the subconscious control of movement and posture, and in the avoidance of potentially damaging stimuli.
4. In a stretch reflex, a muscle contracts in response to stretching of the muscle itself or its tendon.
5. A number of tendon reflexes can be tested clinically. They provide information about the function of segments of the spinal cord and of motor control systems in the brain.

18 Somatic Sensory Pathways

Sensory pathways convey information from a peripheral sensory receptor via lower sensory centers to higher sensory centers in the brain. The pathways for the somatic senses (touch, pain, temperature, and proprioception or position sense) are known as ascending tracts because information is transmitted in an ascending direction from the spinal cord or brainstem to the cerebral cortex, via the thalamus.

Conversely, a motor pathway conveys information from higher centers to muscles or glands. Because of the direction in which information passes, the motor pathways are also known as descending tracts. The descriptions of the ascending and descending tracts reflect the direction of these pathways.

The somatic or general senses comprise the categories (modalities) of touch, pain, temperature, pressure, vibration and proprioception. All are consciously perceived. In addition, there is a subconscious form of proprioception, known as "unconscious proprioception". The senses of vision, hearing, balance, taste and smell are the special senses, described elsewhere, (see pp. 241–284).

Sensory receptors for touch, pressure, vibration and temperature are present in the skin. Receptors for proprioception, the sense of position, lie in muscles, tendons and joints. Pain receptors are widely distributed throughout the body.

The surface of the trunk and limbs can be imagined as being divided into a series of strips. Each strip or dermatome contains sensory receptors that transmit information predominantly to one segment of the spinal cord along the segmental spinal nerve. There is some overlap in the distribution of sensory nerves along the borders of adjacent dermatomes, so that interruption of a single spinal nerve root may cause relatively little sensory impairment.

From the spinal cord the sensory information is conveyed to the brain by ascending sensory pathways, each associated with one or more sensory modalities. Although each tract is fairly specifically associated with its modality, for example touch, there is some intermingling of adjacent tracts at their boundaries and a limited overlap in their functions. Hence, if a tract is interrupted by injury or disease or surgically transected, the sensory information that it carries may not be entirely lost to the patient.

The sensory pathways each consist of a chain of neurons, connected by synapses. Impulses pass from neuron to neuron along the pathway. Neurons are designated first order, second order, etc., according to their position in the chain. For all the senses that reach consciousness, the chain consists of three neurons and terminates in the parietal lobe of the cerebral hemisphere.

Proprioception from muscles that does not reach consciousness, does not conform to this pattern. It goes to the cerebellum and the pathway contains only two neurons. First-order neurons are also referred to as primary sensory neurons. The passage of the impulse across a synapse from one neuron to the next constitutes a synaptic relay. Sensory receptors in the head are innervated by cranial nerves, primarily the trigeminal (V) nerve, but also the facial (VII), glossopharyngeal (IX) and vagus (X) nerves. Ascending tracts from the brainstem accompany those from the spinal cord.

Sensory pathways for conscious sensations are crossed so that sensory information reaches the cerebral hemisphere contralateral to the stimulus. The pathway for unconscious proprioception is uncrossed. Pathways for conscious sensations terminate in the primary sensory cortex, that is, the postcentral gyrus of the parietal lobe, Brodmann's areas 1, 2 and 3. Pathways for unconscious proprioception terminate in the cerebellum.

The cortex of both the postcentral gyrus and the proprioceptive areas of the cerebellum is organized somatotopically, with particular areas of the cortex receiving sensory information from particular areas of the body. In the cerebral cortex the input of sensory information can be visualized as a body image, or homunculus, superimposed on the postcentral gyrus. Body parts with a particularly rich sensory innervation, such as the face and hand, have the largest representation in the cortex, so that they are disproportionately large in the homunculus. Further processing and interpretation of conscious sensory information received in the primary sensory cortex is the function of adjacent somatic sensory association cortex, Brodmann's areas 5 and 7.

- *While there are some diseases that specifically affect one particular tract, some conditions such as infarcts or tumors may damage a wide area of spinal cord or brain tissue containing several tracts and so produce a complex mixture of motor and sensory symptoms.*

- *Damage to sensory pathways may cause loss of sensation (anesthesia), abnormal sensations such as tingling (paresthesia) or increased perception of sensations (hyperesthesia).*

- *The poliomyelitis virus may damage the anterior horn cells in the gray matter of the spinal cord, causing paralysis of muscles. Ascending and descending tracts are not affected.*

- *Vitamin B12 deficiency, which can occur on a vegan diet, causes degeneration of ascending and descending tracts in the spinal cord. The patient's symptoms will depend on which tracts are involved.*

Pain and temperature

Receptors

Cutaneous pain and temperature receptors are free nerve endings in the dermis and epidermis. They also exist in mucous membranes, for example in the oral mucosa and in the cornea, and in the walls of hollow viscera, for example the digestive tract, where they are stimulated by over-distension. The free nerve endings are the terminal branches of the axons of the first-order neurons.

The pathway from the trunk and limbs: the lateral spinothalamic tract

This tract has two components. It is mainly a fast-conducting tract which carries sharp pain sensations such as those felt immediately after an injury. It also contains slow-conducting nerve fibers which carry the sensations of dull aching pain.

The first-order neurons for both pathways lie in the dorsal root ganglia of the spinal nerves. When the receptor is stimulated, sensory information passes along the axon of the first-order neuron into the dorsal horn of the spinal cord. There the axon synapses with a second-order neuron. From this point the fast and slow pathways are separate. For the fast pathway, the second-order neurons' axons cross the midline and ascend in the lateral spinothalamic tract on the opposite side of the body and synapse in the ventral posterolateral nucleus of the thalamus with the third-order neurons. The axons of the third-order neurons pass via the internal capsule to the postcentral gyrus. The course of the slow conducting pathway is similar, except that the third-order neurons lie in the reticular and intralaminar nuclei of the thalamus.

Referred pain is the perception of pain from internal organs (visceral pain) as if it were coming from the outside of the body (somatic pain). For example, pain from the heart may be felt in the chest wall and upper limb, pain from an inflamed appendix is first felt around the umbilicus. First-order neurons' axons from pain receptors in viscera and in superficial structures enter the spinal cord and converge onto the same second-order neurons, whose axons form the spinothalamic tract. From this point onwards somatic and visceral pain are processed together, so that when the sensation reaches consciousness at cortical level the brain cannot distinguish between them. The visceral pain is falsely perceived as superficial.

Some conscious awareness of pain appears to be present at subcortical levels in the pathway, probably in the thalamus. People with severe damage to the somatic sensory cortex can still feel pain, though it is vague and poorly localized.

The primary sensory neurons also have branches that ascend or descend one segment of the cord in the dorsolateral fasciculus (column or tract) of Lissauer before entering the dorsal horn and synapsing with the second-order neurons. Consequently, the tract carrying sensory information to the brain from a particular dermatome may arise one segment above or below the segment actually corresponding to that dermatome. Lesions of the spinal cord may, therefore, abolish sensations from dermatomes below those supplied by the injured segments.

Some axons from Lissauer's tract enter the substantia gelatinosa of the spinal cord and there may be additional synaptic relays in the substantia gelatinosa. This arrangement enables the substantia gelatinosa to act as a "gate" or "filter" regulating the entry of impulses into the spinothalamic tract, thus controlling transmission of painful sensations to consciousness. A second pain control mechanism exists in the periaqueductal gray matter of the midbrain. This system consists of spinomesencephalic fibers which initially accompany the spinothalamic tract, but terminate in the periaqueductal gray matter. Its neurons contain two peptide neurotransmitters, called enkephalins, which are natural analgesics, or endorphins, similar in their actions to morphine. Connections descend from the periaqueductal gray matter to the posterior horn, some synapsing en route in the raphe nuclei of the reticular formation (see Brainstem, p. 165).

The pain control pathways are activated in circumstances of pain and stress, for example on the battlefield or in a serious accident. There are well-documented cases of severely injured people in such situations showing little distress at the time of the injury.

- *"Pain", as defined by The International Association for the Study of Pain, is "an unpleasant sensory and emotional experience associated with actual or potential tissue damage".*

- *"Itch" is conveyed with "pain" by the lateral spinothalamic tract, but the pathway is largely uncrossed.*

- *One cause of pain from phantom limbs following amputation is that nerve axons in the stump are squeezed by scar tissue. The stimulus is perceived by the sensory cortex as not from the stump, but from the missing area of limb. In some patients, areas of cortex deprived of sensory information by the loss of a limb are taken over by surrounding territories. For example, if the hand is lost, the "face" area can spread into the former "hand" area of the cortex.*

- *If pain becomes intractable it may, very rarely, be necessary to obtain relief by cordotomy, an operation in which the lateral spinothalamic tract is cut on the contralateral side to the source of the pain. Due to spinal overlap, the surgeon will cut the cord at a segmental level one or two segments higher than the relevant sensory input.*

- *In syringomyelia, the central canal of the spinal cord expands to create a wide cavity. This expansion causes damage by compressing the decussating lateral spinothalamic fibers in the anterior white commissure of the spinal cord. Pain and temperature sensations from regions of the body supplied by the affected cord segments are abolished.*

The pathway from the head

Sensory receptors for pain and temperature from the face and the top of the head are free nerve endings of fibers in all three divisions of the trigeminal (V) nerve. The facial (VII) nerve carries some pain and temperature fibers from the external ear. The glossopharyngeal (IX) and vagus (X) nerves supply the mucosa of the back of the tongue, pharynx, larynx, auditory tube and middle ear. The scalp behind the vertex of the skull is supplied by cervical spinal nerves. The cranial dura mater has a plentiful supply of pain-sensitive nerve endings supplied by the trigeminal nerve, the vagus nerve and the upper cervical nerves.

The cell bodies of the first-order trigeminal sensory neurons are located in the semilunar or Gasserian ganglion of the trigeminal nerve. The first-order neurons for the facial, glossopharyngeal and vagus nerves lie in the sensory ganglia of those nerves. The ganglia are, therefore, homologous to the dorsal root ganglia of spinal nerves. The central processes of the axons of the first-order neurons descend through the brainstem in the spinal trigeminal tract to the spinal trigeminal nucleus where they synapse with the second-order neurons. The axons of the second-order neurons decussate to the contralateral side and ascend in the ventral trigeminal tract to synapse in the ventral posteromedial nucleus of the thalamus with the third-order neurons. The ventral trigeminal tract or ventral secondary ascending tract of V is analogous to the lateral spinothalamic tract. The axons of the third-order neurons pass through the internal capsule to the postcentral gyrus (Brodmann's areas 1, 2, 3). The pain and temperature pathways from the head are less well understood than the lateral spinothalamic tract from the body. There is some evidence that the ventral trigeminal tract is responsible for the fast transmission of sharp pain sensations and that it is accompanied by a slow-conducting pathway for dull pain, via the reticular formation.

The entry of nerve fibers into the spinal tract and nucleus of the trigeminal nerve is highly organized. It can be described in terms of an imaginary picture of the head being projected onto the nucleus like a slide on a screen. This is called a somatotopic organization and is common in sensory systems. If the nucleus is envisaged as a fingerlike object lying parallel to the neuraxis, then sensations from successive strips of tissue in the head are fed into successive slices of the nucleus. This is called the "onion-skin" concept. It is useful in the diagnosis of lesions in the spinal nucleus or tract. Some functional subdivision also exists in the spinal nucleus. The pars oralis is mainly tactile, though it receives some pain and temperature sensations from the oral cavity and teeth. The pars interpolaris receives touch and some proprioception, and the pars caudalis is principally concerned with pain and temperature from all three divisions of the trigeminal nerve. In addition, in a transverse section of that part of the nucleus connected to the trigeminal nerve itself, three tiers of cells are associated with the ophthalmic, maxillary and mandibular divisions of the nerve, respectively. The distribution of the three divisions on the face can be mapped as three areas, analogous to the dermatomes supplied by spinal nerves. This pattern is used in the interpretation of lesions of the trigeminal nerve itself or its ganglion.

● *Trigeminal neuralgia is a condition in which there is intense pain, of short duration, in the area of distribution of one division of the trigeminal nerve on the face. Between the painful episodes, there are no sensory abnormalities. Its cause is largely unknown. It can sometimes be triggered by other sensory stimuli, such as light touch or cold in the affected area. Many patients can be treated successfully with medication, but surgical treatment may be necessary. Relieving pressure on the trigeminal nerve from branches of the cerebellar arteries running near the nerve can sometimes abolish the pain.*

A diagram demonstrating the sensory input into the spinal tract and nucleus of the trigeminal nerve. *Left:* Onion-skin concept of the longitudinal organization of the nucleus. *Right:* Relationship between a cross-section of the tract and nucleus and the peripheral distribution of the trigeminal nerve.

The colors indicate areas of the face linked to their area of sensory input in the spinal trigeminal nucleus and tract.

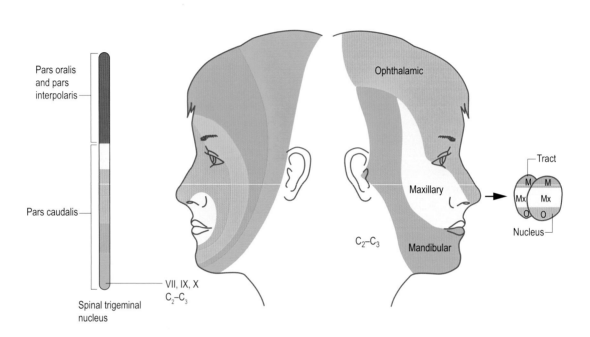

● *In addition to its extensive sensory input, the spinal nucleus of the trigeminal nerve receives some descending connections from the primary sensory and motor cortex of the cerebral hemisphere. The function of these pathways is uncertain, but may be related to modification of sensory processing in the nucleus by the cortex.*

A diagram of the lateral spinothalamic (red) and ventral trigeminothalamic (green) pathways conveying pain and temperature information from the body and head, respectively. Each is shown on one side only for clarity. Fibers from pain and temperature receptors in the head enter in all three divisions of the trigeminal nerve but for clarity only one is drawn.

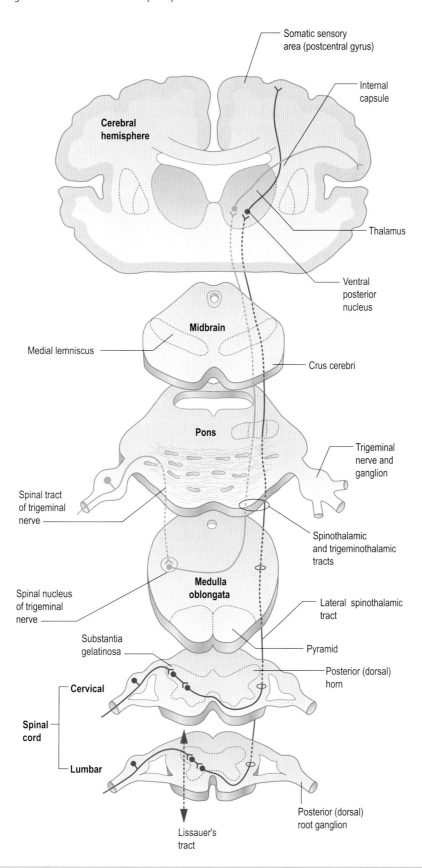

Simple (light or crude) touch and pressure

Receptors

The cutaneous receptors for light touch are varied. They include free nerve endings, nerve endings associated with hair follicles, and nerve endings associated with specialized epidermal cells, the Merkel disks. The pressure receptors are complex structures, the Pacinian corpuscles, in which the nerve endings are enclosed in a multilayered capsule. They are deeply situated in the dermis, and are also found in periosteum, around joints and in mesenteries.

The pathway from the trunk and limbs: the anterior (ventral) spinothalamic tract

Cutaneous receptors for crude touch and pressure are located in the dermal layer of skin. They are innervated by the primary sensory neurons (first-order neurons) which lie in the dorsal root ganglia. When the receptor is stimulated, sensory information passes along the axon of the primary sensory neuron to the dorsal white column where the axons bifurcate. One branch enters the dorsal horn gray matter at the same level while the second branch ascends in the dorsal column ipsilaterally for as many as ten spinal segments. Both branches synapse with second-order neurons in the dorsal horn gray matter. Axons from the second-order neurons decussate and enter the ventral white column where they ascend as the ventral spinothalamic tract. Passing through the brainstem, these axons form part of the spinal lemniscus. This tract ascends to the ventral posterolateral nucleus of the thalamus. Here the neurons synapse with third-order neurons whose axons pass via the internal capsule to the postcentral gyrus (Brodmann's areas 1, 2, 3).

The pathway from the head

The primary (first-order) sensory neurons are situated in the semilunar ganglion of the trigeminal (V) nerve with a few in the geniculate ganglion of the facial nerve (VII) and the superior ganglion of the glossopharyngeal (IX) and vagus (X) nerves (see Pain and temperature, p. 224).

When a receptor supplied by the trigeminal (V) nerve is stimulated, impulses flow along the axon of the primary sensory neuron in the nerve. After the axon traverses the semilunar ganglion, it enters the pons and may synapse with second-order neurons in either the spinal or the principal (chief) sensory nucleus of the trigeminal nerve. The axons of second-order neurons travel as either the crossed (ventral) trigeminothalamic tract or the uncrossed (dorsal) trigeminothalamic tract to synapse in the ventral posteromedial nucleus of the thalamus with the third-order neurons. There is a somatotopic and functional grouping of the third-order neurons. Those processing touch and other somatic sensory information from the mouth lie adjacent to the thalamic neurons of the taste pathway. Axons of the third-order neurons pass through the internal capsule to the primary sensory cortex of the postcentral gyrus.

Fibers in the facial, glossopharyngeal and vagus nerves synapse with second-order neurons in the spinal trigeminal nucleus only, having no input into the principal nucleus. From the spinal nucleus onward, the pathway continues alongside the second-order neurons of the trigeminal pathways.

● *Simple touch is tested clinically by asking the patient to close their eyes, then gently stroking the skin with a piece of cotton and asking the person if they can feel it.*

Fine touch, vibration and conscious proprioception

Receptors

Proprioception is the sense of position or movement. Conscious proprioception is associated with ligaments and joints. The sensory receptors are: free nerve endings, Pacinian corpuscles, which respond to pressure, and Ruffini endings, which respond to stretch.

Fine or discriminating touch is a precise form of touch sensitivity mainly associated with the hands, especially the fingers. The sensory receptors are encapsulated nerve endings known as Meissner's corpuscles which lie in the dermis immediately deep to the epidermis.

The sensors for vibration are the Pacinian corpuscles. These are numerous in the hand. Vibration is not a specific sensory modality but a tactile sense that is discontinuous and rapid.

All three sensations are carried by the same pathway from the trunk and limbs, but travel separately from the head.

● *Fine touch may be assessed clinically by asking the patient to close their eyes and identify objects (e.g. a key) placed in their hand using touch only. Astereognosis is the loss of ability to do so when fine touch pathways are impaired.*

● *Two-point discrimination is the ability to distinguish between two sharp points placed on the skin close together. It is a measure of the level of discriminating touch perception in an area of skin. It is best developed where Meissner's corpuscles are most numerous.*

The pathway from the trunk and limbs: the dorsal (posterior) columns and medial lemniscus

The receptors are innervated by the primary sensory neurons (first-order neurons) which lie in the dorsal root ganglion. When the receptor is stimulated, sensory information passes along the axon of the primary sensory neuron into the ipsilateral dorsal white column where it ascends to the medulla oblongata. Axons from the cervical and upper thoracic levels enter the lateral part of the dorsal column and ascend there as the fasciculus cuneatus whilst axons from the lower thoracic, lumbar and sacral levels enter the medial part of the dorsal column and ascend there as the fasciculus gracilis.

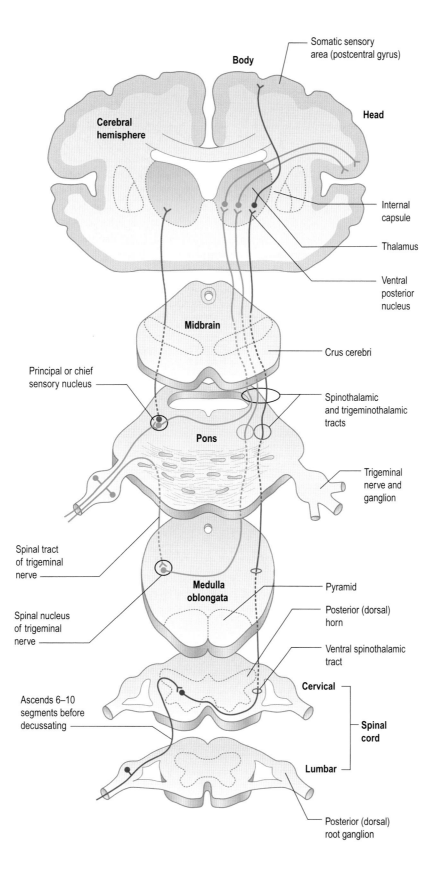

A diagram of the pathways for simple touch and pressure. Pathways conveying simple, light or crude touch and pressure sensations from the body (red) and head (green). The pathways are shown on one side only for clarity. Fibers from touch receptors in the head travel in all three divisions of the trigeminal nerve, but for clarity only one is shown. Uncrossed fibers from the head are shown in blue.

Each fasciculus ascends to its own nucleus in the medulla. Here, the first-order neuron synapses with a second-order neuron whose axon crosses the midline in the sensory decussation and ascends in the contralateral medial lemniscus to the ventral posterolateral nucleus of the thalamus. At this site the second-order neuron synapses with third-order neurons whose axon passes through the internal capsule to the primary sensory cortex, i.e. the postcentral gyrus of the parietal lobe, Brodmann's areas 1, 2 and 3.

The pathways from the head
As already explained, the pathways from the head differ for the sensory modalities.

i) Fine touch and vibration
The face is well supplied with fine touch receptors especially around the lips. When they are stimulated impulses flow in the trigeminal nerve. The first-order neurons lie in the semilunar ganglion. These cells synapse with second-order neurons in the principal or chief sensory nucleus in the pons. The axons of the second-order neurons run in either the ventral (crossed) or dorsal (uncrossed) trigeminothalamic tract to the ventral posteromedial nucleus of the thalamus where they synapse with the third-order neurons. Third-order neuron axons pass via the internal capsule to the postcentral gyrus. The existence of both crossed and uncrossed pathways for crude and fine touch provides for awareness of touch from each side of the head in both cerebral hemispheres.

ii) Conscious proprioception
Proprioceptive axons in the mandibular division of the trigeminal (V) nerve supply the capsule of the temporomandibular joint (TMJ), as well as facial and extra-ocular muscles and the muscles of mastication. The first-order neurons have their cell bodies located in the mesencephalic nucleus of the midbrain. This is an exception to the pattern of first-order sensory neurons being in a ganglion outside the central nervous system. The fibers of the first-order neurons enter the pons in the sensory and motor roots of the trigeminal nerve. In the brainstem they form the mesencephalic tract of the trigeminal (V) nerve. The destination of the central processes is poorly understood, but they are believed to have connections to the contralateral thalamus and to the cerebellum (see below, Unconscious proprioception).

Unconscious proprioception

Receptors
The sensory receptors for unconscious proprioception, the subconscious form of proprioception, are the muscle spindles of skeletal muscles and Golgi tendon organs in tendons.

The pathway from the trunk and limbs: the anterior and posterior spinocerebellar tracts and the cuneocerebellar tracts
The muscle spindles and Golgi tendon organs are innervated by the terminal branches of axons from the first-order neurons in the dorsal root ganglia. Sensory information reaches the cerebellum through three pathways.

i) The anterior (ventral) spinocerebellar tract
This tract transmits unconscious proprioceptive information from the lower limbs and the lower part of the trunk. Axons of the first-order neurons synapse with the second-order neurons in the intermediate zone of the spinal gray matter. These cells also receive afferent fibers from the internuncial neurons of spinal reflexes. Second-order neurons' processes ascend in the lateral funiculus of the spinal cord to the brainstem, where they enter the cerebellum via its superior peduncle and terminate in the vermis. Some fibers in this tract decussate in the spinal cord before ascending.

- If the semilunar ganglion is damaged, all facial sensations on the same side will be lost.

- If one side of the sensory cortex is damaged, pressure and touch on the same side of the face will be unaffected. However, pain and temperature sensations will be lost on the contralateral side.

- Infection of the central nervous system by syphilis may damage the dorsal columns. If the fasciculus cuneatus is affected, conscious proprioception and fine touch from the upper limbs are lost, causing loss of dexterity and astereognosis in the hands.

ii) The posterior (dorsal) spinocerebellar tract
Unconscious proprioception from the lower limb, trunk and upper limb is carried to the ipsilateral side of the cerebellar vermis. First-order neurons enter the spinal cord and synapse with the second-order neurons in Clarke's nucleus, which extends from segment C8 to L3 of the spinal gray matter. Second-order neurons' axons from Clarke's nucleus ascend in the lateral funiculus of the spinal cord to the brainstem, then enter the cerebellum through the inferior peduncle. Some of the cells in Clarke's nucleus are among the largest in the spinal cord, with cell body diameters of up to 50 μm, and axons up to 20 μm thick.

iii) The cuneocerebellar tract
Axons of first-order neurons innervating proprioceptors in the neck and upper limb ascend from segments above C8 in the spinal cord with the fasciculus cuneatus. The second-order neurons lie in the nucleus cuneatus. Their axons enter the cerebellum via the inferior cerebellar peduncle, ipsilaterally.

A diagram of the pathways for fine touch and conscious proprioception. Fine touch from the lumbar and lower thoracic regions (red), the upper thoracic and cervical regions (yellow) and the head (green). With the exception of the head, conscious proprioception is carried by the same pathways. Proprioception from the head (gray), both conscious and unconscious, is also shown. Proprioceptive information from the head is carried only in the mandibular division of the trigeminal (V) nerve, while touch receptors in the head contribute to all three divisions. For clarity, only one is drawn.

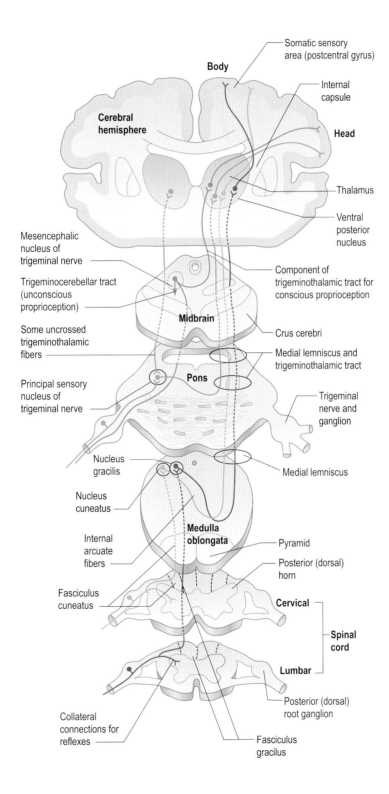

● *Sensory ataxia is uncoordinated movement caused by the loss of conscious proprioception. It is exaggerated when the eyes are closed, causing the patient to overbalance (Romberg's sign).*

The pathway from the head

The pathway for unconscious proprioception from the head follows that for conscious proprioception (see above) to the mesencephalic tract of the trigeminal (V) nerve. Fibers then pass to the cerebellum.

Other sensory tracts

Several other ascending spinal pathways are recognized. These include the spino-reticular, spino-cortical, spino-pontine, spino-vestibular and spino-olivary tracts.

A diagram illustrating the pathways for unconscious proprioception. The anterior (ventral) spinocerebellar tract is shown in red, and the posterior (dorsal) in green. Each is shown on one side only for clarity. Note that because the anterior spinocerebellar tract decussates twice, both tracts project to the ipsilateral side of the cerebellum.

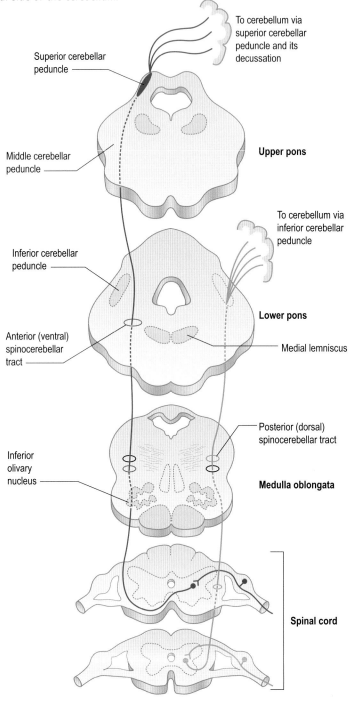

To cerebellum via superior cerebellar peduncle and its decussation

Superior cerebellar peduncle

Upper pons

Middle cerebellar peduncle

To cerebellum via inferior cerebellar peduncle

Inferior cerebellar peduncle

Lower pons

Anterior (ventral) spinocerebellar tract

Medial lemniscus

Posterior (dorsal) spinocerebellar tract

Inferior olivary nucleus

Medulla oblongata

Spinal cord

- *Friederich's ataxia is a degenerative disease affecting the spinocerebellar pathways causing uncoordination of movement and tremor. It first appears in childhood and can lead to severe disability by the early twenties.*

- *The reader is referred to page 195 for further detail on the cerebellum and its connections, and to pages 189–190 for detail of the sensory nuclei of the trigeminal nerve.*

Figures 18.1–18.12 A series of specimens showing the course of the ascending tracts from the spinal cord to the primary sensory cortex.

Fig. 18.1

A transverse section through the upper thoracic levels of the spinal cord to show the position of the ascending tracts. Myelin stain. ×8.3

 1 Central canal
 2 Dorsal (posterior) horn of gray matter
 3 Dorsal (posterior) spinocerebellar tract
 4 Dorsolateral fasciculus (Lissauer's tract)
 5 Dorsolateral sulcus
 6 Fasciculus cuneatus
 7 Fasciculus gracilis
 8 Fasciculi proprii
 9 Lateral horn of gray matter
10 Lateral spinothalamic tract
11 Ventral (anterior) horn of gray matter
12 Ventral (anterior) spinocerebellar tract
13 Ventral (anterior) spinothalamic tract

OXF

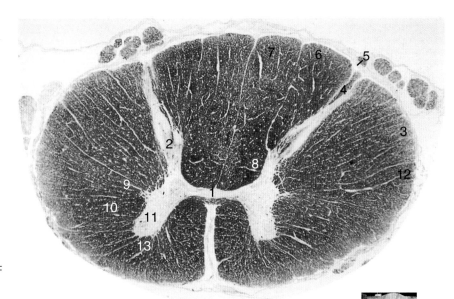

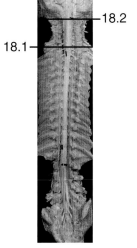

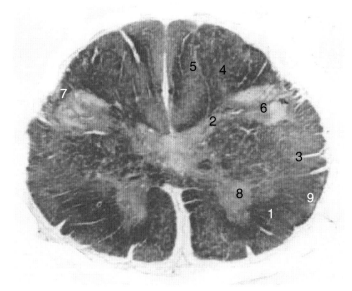

Fig. 18.2

A transverse section through the first cervical segment (C1) of the spinal cord showing the position of the ascending tracts. Solochrome cyanin stain. ×10

1 Anterolateral system (spinothalamic and spinotectal tracts)
2 Dorsal (posterior) horn
3 Dorsal (posterior) spinocerebellar tract
4 Fasciculus cuneatus
5 Fasciculus gracilis
6 Spinal nucleus of trigeminal nerve
7 Spinal tract of trigeminal nerve
8 Ventral (anterior) horn
9 Ventral (anterior) spinocerebellar tract

Dr. A. Fletcher LRI

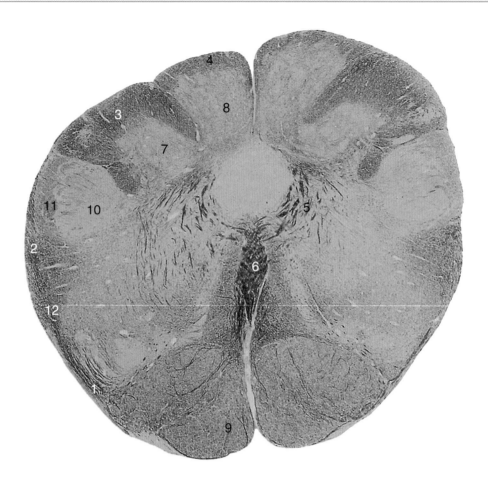

Fig. 18.3
Transverse section through the caudal end of the medulla oblongata showing the internal arcuate fibers passing from the nucleus gracilis and nucleus cuneatus into the medial lemniscus. Weigert stain. ×8.8

1 Anterolateral system (spinothalamic and spinotectal tract)
2 Dorsal (posterior) spinocerebellar tract
3 Fasciculus cuneatus
4 Fasciculus gracilis

5 Internal arcuate fibers
6 Medial lemniscus and its decussation
7 Nucleus cuneatus
8 Nucleus gracilis

9 Pyramid of medulla oblongata
10 Spinal nucleus of trigeminal nerve
11 Spinal tract of trigeminal nerve
12 Ventral (anterior) spinocerebellar tract

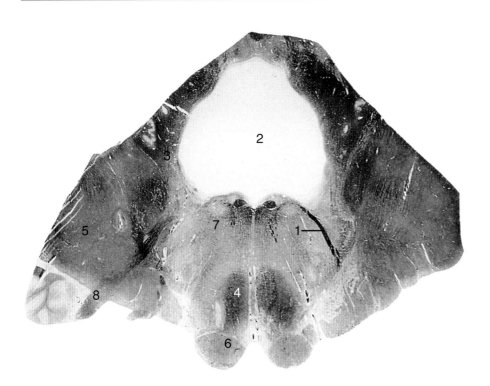

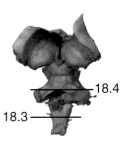

Fig. 18.4
Transverse section through the junction between the medulla oblongata and the pons showing the midline position and vertical orientation of the medial lemniscus. Weigert stain. ×3.4

1 Facial nerve (VII)	**4** Medial lemniscus	**7** Reticular formation
2 Fourth ventricle	**5** Middle cerebellar peduncle	**8** Vestibulocochlear nerve (VIII)
3 Inferior cerebellar peduncle	**6** Pyramid of medulla oblongata	MHMS

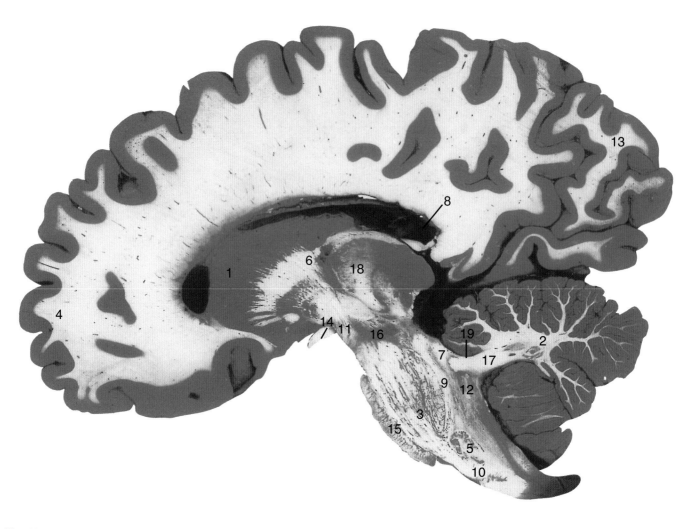

Fig. 18.5
A longitudinal thick slice through the brain showing the medial lemniscus ascending through the brainstem. Mulligan stain. ×1

1 Caudate nucleus
2 Cerebellum
3 Corticospinal tract
4 Frontal lobe
5 Inferior olivary nucleus
6 Internal capsule
7 Lateral lemniscus
8 Lateral ventricle
9 Medial lemniscus
10 Medulla oblongata

11 Midbrain
12 Motor, principal sensory and mesencephalic nuclei of trigeminal nerve
13 Occipital lobe
14 Optic chiasma
15 Pons
16 Substantia nigra
17 Superior cerebellar peduncle
18 Thalamus
19 Ventral (anterior) spinocerebellar tract

Fig. 18.6
A transverse section of pons at the level of the facial and abducens nerves showing the ascending tracts. Weigert stain. ×2.75

1 Abducens nerve (VI)
2 Abducens nucleus
3 Anterolateral system (spinothalamic and spinotectal tracts)
4 Corticospinal tract
5 Facial nerve (VII)
6 Fourth ventricle
7 Medial lemniscus
8 Middle cerebellar peduncle
9 Reticular formation
10 Spinal nucleus of trigeminal nerve
11 Transverse pontine fibers
12 Trigeminal nerve (V) (spinal tract)
13 Ventral (anterior) spinocerebellar tract
14 Vestibular nuclei

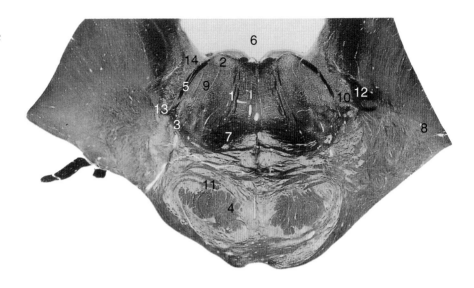

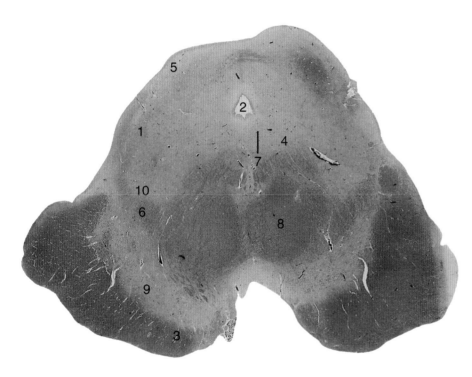

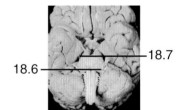

Fig. 18.7
A transverse section through the midbrain showing the medial lemniscus, anterolateral system and trigeminothalamic tracts. Myelin stain. ×3.9

1 Anterolateral system (spinothalamic and spinotectal tracts)
2 Cerebral aqueduct
3 Crus cerebri
4 Dorsal trigeminothalamic tract
5 Inferior colliculus
6 Medial lemniscus
7 Oculomotor nucleus
8 Red nucleus
9 Substantia nigra
10 Ventral trigeminothalamic tract

Figures 18.8–18.10 Sections showing the ventral posterior nuclei of the thalamus.

Fig. 18.8
A coronal section through one cerebral hemisphere and half the diencephalon and brainstem showing the thalamus in relation to the internal capsule. Higher magnification at asterisk in Figure 18.12. Solochrome cyanin and nuclear fast red stain. ×0.65

1	Caudate nucleus	**9**	Midbrain
2	Corpus callosum	**10**	Parietal lobe
3	Crus cerebri	**11**	Pons
4	Hippocampus	**12**	Primary sensory cortex
5	Insula	**13**	Red nucleus
6	Internal capsule	**14**	Substantia nigra
7	Lateral ventricle	**15**	Temporal lobe
8	Lentiform nucleus	**16**	Thalamus

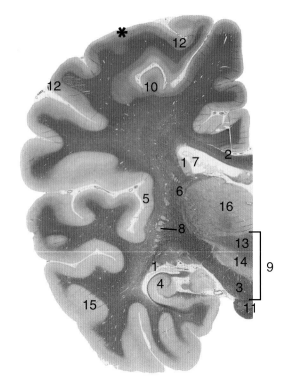

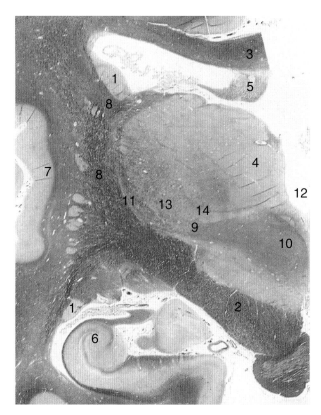

Fig. 18.9
An enlargement of the thalamus from Figure 18.8 showing the ventral posterolateral and ventral posteromedial nuclei. Solochrome cyanin and nuclear fast red stain. ×1.6

1	Caudate nucleus	**9**	Medial lemniscus, spinothalamic and trigeminothalamic tracts
2	Cerebral peduncle		
3	Corpus callosum	**10**	Red nucleus
4	Dorsomedial nucleus of thalamus	**11**	Reticular nucleus of thalamus
		12	Third ventricle
5	Fornix	**13**	Ventral posterolateral nucleus of thalamus
6	Hippocampus		
7	Insula	**14**	Ventral posteromedial nucleus of thalamus
8	Internal capsule		

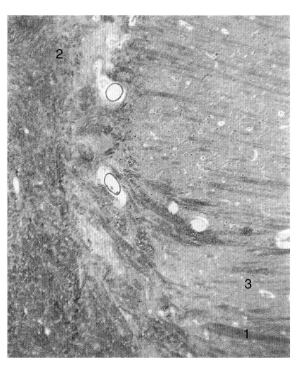

Fig. 18.10
A high magnification view of ascending tract fibers entering the ventral posterolateral nucleus. Solochrome cyanin and nuclear fast red stain. ×20

1 Ascending tract fibers
2 Internal capsule
3 Ventral posterolateral nucleus

Figures 18.11 and 18.12 The primary sensory cortex.

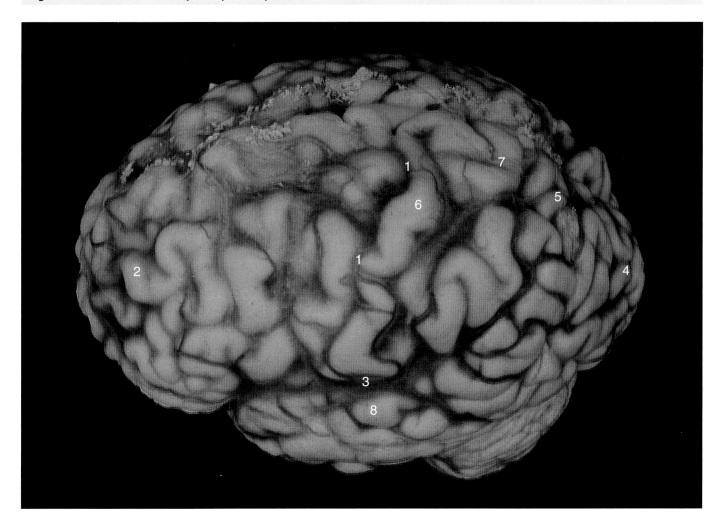

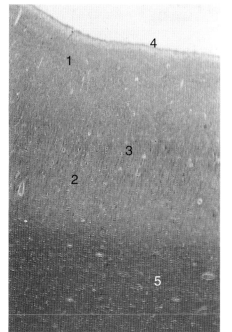

Fig. 18.11
A lateral view of the cerebral hemisphere showing the postcentral gyrus.
×0.97

1 Central sulcus
2 Frontal lobe
3 Lateral sulcus
4 Occipital lobe
5 Parietal lobe
6 Postcentral gyrus
7 Sensory association cortex
8 Temporal lobe

Fig. 18.12
A histological section of part of the postcentral gyrus from Figure 18.8 (asterisk) showing the bands of Baillarger, produced by incoming afferent fibers from the thalamus. Solochrome cyanin and nuclear fast red stain. ×25

1 Cortex
2 Inner band of Baillarger
3 Outer band of Baillarger
4 Pia mater
5 White matter

Summary

1. Touch, pain, pressure, temperature and proprioception are known as the general or somatic senses.
2. Touch, pain, pressure and temperature are consciously perceived.
3. Proprioception is the sense of body position, whether conscious or subconscious.
4. Ascending tracts convey information about the somatic senses from sensory receptors throughout the body, via the spinal cord to the brain.
5. An ascending tract consists of a chain of neurons and their connections and may decussate (cross the neuraxis) as it ascends.
6. Each tract specializes in the transmission of one or more types (modalities) of sensation.
7. The tracts for conscious sensations end in the primary sensory cortex (postcentral gyrus) of the parietal lobe. Unconscious proprioceptive pathways end in the cerebellum.
8. Pain and temperature are carried by the lateral spinothalamic tract, crude touch and pressure by the anterior spinothalamic tract, fine touch and conscious proprioception by the dorsal columns and unconscious proprioception by the spinocerebellar tracts.
9. Trigeminothalamic and trigeminocerebellar tracts convey somatic sensory information from the head.
10. High-level processing and interpretation of conscious sensations are carried out in the sensory association cortex of the parietal lobe.

19 Vision

The visual pathways

Vision is a complex phenomenon involving not only the eye itself, but also the visual pathway connecting the eye to the cerebral cortex and associated pathways for visual reflexes. The retina develops as an outgrowth of the embryonic forebrain (diencephalon), and interacts with surrounding tissues, inducing them to form the other parts of the eye.

The cornea, lens and vitreous body are transparent and focus light onto the retina. The iris and ciliary body are muscular and pigmented. The choroid is a vascular nutritive layer and the sclera is a firm protective coat.

The retina contains the photoreceptive rods and cones and is the only component of the eye actually sensitive to light. Rods are more numerous than cones. The average human retina contains 92 million rods but only 4.6 million cones. Rods are peripherally situated, function best in dim light, and cannot resolve detail or perceive color. Cones are more centrally situated, especially concentrated in the macula lutea. The most sensitive part of the macula lutea is known as the fovea, where cones reach their maximum density of 199 000 per square millimeter. They function in bright light and give high acuity and color vision.

Rods and cones contain visual pigments, which undergo chemical change when exposed to light. They are unique among sensory receptors in that their activity is inhibited, rather than increased, when they are stimulated. The response of rods and cones to light initiates the transmission of information through the visual pathway. Photoreceptors synapse with the retinal bipolar cells and these in turn synapse with the retinal ganglion cells. Horizontal and amacrine cells are retinal interneurons, found in the same layer as bipolar cells in the inner nuclear layer. They enable neighboring bipolar or ganglion cells to interact. Amacrine cells are a specialized type of multipolar neuron. They have no axons. Their dendrites all lie on the same side of the cell body and can conduct impulses in any direction.

Unmyelinated ganglion cell axons converge across the retinal surface to the optic disk. They then become myelinated as they leave the eye to form the optic nerve. Each optic nerve contains about one million fibers. It is not a true nerve but a drawn-out brain tract, hence its supporting cells are neuroglia (including oligodendrocytes) and not Schwann cells. One to two per cent of retinal ganglion cells are not connected to rods or cones. They are directly stimulated by light and are connected to the suprachiasmatic nucleus of the hypothalamus. This pathway has been linked to the control of diurnal rhythms such as sleeping and waking.

Left and right optic nerves meet at the optic chiasma. Fibers from the nasal side of each retina decussate into the contralateral optic tract, while fibers from the temporal side continue in the ipsilateral optic tract. About 90% of optic tract fibers end by synapsing with neurons in the lateral geniculate body. The remaining 10% enter the midbrain and pass both to the superior colliculus and pretectal area (see p. 255).

Cells in the lateral geniculate body are arranged in six layers. Each layer receives contralateral or ipsilateral optic tract fibers but not both. From the lateral geniculate body the visual pathway continues as the visual radiation or the geniculocalcarine tract. Visual pathway fibers entering the cortex form a band, the stria of Gennari. The fibers end in the striate cortex (Brodmann's area 17), which is the primary visual cortex located along the lips of the calcarine fissure in the occipital lobe.

Impulses from the macula lutea are received in the most posterior part of the depths and borders of the calcarine fissure. Neurons in the primary visual cortex are aligned in columns with alternate columns receiving pathways from left and right retinae. Visual information received in the primary visual cortex is further processed and interpreted in visual association cortex, also known as secondary and tertiary visual cortex. This surrounds the primary visual cortex (V1). It forms Brodmann's areas 18 and 19 in the occipital lobe and cuneus, and extends rostrally into the fusiform or occipitotemporal gyrus on the inferior aspect of the temporal lobe. Within the association cortex are regions designated V2 to V5, specializing in different aspects of vision such as color, movement, contrast, shape and recognition of specific objects such as faces. Up to 10% of the nerve fibers of the visual pathway go directly to the association cortex, bypassing V1. This connection may explain why some blind people are able to detect moving objects even though they may not consciously "see" them. Surprisingly, the primary visual cortex is stimulated by touch when blind people read Braille. Recall of previous visual experience is an important factor in interpreting new visual information. It involves the prefrontal cortex of the frontal lobe. This higher-level processing results in a delay of about 80 milliseconds between retinal imaging and conscious interpretation. Finding your way from place to place in your environment activates the hippocampus and inferior parietal cortex in addition to the visual cortex.

At rest, the two eyes face forwards so that their visual fields overlap, giving binocular vision. They are moved in the orbits by six extraocular muscles, supplied by the oculomotor (III), trochlear (IV) and abducens (VI) nerves. In the frontal lobe, there is a cortical center for the control of eye movements. While viewing a scene or object, the eyes make constant tracking movements to keep the image in the central part of the retina. The medial longitudinal fasciculus (bundle) connects the nuclei of the oculomotor, trochlear and abducens nerves together, so that the actions of the extraocular muscles can be coordinated.

Works of art that create an illusion of movement activate movement-sensitive areas in the visual association cortex.

Artists differ from the general population in the speed of their eye movements and in the pattern of brain activity when they are drawing. It is not known whether these differences are inborn or learned.

● *If a person views a visual stimulus, for example a pattern on a screen, electrical activity called the "visual evoked potential" can be recorded by electrodes stuck to the scalp.*

● *Decussating fibers in the optic chiasma may be compressed by hypophyseal tumors. Vision from the lateral half of both visual fields is lost (bitemporal hemianopia).*

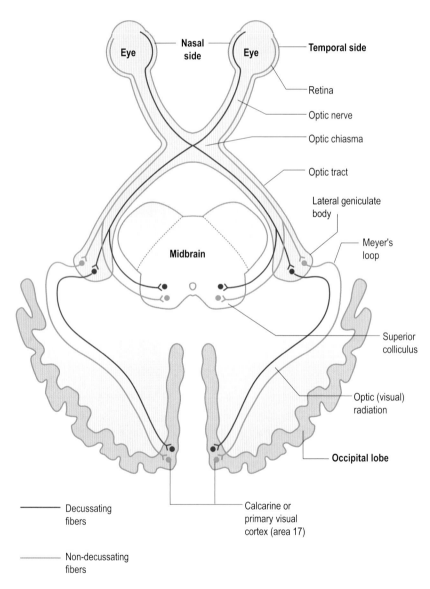

A diagram showing the course of decussating and non-decussating fibers in the visual pathway, and collateral pathways to the superior colliculus.

✳ Only fibers destined for the lower half of area 17 form Meyer's loop.

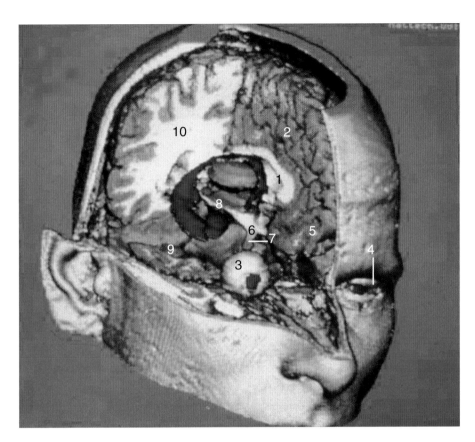

Fig. 19.1
Cutaway three-dimensional computer reconstruction of the head to show the eye in relation to the brain.

1 Corpus callosum
2 Cortex
3 Eyeball

4 Eyelid
5 Frontal lobe
6 Optic chiasma

7 Optic nerve
8 Optic tract
9 Temporal lobe

10 White matter

Prof. F. W. Zonneveld UUH

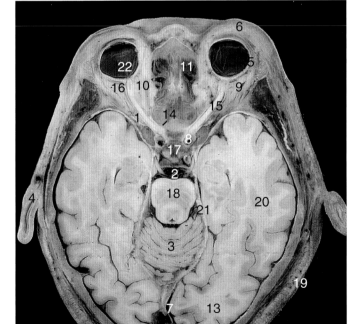

Fig. 19.2
Horizontal section through the head to show the eye *in situ*. ×0.56

1 Apex of orbit
2 Basilar artery
3 Cerebellum
4 Ear
5 Eye
6 Eyelid
7 Falx cerebri
8 Internal carotid artery
9 Lateral rectus artery
10 Medial rectus muscle
11 Nasal cavity
12 Occipital bone
13 Occipital lobe
14 Optic canal
15 Optic nerve (II)
16 Orbital fat
17 Position of pituitary gland
18 Pons
19 Scalp
20 Temporal lobe
21 Tentorium cerebelli
22 Vitreous body

UN

Figures 19.3 and 19.4 frontal and coronal MRI scans to illustrate the anatomy of the orbit.

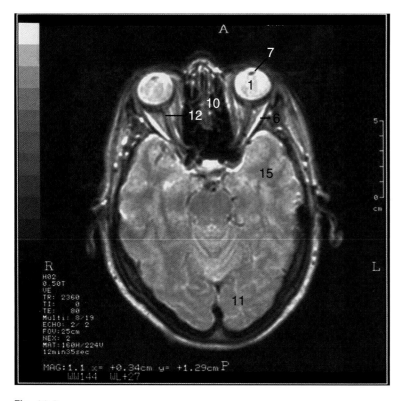

Fig. 19.3
Frontal MRI scan.

Dr. R. Abbott LRI

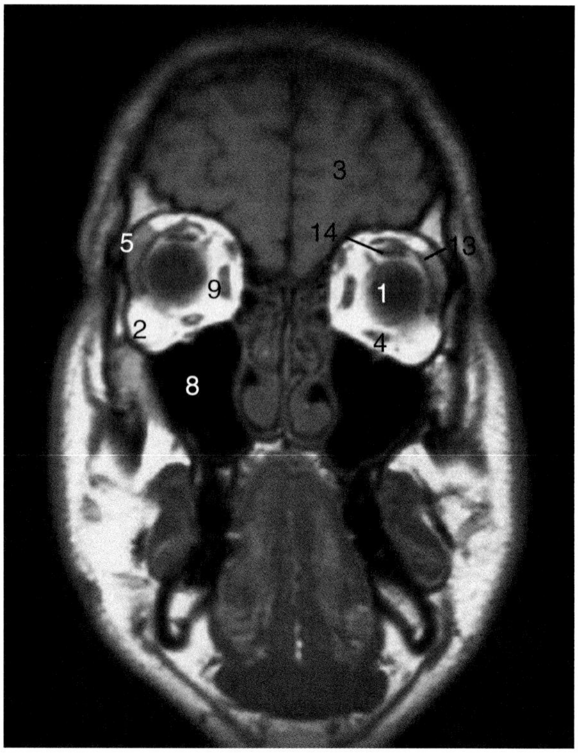

Fig. 19.4
Coronal MRI scan.

Dr. R. Abbott LRI

 1 Eyeball
 2 Fat in orbit
 3 Frontal lobe
 4 Inferior rectus muscle
 5 Lachrymal gland
 6 Lateral rectus muscle
 7 Lens
 8 Maxillary sinus

 9 Medial rectus muscle
10 Nasal cavity
11 Occipital lobe
12 Optic nerve
13 Superior oblique muscle
14 Superior rectus muscle
15 Temporal lobe

● *Damage to the nuclei of the oculomotor (III), trochlear (IV) and abducens (VI) nerves, or to the nerves themselves, will paralyze the extraocular muscles and may cause diplopia by disturbing the normal overlap of the visual fields.*

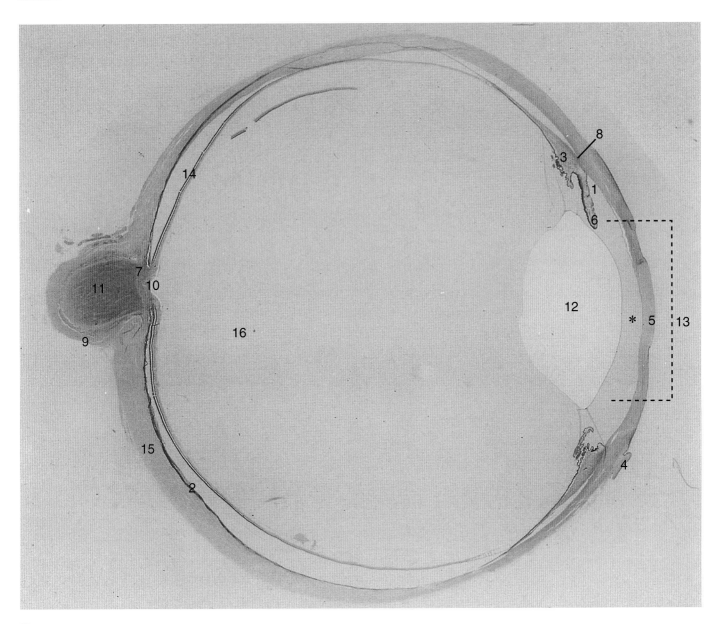

Fig. 19.5
A low power photomicrograph of a histological section through the whole eye to show its component parts. Celloidin section, hematoxylin and eosin stain. ×6.9 This section is from the eye of a patient who had received a corneal graft.

1 Angle	**7** Lamina cribrosa	**13** Pupil
2 Choroid and pigment epithelium	**8** Limbus or corneoscleral junction	**14** Retina
3 Ciliary body	**9** Meningeal coverings of optic nerve	**15** Sclera
4 Conjunctiva	**10** Optic disk	**16** Vitreous body
5 Cornea	**11** Optic nerve (II)	
6 Iris	**12** Position of lens (lost in sectioning)	* The asterisk is in the anterior chamber

Dr. J. Southgate

● *In the retina, layers or structures nearest to the interior of the eyeball are described as "inner", e.g. inner plexiform layer. Layers nearer to the exterior are described as "outer", e.g. outer nuclear layer.*

● *The central artery of the retina is an end artery. It supplies the innermost layers of the retina, outer layers being nourished by the choroidal vessels.*

Figures 19.6–19.8 Histological sections showing the structure of the retina. They share the following labels:

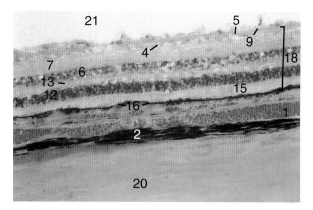

Fig. 19.6
Low power photomicrograph of a paraffin wax section through the choroid, sclera and retina, to show the retinal layers. Masson's trichrome stain. ×113

OXF

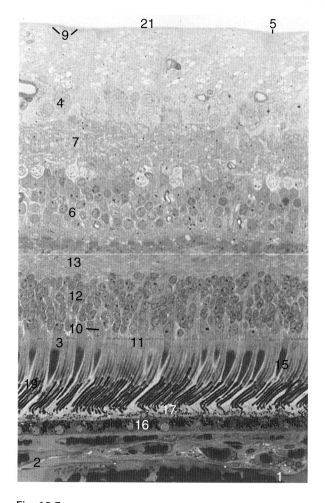

Fig. 19.7
Medium power photomicrograph of a plastic section through the retina of a 19-year-old. Toluidine blue stain. ×489

Prof. J. Marshall

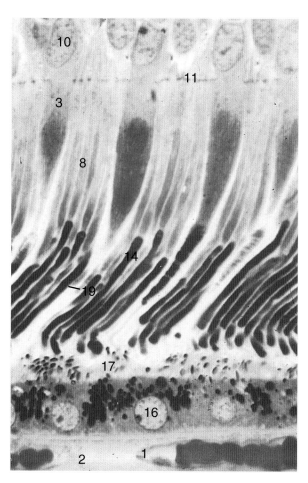

Fig. 19.8
High power photomicrograph of a plastic section through the retina showing details of the pigment epithelium and photoreceptors. Toluidine blue stain. ×1947

Prof. J. Marshall

1 Blood vessel	**12** Outer nuclear layer
2 Choroid	**13** Outer plexiform layer
3 Cone	**14** Outer segment
4 Ganglion cell layer	**15** Photoreceptor layer
5 Inner limiting membrane	**16** Pigment epithelium
6 Inner nuclear layer	**17** Processes of pigment
7 Inner plexiform layer	epithelial cells
8 Inner segment	**18** Retina
9 Nerve fiber layer	**19** Rod
10 Nucleus of photoreceptor cell	**20** Sclera
11 Outer limiting "membrane"	**21** Vitreous body

● *The outer limiting "membrane" is a line of deeply staining cell-to-cell adhesions. The inner limiting membrane is similar to a basement membrane.*

Figures 19.9–19.12 Structure of the optic nerve.

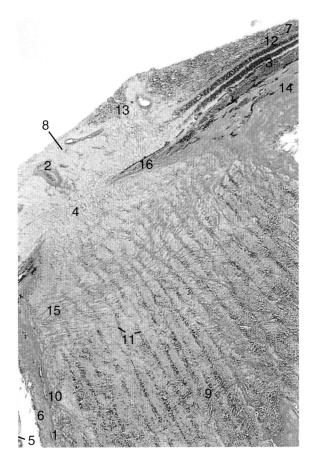

Fig. 19.9
A low power photomicrograph showing the exit of the optic nerve from the eye. Masson's trichrome stain. ×56

 1 Arachnoid mater and subarachnoid space
 2 Central retinal vessels
 3 Choroid
 4 Choroidal part of lamina cribrosa
 5 Dura mater lining optic foramen
 6 Dural sheath of optic nerve
 7 Nerve fiber layer of retina
 8 Optic disk
 9 Optic nerve (II)
10 Pia mater
11 Pial septa in optic nerve
12 Retina
13 Retinal part of optic nerve head
14 Sclera
15 Scleral part of lamina cribrosa
16 Spur of collagenous tissue between choroid and lamina cribrosa

OXF

● *Individual nerve fiber bundles within the optic nerve are separated by pial septa and ensheathed by layers of glial cells. Glial cells also lie within the bundles, between the nerve fibers.*

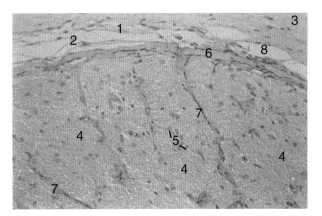

Fig. 19.10
A transverse section showing the meningeal coverings of the optic nerve. Hematoxylin and eosin stain. ×57

1 Arachnoid mater   5 Neuroglial nuclei
2 Arachnoid trabeculae   6 Pia mater
3 Dura mater   7 Pial septa
4 Nerve fiber bundles   8 Subarachnoid space

OXF

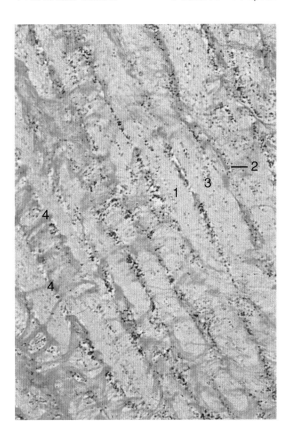

Fig. 19.11
A longitudinal section of optic nerve showing the distribution of neuroglial cells. Masson's trichrome stain. ×112

1 Nerve fiber bundle
2 Neuroglial nuclei around fiber bundle
3 Neuroglial nuclei within fiber bundle
4 Pial septa

OXF

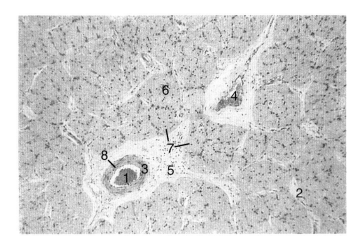

Fig. 19.12
Section showing the central retinal artery and vein inside the optic nerve. Hematoxylin and eosin stain. ×199

1 Blood cells in vessel lumen
2 Capillary
3 Central retinal artery
4 Central retinal vein
5 Fibroblast nuclei
6 Neuroglial cell nuclei
7 Optic nerve fiber bundles
8 Smooth muscle of arterial wall

Dr. J. Southgate

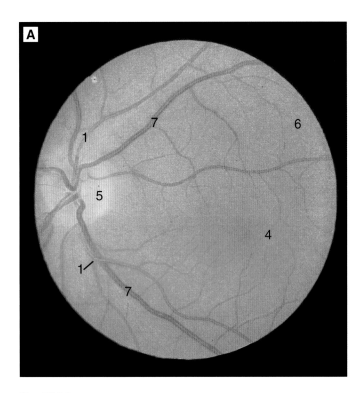

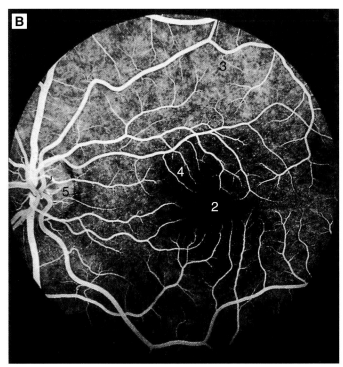

Fig. 19.13
Preparations showing the blood supply to the retina. The normal retinal circulation compared through an ophthalmoscope and in a fluorescein angiogram. **A** Visual photograph. **B** Fluorescein angiogram.

1 Branches of central retinal artery
2 Capillary-free zone (macula)
3 Choroidal fluorescence
4 Macular area

5 Optic disk
6 Retina
7 Tributaries of central retinal vein

Prof. A. Fielder and Mr. H. Harris

● A rise in the intracranial pressure is a feature of many neurological diseases, for example tumor or hemorrhage. If untreated, it can cause serious brain damage or even death. The optic nerve is surrounded by an extension of the subarachnoid space. The optic disk will bulge into the eye if the intracranial pressure increases. This phenomenon is known as papilledema. Thus, while direct measurement of the intracranial pressure is impractical, a rise can be detected by examining the eye through an ophthalmoscope.

Figures 19.14–19.15 Dissections and histological preparations showing the visual pathway.

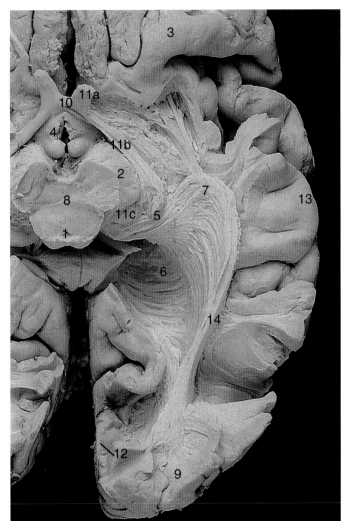

Fig. 19.14
The brain dissected from below to show the pathway from the optic nerve to the occipital lobe. ×1.2

1 Cerebral aqueduct (of Sylvius)
2 Cerebral peduncle
3 Frontal lobe
4 Hypothalamus
5 Lateral geniculate body
6 Lateral ventricle wall
7 Meyer's loop
8 Midbrain
9 Occipital lobe
10 Optic chiasma
11a Optic nerve, 11b Optic tract, 11c Tectal tract
12 Primary visual or calcarine cortex
13 Temporal lobe
14 Visual radiation

● *Meyer's loop consists of visual radiation fibers looping anteriorly around the lateral ventricle in the temporal lobe.*

Fig. 19.15
A paraffin wax section of diencephalon and midbrain showing the optic chiasma. Weigert stain. ×2

This section has been orientated to match that of the optic chiasma and tract in the dissection shown in Figure 19.26.

1 Cerebral aqueduct becoming third ventricle
2 Cerebral peduncle
3 Fornix
4 Hypothalamus
5 Lateral geniculate body
6 Medial geniculate body
7 Optic chiasma
8 Optic nerve
9 Optic tract
10 Pulvinar of thalamus
11 Red nucleus
12 Superior colliculus

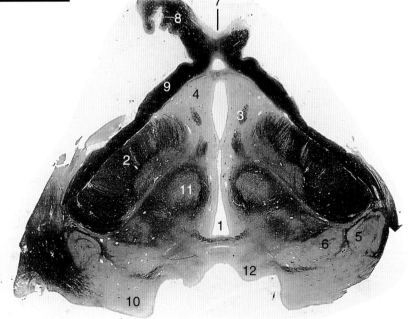

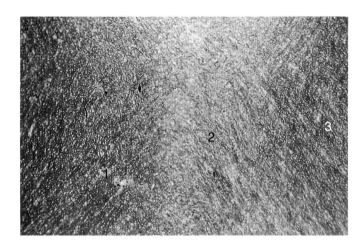

Fig. 19.16
A histological section showing decussating fibers in the optic chiasma. Weigert stain. ×65

1 Blood vessel
2 Decussating fibers
3 Non-decussating fibers

Fig. 19.17
A histological section showing the structure of the lateral geniculate body. Weigert stain. ×11

1 Cerebral peduncle
2 Hilum of lateral geniculate body
3 Lateral geniculate body
4 Medial geniculate body
5 Optic tract
6 Pulvinar
7 Retrolentiform part of internal capsule
8 Visual radiation
9 I–VI cellular layers of lateral geniculate body

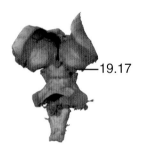

—19.17

● *In the lateral geniculate body, layers I and II are known as the magnocellular layers because of the large size of their cells. The cells of layers III to VI are smaller. These are the parvocellular layers (from the Latin magnus = large, parvus = small).*

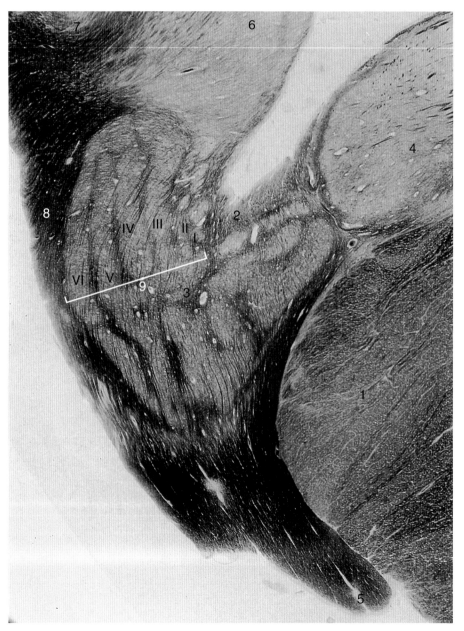

Figures 19.18–19.22 Dissections, functional MRI image and histological preparations to show the visual pathway between the lateral geniculate body and the primary visual cortex in the occipital lobe.

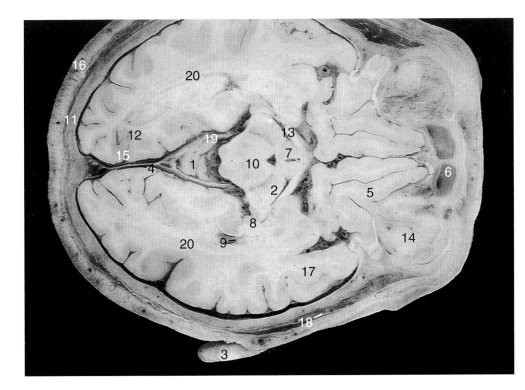

Fig. 19.18
A horizontal section through the head showing the visual radiation (optic radiation, geniculocalcarine tract). ×0.72

 1 Cerebellum
 2 Cerebral peduncle
 3 Ear
 4 Falx cerebri
 5 Frontal lobe
 6 Frontal sinus
 7 Hypothalamus
 8 Lateral geniculate body
 9 Lateral ventricle
10 Midbrain
11 Occipital bone
12 Occipital lobe
13 Optic tract
14 Orbit
15 Primary visual (calcarine) cortex
16 Scalp
17 Temporal lobe
18 Temporalis muscle
19 Tentorium cerebelli
20 Visual radiation

UN

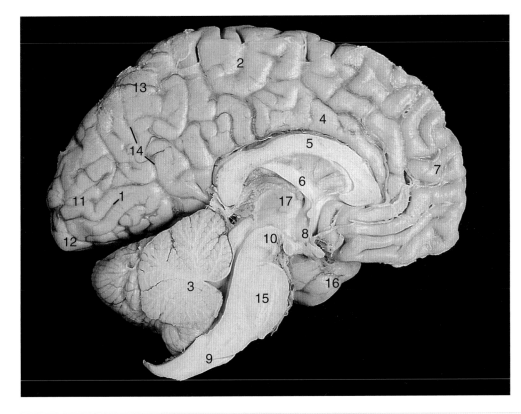

Fig. 19.19
A sagittal section of the brain showing the calcarine sulcus and the primary visual cortex on the medial aspect of the occipital lobe. ×0.76

 1 Calcarine sulcus
 2 Central sulcus
 3 Cerebellum
 4 Cingulate gyrus
 5 Corpus callosum
 6 Fornix
 7 Frontal lobe
 8 Hypothalamus
 9 Medulla oblongata
10 Midbrain
11 Occipital lobe
12 Occipital pole
13 Parietal lobe
14 Parieto-occipital sulcus
15 Pons
16 Temporal lobe
17 Thalamus

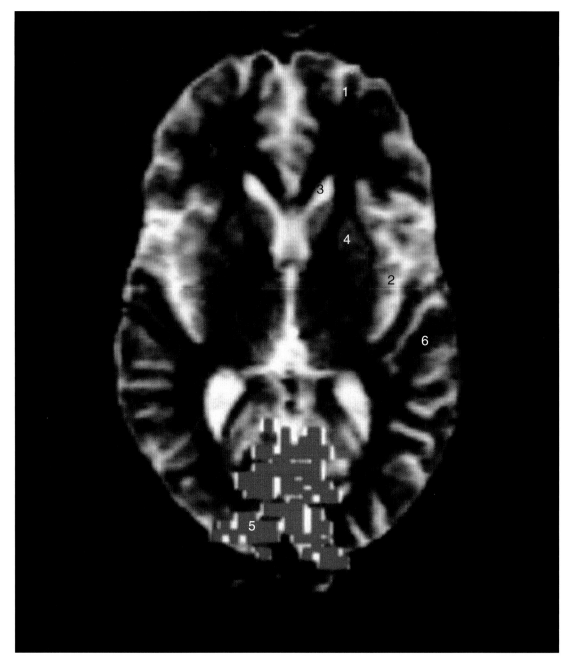

Fig. 19.20
Functional MRI image to illustrate the visual cortex in the occipital lobe. Areas colored red indicate neural activity in the primary visual cortex and surrounding association cortex as the subject performs a visual task.

1 Frontal lobe	**4** Lentiform nucleus
2 Insula	**5** Occipital lobe
3 Lateral ventricle	**6** Temporal lobe

Dr. S. C. R. Williams IP

- *Association tracts connect the visual association cortex to the angular gyrus of its own side; other fibers connect one angular gyrus to the one on the opposite side by passing through the corpus callosum. These pathways are essential for reading.*

- *The fusiform gyrus (see p. 111) is part of the visual association cortex concerned with face recognition. In the majority of people this function is closely localized in the fusiform gyrus. In people with autism and Asperger's syndrome, localization of face recognition is more diffuse. There may be difficulty in interpreting facial expressions.*

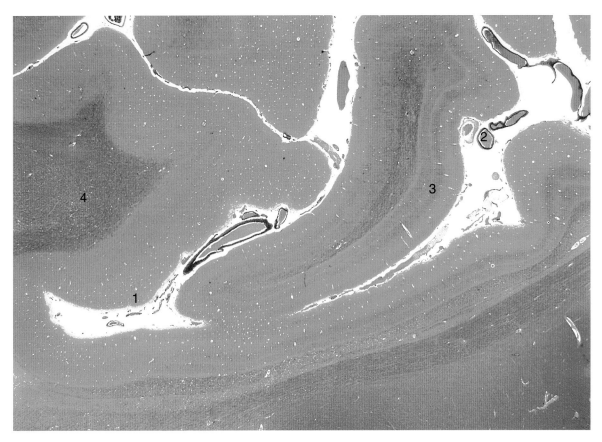

Fig. 19.21
Low power photomicrograph of part of a horizontal section through the primary visual cortex to show cortex, white matter and posterior cerebral vessels. Solochrome cyanin and light green stain. ×5.3

1 Cortex
2 Posterior cerebral vessels
3 Stria of Gennari (Gennari's white line)
4 White matter

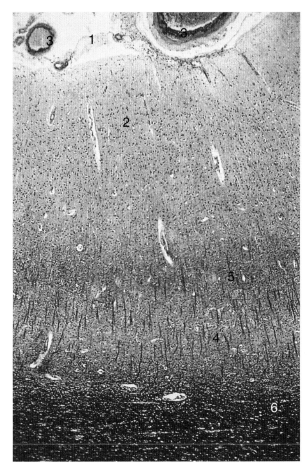

Fig. 19.22
A histological section through the full thickness of the primary visual cortex to show the stria of Gennari. Myelin stain. ×34

1 Arachnoid mater
2 Cortex
3 Posterior cerebral vessels
4 Projection fibers from visual radiation
5 Stria of Gennari
6 White matter

CAM

● *Franceso Gennari (1750–1796?) discovered and described the stria named after him while still a medical student in Italy.*

Summary

1. The retina is the only part of the eye that is actually sensitive to light. Images focused on the retina stimulate photoreceptors.
2. The optic nerve arises from the ganglion cells of the retina and connects the retina via the visual pathway to the visual cortex of the occipital lobe.
3. At the optic chiasma, half of the fibers in each optic nerve decussate.
4. After the decussation on each side, the pathway is known as the optic tract which terminates at the lateral geniculate body.
5. At the lateral geniculate body, some fibers leave the visual pathway for the superior colliculus. These connections are involved in visual reflexes.
6. From the lateral geniculate body, the visual pathway continues as the visual or optic radiation to the occipital lobe.
7. In the occipital lobe, the pathway terminates in the calcarine cortex.
8. The calcarine cortex is known as the primary visual cortex.
9. The remainder of the occipital lobe, and the occipitotemporal gyrus, constitute visual association cortex where visual information is interpreted.
10. Eye movements are controlled by the extraocular muscles.
11. The extraocular muscles are supplied by the oculomotor, trochlear and abducens nerves. The actions of the individual muscles are coordinated via the medial longitudinal fasciculus.

Structures associated with the visual pathway

At the rostral end of the midbrain lie two important visual structures, the superior colliculus and the pretectal area. Both receive fibers from the optic tract that do not pass to the lateral geniculate body, i.e. about 10% of the fibers of the optic tract.

The superior colliculus has evolved from the optic lobe, which is a part of the midbrain, and in lower vertebrates is the highest visual center. This is reflected in its varied connections to other parts of the brain, including the cerebral cortex and other sensory systems. The superior colliculus has a cortex composed of several layers of cells. It controls visual reflexes, such as the coordinated movements of the eyes in tracking moving objects or in scanning a static scene.

The pretectal area, including the pretectal nucleus, is an extensive, complex region with many nuclei in front of the superior colliculus. One of these, the olivary pretectal nucleus, controls the light reflex, adjusting pupil size to environmental light levels. At least three pretectal nuclei receive some input from the eyes.

Figures 19.23–19.24 Dissections and histological preparations showing the superior colliculus and pretectal area.

Fig. 19.23

The brainstem viewed from the dorsal surface to show the superior and inferior colliculi. ×1.5

1 Fourth ventricle
2 Inferior colliculus
3 Lingula of cerebellum
4 Medulla oblongata
5 Midbrain
6 Middle cerebellar peduncle
7 Pons
8 Superior cerebellar peduncle
9 Superior colliculus
10 Trochlear nerve (IV)

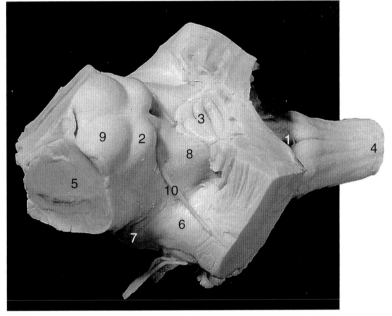

Fig. 19.24

Sagittal histological section of brainstem showing the superior and inferior colliculi and the pretectal area. Solochrome cyanin and nuclear fast red stain. ×1.99

1 Brachium of superior colliculus
2 Cerebral aqueduct
3 Corticospinal fibers
4 Crus cerebri
5 Fourth ventricle
6 Inferior colliculus
7 Inferior olivary nucleus
8 Medulla oblongata
9 Midbrain
10 Pons
11 Posterior column nuclei
12 Pretectal area
13 Superior cerebellar peduncle
14 Superior colliculus
15 Superior medullary velum
16 Tegmentum
17 Trigeminal nerve fibers (V)

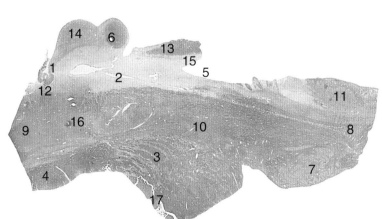

Fig. 19.25
A coronal section through the tectum of the midbrain showing the superior colliculus. Weigert stain. ×5.5

1 Brachium of inferior colliculus
2 Central gray matter
3 Cerebral aqueduct
4 Commissure of superior colliculus
5 Medial lemniscus
6 Oculomotor nerve fibers
7 Oculomotor nucleus
8 Reticular formation
9 Spinothalamic tract
10 Superior colliculus
11 Strata of superior colliculus

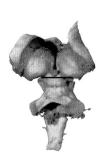

● *As well as visual input into its superficial layer, the superior colliculus receives auditory and somatosensory connections into its deep strata. It gives rise to the tectospinal tract, an extrapyramidal motor pathway (see p. 293). It is a sensory/motor integrating center, particularly in relation to orientating stimuli, such as turning the head towards a sudden sound or flash of light.*

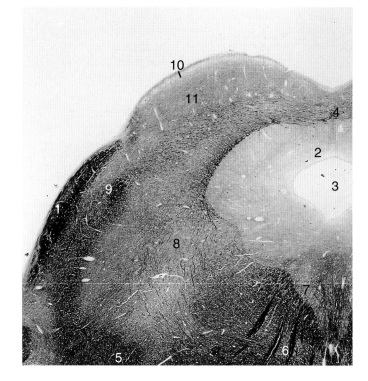

Fig. 19.26
A coronal section through part of the transition between midbrain and diencephalon showing the position and relationships of the pretectal area. Myelin stain and counterstain. ×3.25

1 Central gray matter
2 Cerebral aqueduct/third ventricle transition
3 Crus cerebri
4 Fornix
5 Habenular commissure
6 Habenulopeduncular tract
7 Hypothalamus
8 Lateral geniculate body
9 Mamillothalamic tract
10 Medial geniculate body
11 Optic radiation
12 Optic tract
13 Pineal organ
14 Posterior commissure
15 Pretectal area including pretectal nucleus
16 Pulvinar of thalamus

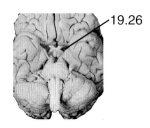

19.26

MHMS

● *The pupillary sphincter muscle of the eye is controlled by the Edinger-Westphal (parasympathetic) portion of the oculomotor nucleus. In the light reflex the pupillary sphincter muscle contracts, constricting the pupil, when a bright light is shone into the eye. Normally, both pupils constrict even if only one eye is illuminated (consensual light reflex), because each pretectal area is connected to the Edinger-Westphal nucleus on both sides.*

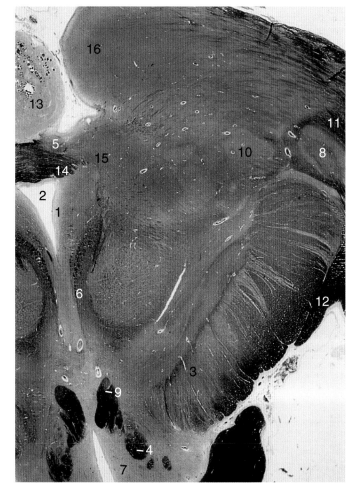

Summary

1. The superior colliculi and the pretectal area lie at the rostral end of the midbrain.
2. They are connected to the retina via the optic tract. Together they receive about 10% of its nerve fibers.
3. The superior colliculi control visual reflexes, for example coordinated eye movements in tracking a moving object.
4. The pretectal area controls pupillary reflexes, such as the light reflex.

20 Hearing and Language

Hearing and Language

The auditory (VIII) nerve transmits information to the brain from the auditory and vestibular apparatus of the inner ear; each apparatus is supplied with its own division of the nerve. The auditory pathway will be dealt with in this section and the vestibular in the next.

The auditory pathway is initiated when hair cells in the cochlea (inner ear) are stimulated. Throughout this pathway GABA and glycine are the most important neurotransmitters. Sound is transmitted as vibrations by the external to the middle ear which sets up pressure waves that travel at 1550 m/sec through the fluids of the cochlea (endolymph and perilymph) and this fluid movement stimulates the hair cells.

The hair cells are innervated by bipolar primary sensory neurons whose cell bodies are located in the spiral ganglion in the cochlea. The central processes of these cells run in the cochlear division of the vestibulocochlear (VIII) nerve to the pontomedullary junction. On entering the brainstem they separate into two divisions, some passing to the dorsal cochlear nucleus and some to the ventral cochlear nucleus. From the cochlear nuclei the auditory pathway becomes diverse and sensory information is carried by a variety of routes to the primary auditory cortex in the temporal lobe (Brodmann's areas 41 and 42). It is important to note that each auditory cortex will receive fibers from the left and right cochlear nuclei. This means that if one auditory cortex is damaged hearing will still occur from both ears.

The dorsal and ventral cochlear nuclei are connected to the inferior colliculus by the lateral lemniscus. Some axons from the cochlear nuclei ascend in the lateral lemniscus on their own side while others decussate in the trapezoid body and ascend in the contralateral lateral lemniscus. Other axons have an additional synapse in the superior olivary nucleus before entering the lateral lemniscus either with or without decussating. To mediate auditory reflexes internuncial (messenger) neurons connect the nucleus of the inferior colliculus to various motor centers. For example, when startled by a loud noise, the eyes close and the body jumps in response.

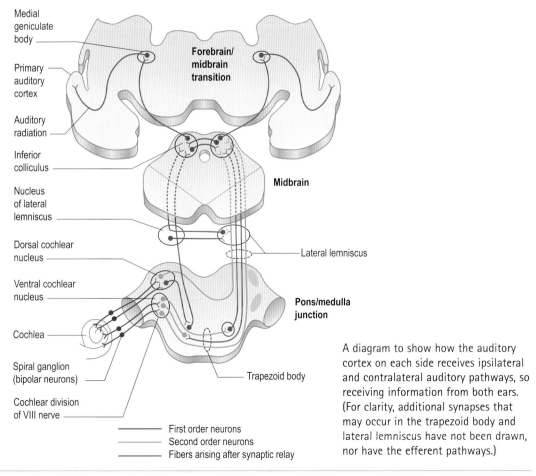

Medial geniculate body
Primary auditory cortex
Auditory radiation
Inferior colliculus
Nucleus of lateral lemniscus
Dorsal cochlear nucleus
Ventral cochlear nucleus
Cochlea
Spiral ganglion (bipolar neurons)
Cochlear division of VIII nerve

Forebrain/midbrain transition
Midbrain
Lateral lemniscus
Pons/medulla junction
Trapezoid body

First order neurons
Second order neurons
Fibers arising after synaptic relay

A diagram to show how the auditory cortex on each side receives ipsilateral and contralateral auditory pathways, so receiving information from both ears. (For clarity, additional synapses that may occur in the trapezoid body and lateral lemniscus have not been drawn, nor have the efferent pathways.)

259

The nuclei of the inferior colliculi are also connected to one another by commissural fibers. From the nucleus of the inferior colliculus, fibers pass via the brachium of the inferior colliculus to the medial geniculate body where they synapse with neurons. The axons of these neurons form the auditory radiations which end in the cortex of the superior temporal gyrus. This is known as the primary auditory cortex (Brodmann's areas 41 and 42). Because of the multiple decussations of fibers at several points along the auditory pathway, hearing is bilaterally represented at cortical and subcortical levels in the pathway. The brain can compare both the time of arrival of a sound at each ear, and its intensity. This information is used to determine the direction from which a sound comes. The superior olivary nucleus is important in direction-finding, as well as other aspects of auditory perception. The olivocochlear bundle is an efferent component of the auditory pathway. It runs from the superior olivary nucleus to the cochlea. It improves the perception of low-intensity sounds by influencing hair cell sensitivity.

The inner ear can be injured by very loud sound. The level of damage depends on both the intensity of the sound and its duration. Two mechanisms exist that help to protect the inner ear from noise damage. Movements of the tympanic membrane and the auditory ossicles can be restrained by reflex contraction of the tensor tympani and the stapedius muscle of the middle ear, thus reducing the intensity of the pressure wave inside the cochlea. The pathway for these reflexes is a connection from the ventral cochlear nuclei to the nuclei of the trigeminal and facial nerves, via the superior olivary nucleus. The tensor tympani muscle is supplied by the mandibular division of the trigeminal nerve; the facial nerve supplies stapedius.

Surrounding the primary auditory cortex in the temporal lobe lies the auditory association cortex, for the interpretation of sounds, including the sounds of the human voice. A localized area of primary auditory cortex lying alongside the superior temporal sulcus is specifically stimulated by vocal sounds, both speech and non-speech sounds, such as that of a baby crying. During speech the auditory cortex constantly monitors the sounds produced by the speaker. This helps to ensure fluency.

Language is one of the most complex aspects of human behavior and brain function. As well as the production of speech sounds, language involves higher cognitive functions including verbal memory, word recognition and interpretation, and mechanisms for arranging words in grammatical structures such as sentences. A number of cortical regions related to linguistic functions have been identified in the temporal lobe, the parietal lobe and the frontal lobe. Two well-defined speech areas are Broca's area (Brodman's areas 44/45) in the frontal lobe and Wernicke's area (part of Brodman's area 22) in the temporal lobe. The prefrontal cortex of the frontal lobe is active in high-level language processing such as analyzing the meaning of words. In most people, language functions, including spoken, written and sign language are controlled by the left cerebral hemisphere.

The posterior part of the insula is connected to the primary auditory cortex. Speech and speech-like facial expressions evoke neural activity in the insula and in the amygdaloid nucleus. Since both these areas are components of the limbic system (see p. 319), their connections correlate the expression and communication of emotions with the use of language.

- *In conduction (middle ear) deafness a vibrating tuning fork can only be partly heard (or not at all) unless placed on the patient's skull, bypassing the middle ear. In sensorineural deafness a vibrating tuning fork can only be partly heard (or not at all) when placed on the skull.*

- *Auditory areas of the temporal lobe cortex are activated when deaf people lip-read or use sign language.*

- *Cochlear atrophy is one of the most common causes of deafness in the elderly.*

- *One cause of congenital deafness is maternal infection with rubella.*

- *Large doses of antibiotics (neomycin and streptomycin) may cause deafness and vestibular disturbances.*

- *The unit of "loudness" (sound intensity), based on the pressure exerted by the sound wave as it passes through the air, is the decibel. As defined by the National Physical Laboratory, Teddington, UK, the quietest sound audible by a young adult is defined as 0 decibels. Sound levels above 120 decibels are painful. At 140 decibels the organ of Corti is destroyed. The intensities of some common noises in the modern environment are shown in the table.*

The intensity in decibels of some common sounds

Rustling leaves	15	
Quiet speech	30–40	
Loud speech	60	
Dishwasher	75	
Lawnmower	85–100	
Heavy traffic	90	} damaging if exposure prolonged
Rock band	100–110	
Jet engine starting	140	severe immediate damage

Fig. 20.1
A CT scan image showing the position of the petrous temporal bone.

1 Cerebellum
2 External ear
3 Mastoid air cells
4 Middle ear cavity
5 Occipital bone
6 Orbit
7 Petrous temporal bone (red triangle approximates to its outline)
8 Sphenoidal sinus
9 Temporal bone
10 Temporal lobe

Dr. R. Abbott LRI

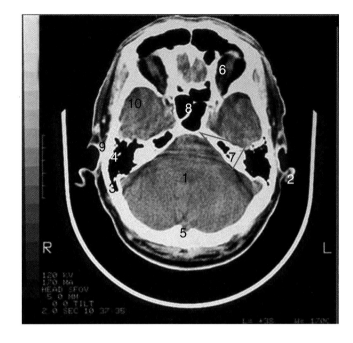

Fig. 20.2
A model of the ear viewed obliquely. ×0.25

1 Auditory (Eustachian) tube
2 Auricle (pinna) ⎫
3 External auditory meatus ⎬ External ear
4 Cochlea
5 Incus
6 Inner ear
7 Internal carotid artery
8 Malleus
9 Middle ear
10 Semicircular canals
11 Skin
12 Statoacoustic (vestibulocochlear, VIII) nerve
13 Temporal bone (petrous part)
14 Temporal bone (squamous part)
15 Tympanic membrane

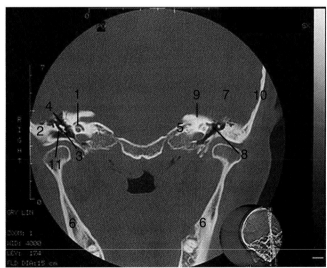

Fig. 20.3
A high bone definition CT scan image of the temporal bone demonstrating some features of the middle and inner ear. The two sides appear different because the patient's head was not perfectly aligned with the plane of the scan.

1 Cochlea
2 External ear
3 Handle of malleus
4 Head of malleus
5 Inner ear
6 Mandible
7 Middle cranial fossa
8 Middle ear cavity
9 Petrous temporal bone
10 Squamous part of temporal bone
11 Tympanic membrane

Dr. R. Abbott LRI

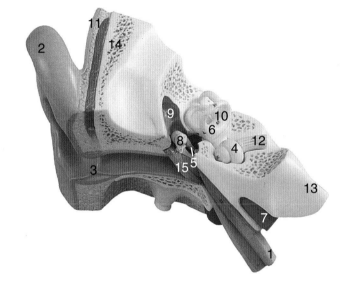

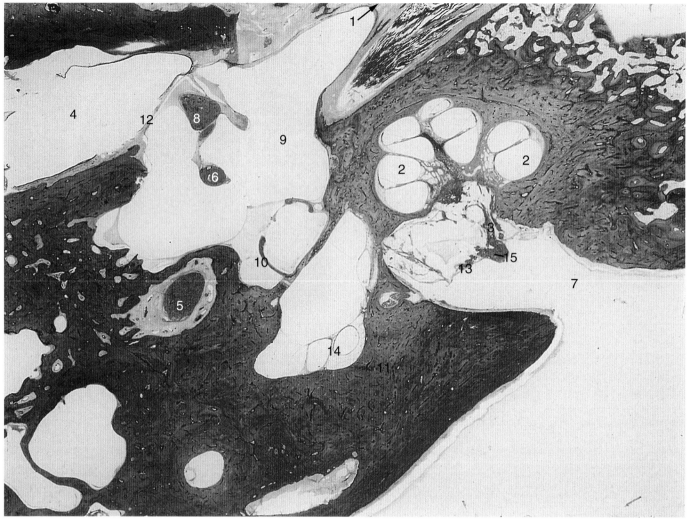

Fig. 20.4
A horizontal section through the temporal bone showing the external, middle and inner ear. Hematoxylin and eosin stain. ×6.9

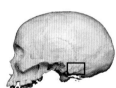

 1 Auditory (Eustachian) tube (direction, arrow)
 2 Cochlea
 3 Cochlear nerve
 4 External auditory meatus
 5 Facial nerve
 6 Incus
 7 Internal auditory meatus
 8 Malleus
 9 Middle ear
10 Stapes
11 Temporal bone
12 Tympanic membrane
13 Vestibular nerve
14 Vestibule
15 Vestibulocochlear nerve (VIII)

Mr. N. Badham

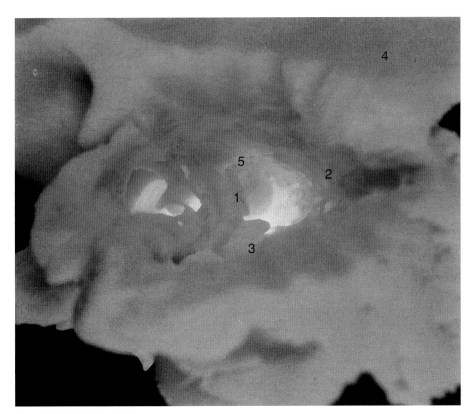

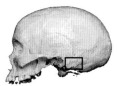

Fig. 20.5
The temporal bone dissected open to illustrate the orientation of the semicircular canals. The lateral wall of the temporal bone has been removed as well as the middle ear. ×2.4

1 Lateral semicircular canal
2 Petrous temporal bone
3 Posterior semicircular canal
4 Squamous temporal bone
5 Superior semicircular canal

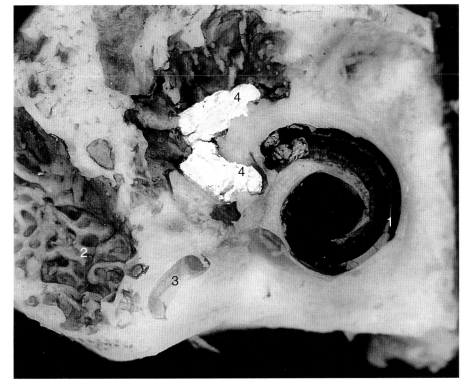

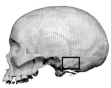

Fig. 20.6
The petrous temporal bone dissected to demonstrate the spiral form of the cochlea in the inner ear. The bony cochlea has been opened and the membranous cochlear duct stained with osmium tetroxide. ×4.3

1 Cochlear duct
2 Cancellous bone
3 Semicircular canal
4 Supporting material

Dr. M. Ingle Wright

Figures 20.7–20.11 Histological preparations of the inner ear.

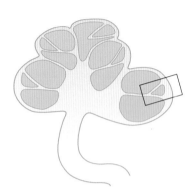

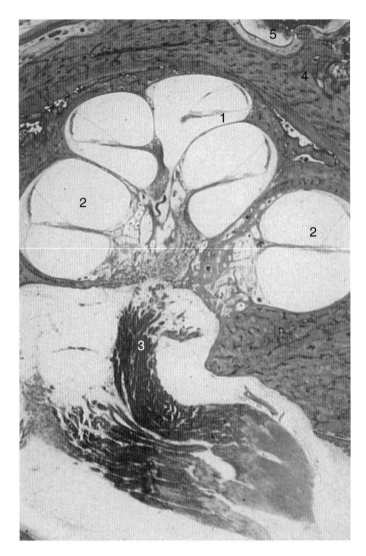

Fig. 20.7
A section and accompanying diagram through the cochlea and cochlear nerve. Hematoxylin and eosin stain. ×12.5

1 Basilar membrane
2 Cochlea
3 Cochlear nerve (VIII)
4 Temporal bone
5 Vestibule

Dr. M. Ingle Wright

Fig. 20.8
A radial section through one turn of the fetal cochlea showing the cochlear duct, organ of Corti and tectorial membrane. A higher magnification as indicated in the diagram above. Hematoxylin and eosin stain. ×80

1 Cells of Hensen
2 Cochlear duct
3 Cochlear nerve (VIII)
4 Organ of Corti
5 Scala tympani
6 Scala vestibuli
7 Spiral ligament
8 Tectorial membrane
9 Vestibular membrane

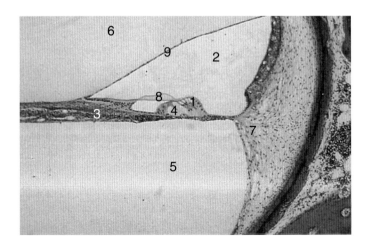

Mr. N. Badham

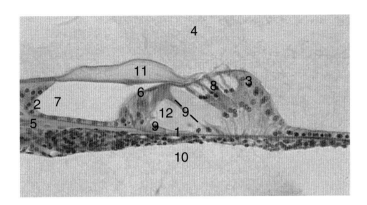

Fig. 20.9
A higher magnification of the organ of Corti. ×325

1 Basilar membrane
2 Border cells
3 Cells of Hensen
4 Cochlear duct
5 Cochlear nerve
6 Inner hair cell
7 Internal spiral sulcus
8 Outer hair cells
9 Pillar cells
10 Scala tympani
11 Tectorial membrane
12 Tunnel

Mr. N. Badham

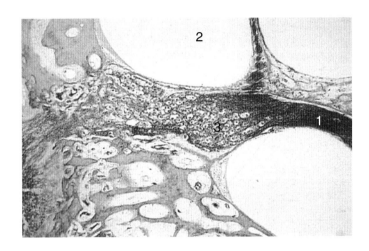

Fig. 20.10
The adult spiral ganglion and auditory (VIII) nerve. Hematoxylin and eosin stain. ×81

1 Auditory nerve (VIII)
2 Cochlea
3 Spiral ganglion

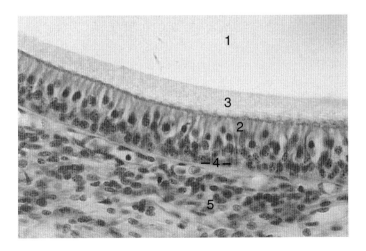

Fig. 20.11
A histological section through the macula of the fetal vestibule. Hematoxylin and eosin stain. ×262

1 Endolymph-filled lumen of vestibule
2 Hair cells
3 Otolithic membrane
4 Supporting cells
5 Wall of the vestibule

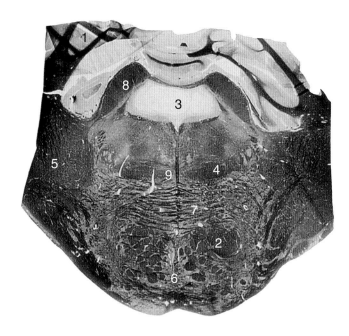

Fig. 20.12
The trapezoid body in the pons. Weigert stain. ×2.5

1 Cerebellum
2 Corticospinal tract
3 Fourth ventricle
4 Medial lemniscus
5 Middle cerebellar peduncle
6 Pons
7 Pontine nuclei
8 Superior cerebellar peduncle
9 Trapezoid body

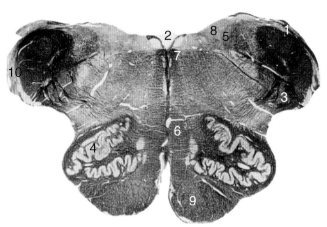

Fig. 20.13
A transverse section of the mid-medulla oblongata demonstrating the cochlear nuclei and the medial and inferior vestibular nuclei. Weigert stain. ×3.6

1 Dorsal cochlear nucleus
2 Fourth ventricle
3 Inferior cerebellar peduncle
4 Inferior olivary nucleus
5 Inferior vestibular nucleus and vestibulospinal tract
6 Medial lemniscus
7 Medial longitudinal fasciculus
8 Medial vestibular nucleus
9 Pyramid
10 Ventral cochlear nucleus

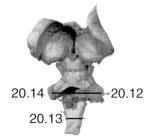

Fig. 20.14
A transverse section of the pons showing the position of the superior olivary nucleus and superior and lateral vestibular nuclei and their relations. Weigert stain. ×3.3

1 Abducens nerve (VI)
2 Abducens nucleus
3 Central tegmental tract
4 Cerebellum
5 Corticospinal tract
6 Facial nerve (VII)
7 Facial nucleus
8 Fourth ventricle
9 Medial lemniscus
10 Middle cerebellar peduncle
11 Pons
12 Spinal tract and nucleus of V
13 Superior olivary nucleus
14 Superior and lateral vestibular nuclei

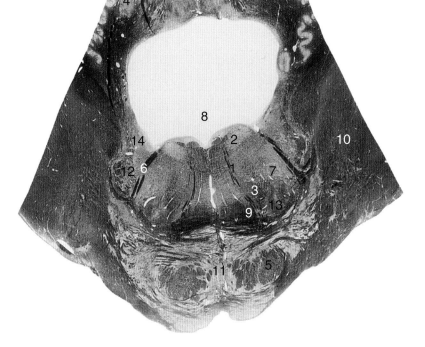

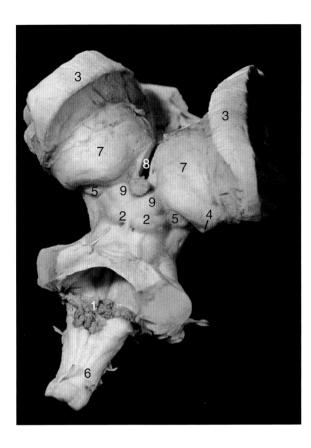

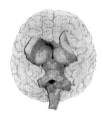

Fig. 20.15

A dissection of the brainstem and diencephalon showing the inferior colliculi and medial geniculate bodies. Dorsal surface view. ×1

1 Choroid plexus of fourth ventricle
2 Inferior colliculus
3 Internal capsule
4 Lateral geniculate body
5 Medial geniculate body
6 Medulla oblongata
7 Thalamus
8 Third ventricle
9 Superior colliculus (plural = colliculi)

Fig. 20.16

A transverse thick slice through the upper third of the pons showing the lateral lemniscus and inferior colliculus. Mulligan stain. ×1.3

1 Cerebellum	8 Medial longitudinal fasciculus
2 Corticospinal tract	9 Middle cerebellar peduncle
3 Fourth ventricle	10 Parietal lobe
4 Inferior colliculus	11 Reticular formation
5 Lateral lemniscus	12 Superior cerebellar peduncle
6 Lateral ventricle	13 Transverse pontine fibers
7 Medial lemniscus	

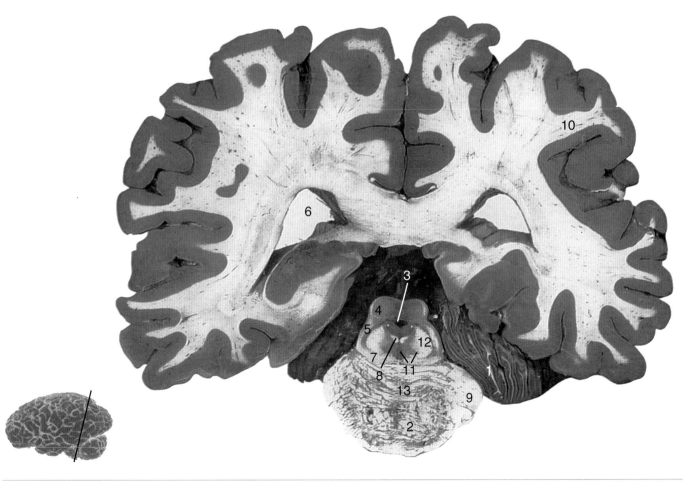

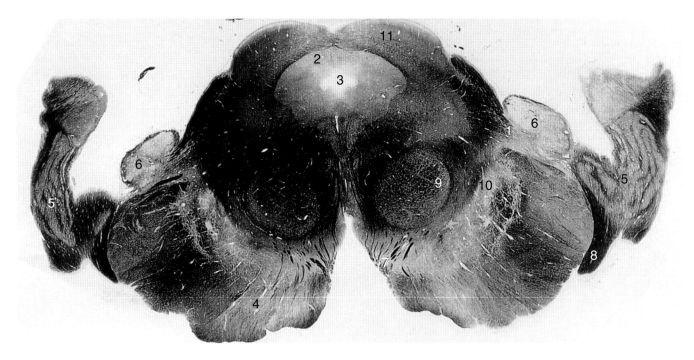

Fig. 20.17
A transverse section through the rostral end of
the midbrain showing the medial geniculate
body and the brachium of the inferior colliculus.
Weigert stain. ×3.4

 1 Brachium of inferior colliculus
 2 Central gray matter
 3 Cerebral aqueduct
 4 Crus cerebri
 5 Lateral geniculate body
 6 Medial geniculate body
 7 Oculomotor nerve (III)
 8 Optic tract
 9 Red nucleus
10 Substantia nigra
11 Superior colliculus

Fig. 20.18
A higher magnification view of a portion of an
adjacent section to Figure 20.17 showing the left
medial geniculate body. Weigert stain. ×14.3

1 Cerebral peduncle
2 Lateral geniculate body
3 Medial geniculate body
4 Midbrain
5 Substantia nigra
6 Thalamus

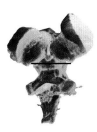

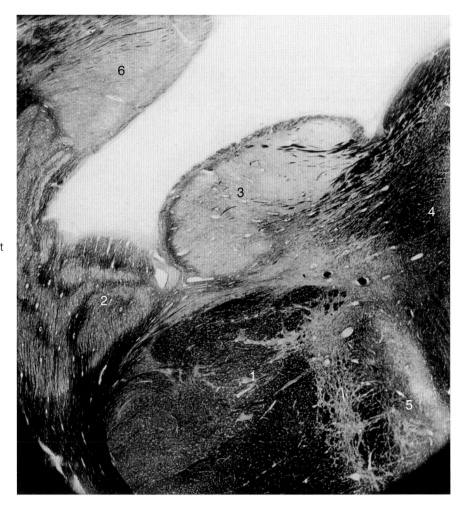

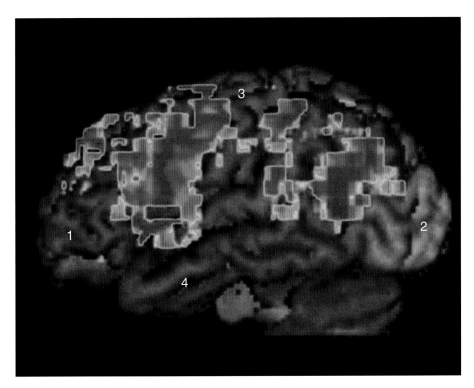

Fig. 20.19
A composite fMRI scan from five right-handed male subjects showing language processing areas in the left cerebral hemisphere. Active areas are shown by red and yellow pixels in the frontal and parietal lobes.

1 Frontal lobe
2 Occipital lobe
3 Parietal lobe
4 Temporal lobe

Dr. S. C. R. Williams IP

- *Language processing in men is mainly restricted to the left hemisphere, while in women it takes place in both cerebral hemispheres. This may be one reason why women sometimes recover better than men after a stroke affecting language-related areas on the left.*

- *In bilingual people, separate portions of cortex within Broca's area (Brodman's areas 44/45) are active during the speaking of each language. If the second language is learned early in childhood the areas are close together, but if it is acquired in later life the areas are widely separated.*

- *Memory for music is located in the prefrontal cortex of the frontal lobe.*

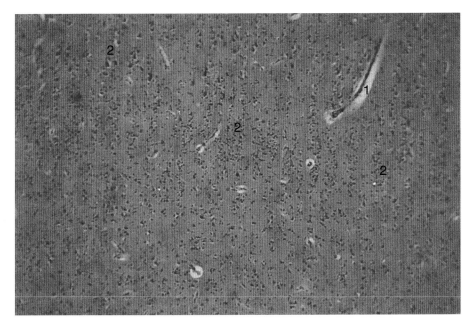

Fig. 20.20
The auditory cortex of the temporal lobe illustrating the parallel columns of cells. Hematoxylin and eosin stain. ×110

1 Blood vessel
2 Columns of neurons

Summary

1. The organ of hearing is the cochlea, part of the inner ear.
2. Sound is transmitted to the cochlea by the external and middle ears.
3. The cochlea is filled with fluids, the endolymph and perilymph. Sound waves are converted into pressure waves moving through the fluids.
4. Movement stimulates the hair cells in the cochlea.
5. The cochlea is innervated by the cochlear division of the vestibulocochlear (VIII) nerve.
6. The auditory pathway begins at the cochlea and ends in the primary auditory cortex in the temporal lobe.
7. The primary auditory cortex receives input on each side from both ears.
8. Sounds are interpreted by the auditory association cortex.
9. Structurally and functionally, the auditory system is connected to areas of cortex involved in the production and understanding of speech.

21 Equilibrium

The sense of equilibrium has a threefold function: as a form of proprioception providing conscious awareness of position and balance, to maintain posture and to keep the image falling on the retina steady.

The three receptor organs for equilibrium are found in the inner ear. They are located in all three spatial planes and are called the utricle, saccule and the semicircular canals. Like the cochlea (see p. 259) they contain two fluids, the endolymph and the perilymph. Projecting into the endolymph are hair cells which are sensitive to the movements of the endolymph. The hair cells have apical projections, called stereocilia. Each cell's stereocilia point at a slightly different angle to those of its neighbors. Each position of the head stimulates a different group of hair cells, and so generates a unique pattern of nerve impulses. The saccule and utricle respond to gravity, signaling orientation, and to linear motion, e.g. moving forward or backward. The semicircular canals respond when the head or whole body is rotated.

From the inner ear the stimulus is transmitted to the vestibular bipolar ganglion situated in the internal acoustic meatus where the primary neuron cell bodies are aggregated. Their axons enter the brainstem at the pontomedullary junction. Most terminate in four vestibular nuclei in the area acoustica of the floor of the fourth ventricle. Others go directly to the cerebellum. The vestibular nuclei have six major connections, vestibulocerebellar, vestibulospinal, vestibulo-ocular, vestibulocortical, accessory and vestibuloreticular, and feedback connections to the vestibule itself.

Vestibulocerebellar connections

This is a cerebellar–vestibular feedback mechanism. The axons from the vestibular ganglion terminate in the superior and lateral vestibular nuclei. Second-order neurons pass via the inferior peduncle to the flocculonodular lobe of the archicerebellum. Some first-order neurons pass directly to this area.

The feedback stimulus travels to the fastigial nucleus and inferior peduncle, and hence to the vestibular nuclei of both sides.

Vestibulospinal tracts

The axons of neurons in the lateral vestibular nucleus descend ipsilaterally as the lateral vestibulospinal tract and synapse on lower motor neurons. The axons of neurons in

the superior, medial and inferior vestibular nuclei, both crossed and uncrossed, descend as the medial vestibulospinal tracts to synapse on lower motor neurons. The function of the vestibulospinal tracts is to control reflex contractions of muscles in the neck and trunk that maintain posture and equilibrium.

Vestibulo-ocular tracts

Besides maintaining the body equilibrium, the vestibular system also plays a role in regulating eyeball movements, to maintain a steady image of the visual field on the retina even when the body is moving. This tract functions when one's eyes are "fixed" on an object and the head turns. Just before the medial vestibulospinal tract descends, it branches and some axons ascend as the medial longitudinal fasciculus in the pons and midbrain where they synapse in the nuclei associated with eyeball movements (oculomotor III, trochlear IV and abducens VI). The vestibular system is also connected to motor neuron pools responsible for head and neck movements.

Vestibulocortical connections

Vestibular connections to the thalamus and cerebral cortex are responsible for conscious perception of spatial position and balance. There is some uncertainty about the morphology of the vestibulocortical pathways. Like other ascending sensory tracts, they have a synaptic relay in the thalamus. Two probable vestibulothalamic pathways have been identified; one accompanies the auditory pathway, the other runs via the reticular formation. From the thalamus, the vestibulocortical pathway runs to a small area of cortex in the parietal lobe, near to the most inferior portion of the primary somatic sensory cortex, i.e. the part receiving sensory pathways from the head. Functional MRI scanning studies also indicate connections to the sensory association cortex and to the insula. Such connections suggest that the brain integrates balance and movement sensations into the spatial "map" of the environment provided by the senses of touch and proprioception.

Accessory pathway

In addition to the feedback mechanism of the vestibulocerebellar connections, there is another pathway.

The fastigial nucleus is connected to the descending reticular areas and nuclei of the brainstem. These discharge via the multisynaptic reticulospinal tract to the lower motor neurons. Connections from the vestibular nuclei to visceral control centers in the reticular formation also exist. Certain movements overstimulate these pathways and create the sensations of nausea and disorientation experienced in motion sickness.

● *Equilibrium is one of the earliest senses to evolve in vertebrates. Fishes possess semicircular canals whose structure is almost identical to those of the human ear.*

● *Sound does not stimulate the vestibule because the pressure wave in the cochlea generated by sound affects all parts of the vestibule equally. There is no deflection of the stereocilia, so the hair cells are not stimulated.*

● *The lateral vestibular nucleus is also known as Deiters' nucleus after Professor Otto Friedrich Karl Deiters (1834–1863) of Bonn, Germany. Although he lived only to the age of 29 he discovered many features of the inner ear, including the hair cells.*

● *Nystagmus (the abnormal and constant movement of the eyes) and dizziness are common symptoms of vestibular injury.*

● *Lesions of the vestibular system often result in disturbances of walking and equilibrium.*

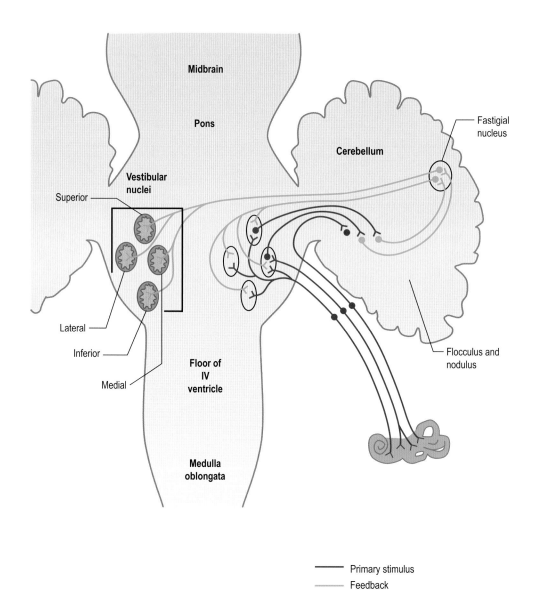

Diagram showing the vestibulocerebellar connections of the vestibular pathway. They are shown on one side only for clarity.

Summary

1. The sense organs for equilibrium are the semicircular canals, saccule and utricle of the inner ear. Collectively these structures are known as the vestibule.
2. They are innervated by the vestibular division of the vestibulocochlear (VIII) nerve.
3. The vestibular nerve is connected to four vestibular nuclei in the brainstem and to the cerebellum.
4. Connections from the vestibular nuclei go to the cerebellum, spinal cord, thalamus, reticular formation, nuclei of cranial nerves III, IV and VI, and back to the vestibule.
5. The vestibular pathways have three functions: proprioception, posture and stability in the visual system.
6. Common disorders of vestibular function include vertigo and motion sickness.

22 Smell

Smell can trigger various responses, both emotional and reflex (for example, the smell of bread baking evokes pleasure and induces salivation). Smell, as well as taste, plays a major role in our perception of substances in the mouth. Sniffing actively brings airborne odor-bearing molecules into the nose, where they dissolve in the mucus covering the nasal mucous membrane. Only a small area, the olfactory epithelium, is sensitive to smell.

The yellowish-brown olfactory epithelium is located in the upper nasal cavity. Within the epithelium are bipolar olfactory receptor neurons which have apical microvilli. Receptor molecules on the microvilli bind specific odoriferent ("smell bearing") molecules. In the process, the cells are stimulated. The axons of these first-order unmyelinated bipolar neurons collect together into approximately 20 nerve bundles and pass up through the cribriform plate of the ethmoid bone into the olfactory bulb where they synapse with second-order neurons. The second-order axons form the olfactory tract. The tract passes posteriorly and upon reaching the anterior perforated substance of the frontal lobe bifurcates to form the medial and lateral olfactory tracts or striae.

The axons of the medial olfactory stria terminate in two ways: in the anterior perforated substance and paraolfactory (septal) area; or some enter the anterior commissure and cross to the contralateral septal area.

The axons of the lateral olfactory stria terminate in the uncus (prepyriform area) of temporal lobe cortex. This is not numbered as one of Brodmann's areas because it comprises the three-layered allocortex, not six-layered neocortex, with which Brodmann's study was concerned. Olfactory tract fibers also end in the amygdaloid nucleus (periamygdaloid area). Neuronal connections from the primary olfactory cortex pass to the secondary olfactory cortex (entorrhinal area of the parahippocampal gyrus: Brodmann's area 28), lateral preoptic area, amygdaloid nucleus and medial forebrain bundle. These cortical areas are responsible for the interpretation of smell.

Tertiary olfactory cortex lies on the inferior aspect of the frontal lobe in the orbital gyri. It is activated by the act of "sniffing", even if no odor is present, as well as by smells. Olfactory perception is predominantly lateralized to the right cerebral hemisphere.

Olfactory areas of the cerebral cortex have extensive connections with the hypothalamus. These, and also a pathway involving the habenular nuclei, form the basis for reflex visceral responses to olfactory stimuli controlled by the autonomic nervous system, for example salivating at the smell of food, vomiting in response to unpleasant odors. Between the stimulus (the odor) and the response (increased visceral activity) the pathways are anatomically complex, often involving many synaptic relays, and are not always well understood. The major and best described ones are listed below and illustrated in the diagrams (see pp. 276 & 279).

1. From the amygdaloid nucleus to the hippocampus, then via the fornix to the hypothalamus.
2. From the amygdaloid nucleus to the hypothalamus by a connecting tract, the stria terminalis.
3. From the septal area to the hypothalamus. The hypothalamus itself is not directly linked to viscera. It is connected by reflex-discharge pathways to the reticular formation and visceral motor cranial nerve nuclei in the brainstem through which viscera are innervated. The most important of these tracts are the mamillotegmental tract and the dorsal longitudinal fasciculus.

The emotional reaction to many olfactory stimuli is evidence of links between the olfactory pathways and the limbic system (see p. 319).

The septal area is connected to the cingulate gyrus through the cingulum, and to the hippocampus. The entorhinal area (Brodmann's area 28) is also linked to the hippocampus. Indirectly, the olfactory system is also connected to the cingulate gyrus by a complex pathway from the hypothalamus, mamillothalamic tract and anterior thalamic nuclei.

- *The olfactory receptor neurons are one of the rare sites in which damaged neurons can be replaced by cell division.*

- *The human nose can distinguish approximately 2000 different odors. Individual cells sensitive to particular odors have not been identified in either the olfactory epithelium or the olfactory bulb. Specificity seems to lie in the different patterns of cells in the olfactory bulb activated by different odor molecules.*

- *Dogs' noses are so sensitive that they can distinguish the smells of T-shirts worn by different people, even non-identical twins. Identical twins have identical body smells.*

- *There are seven primary odors (musky, floral, peppermint, pungent, putrid, camphor, ether-like) that combine to produce all other known odors.*

- *Anosmia is the loss of smell due to damage to the receptor cells, olfactory bulb or tract.*

● *Temporal lobe lesions in the area of the amygdala and uncus often produce olfactory hallucinations.*

● *The insula is believed to be connected to the lateral olfactory gyrus.*

● *Pheromones are chemicals that have no consciously detectable odor when inhaled, but can elicit powerful responses. In many animals they are used to signal physiological or emotional states such as aggression or readiness to mate. The pheromone receptor is the vomeronasal organ, also known as Jacobson's organ, in* the floor of the nasal cavity. Its neural connections are little known, but it may be linked to the hypothalamus. Because it was once believed that smell was unimportant in humans, it was thought that we did not make use of pheromones. However, recent discoveries have demonstrated the existence of the vomeronasal organ and an important role for pheromones in human behavior.

● *For illustrations of the hypothalamus, autonomic nuclei in the brainstem and the limbic system, see pp. 154–156, 191 and 319.*

Diagram of the olfactory projection to the cerebral cortex. Pathways shown on one side only for clarity.

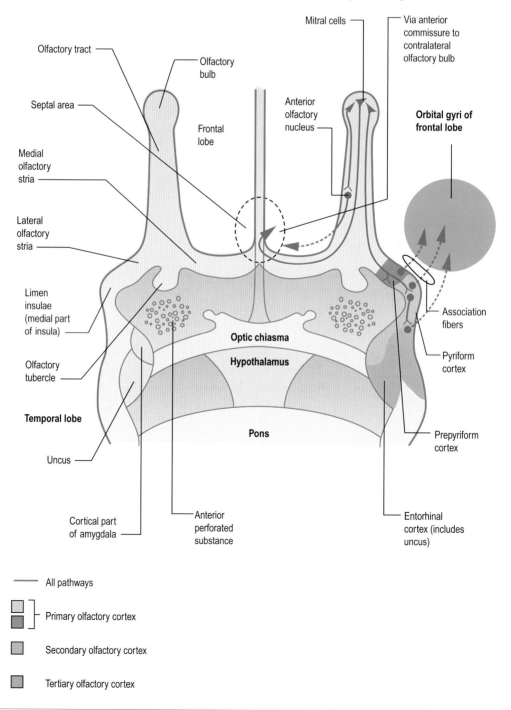

Mitral cells

Via anterior commissure to contralateral olfactory bulb

Olfactory tract

Olfactory bulb

Septal area

Frontal lobe

Anterior olfactory nucleus

Orbital gyri of frontal lobe

Medial olfactory stria

Lateral olfactory stria

Limen insulae (medial part of insula)

Association fibers

Olfactory tubercle

Optic chiasma

Hypothalamus

Pyriform cortex

Temporal lobe

Pons

Prepyriform cortex

Uncus

Cortical part of amygdala

Anterior perforated substance

Entorhinal cortex (includes uncus)

—— All pathways

Primary olfactory cortex

Secondary olfactory cortex

Tertiary olfactory cortex

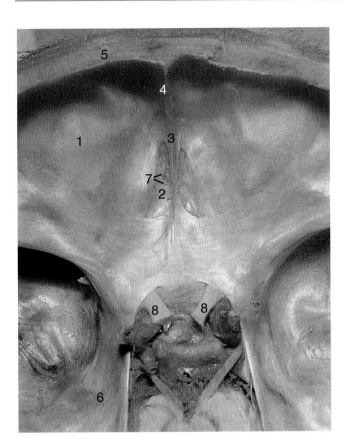

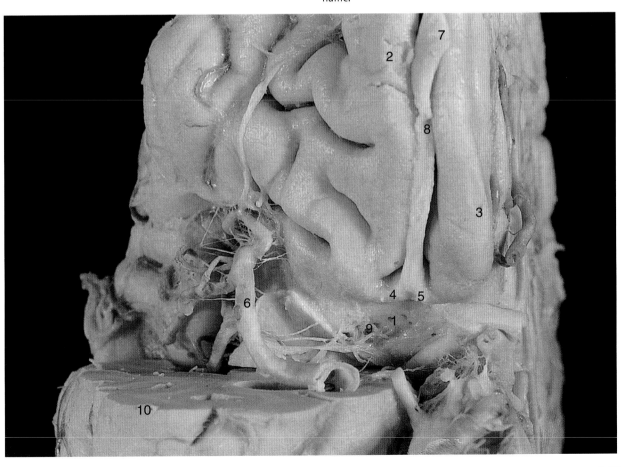

Fig. 22.1
The floor of the anterior cranial fossa showing the cribriform plate and the olfactory nerves passing through. ×1

1 Anterior cranial fossa
2 Cribriform plate
3 Crista galli
4 Falx cerebri
5 Frontal bone
6 Middle cranial fossa
7 Olfactory nerves
8 Optic nerves

Fig. 22.2
The frontal lobe on one half of the brain as seen from below with part of the temporal lobe removed. Note the olfactory tract and its bifurcation into the medial and lateral olfactory striae. ×2.3

1 Anterior perforated substance
2 Frontal lobe
3 Gyrus rectus
4 Lateral olfactory stria
5 Medial olfactory stria
6 Middle cerebral artery
7 Olfactory bulb
8 Olfactory tract
9 Striate arteries*
10 Temporal lobe (partly removed)

* Branches of the striate arteries pulled out during dissection leave holes in the anterior perforated substance. This gives the area its name.

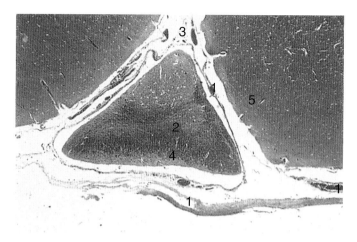

Fig. 22.3
A transverse section of the olfactory tract. Solochrome cyanin and nuclear fast red stain. ×25

1 Blood vessels
2 Nucleus olfactorius anterior (gray matter)
3 Olfactory sulcus
4 Olfactory tract
5 Orbital surface of frontal lobe

Miss L. Ward LRI

Fig. 22.4
Transverse section of the anterior perforated substance. Luxol fast blue and cresyl violet stain. ×25

1 Anterior perforated substance
2 Blood vessels
3 Island of Calleja
4 Olfactory tract

● *Cell bodies in the anterior perforated substance form groups called islands of Calleja.*

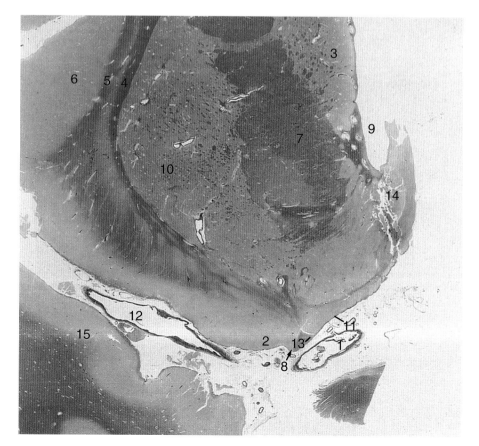

Fig. 22.5
A coronal section of the olfactory tract lying on the anterior perforated substance and dividing into the medial and lateral olfactory striae. Solochrome cyanin and nuclear fast red stain. ×3.5

1 Anterior cerebral artery
2 Anterior perforated substance
3 Caudate nucleus
4 External capsule
5 Extreme capsule
6 Insula
7 Internal capsule
8 Lateral olfactory stria (origin of) (arrow)
9 Lateral ventricle
10 Lentiform nucleus
11 Medial olfactory stria
12 Middle cerebral artery
13 Olfactory tract
14 Septal area
15 Temporal lobe

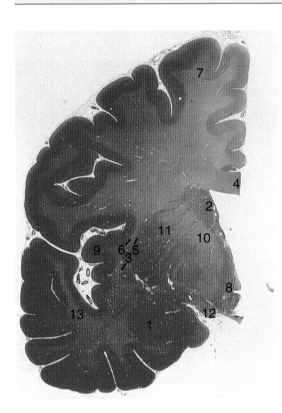

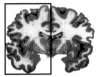

Fig. 22.6
Coronal section through one cerebral hemisphere showing the amygdaloid nucleus. Carmine stain. ×0.72

1 Amygdaloid nucleus
2 Caudate nucleus
3 Claustrum
4 Corpus callosum
5 External capsule
6 Extreme capsule
7 Frontal lobe
8 Hypothalamus
9 Insula
10 Internal capsule
11 Lentiform nucleus
12 Optic tract
13 Temporal lobe

Diagram showing connections from the olfactory pathway to the hypothalamus, brainstem and limbic system for autonomic and emotional responses to smells.

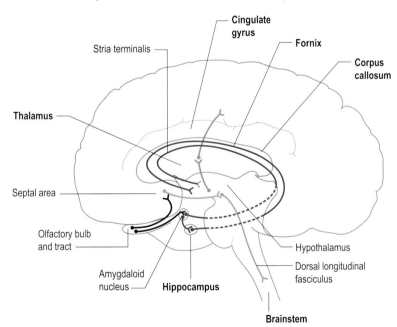

——— Connections to the hypothalamus via the stria terminalis and fornix, for autonomic and emotional responses

——— Direct connections from the septal area to the hypothalamus

——— From the hypothalamus to the brainstem via the dorsal longitudinal fasciculus, for reflexes, e.g. salivation

——— Via the mamillothalamic tract to the thalamus, thence to the cingulate gyrus

Summary

1. Smell is a chemical sense triggered by molecules in the air.
2. The sensory receptors lie in the olfactory epithelium of the nasal cavity.
3. Olfactory nerves pass up through the cribriform plate to the olfactory bulb.
4. The olfactory tract is connected to olfactory cortex in the frontal and temporal lobes.
5. The olfactory system is linked to the hypothalamus and the limbic system. This link provides an anatomical basis for the physiological or emotional responses that smells may generate.

23 Taste

The overall sensation of taste is a complex of true taste, smell, texture and temperature. The true taste sensations include sourness, saltiness, sweetness, bitterness and other tastes (for example, metallic). Sweet tastes are associated with organic molecules such as sugars and alcohols, bitter tastes with organic substances, many of which are poisonous, salty tastes with ionic solutions, especially sodium, e.g. sodium chloride, and sour tastes with hydrogen ions in solution. Approximately 200 different tastes can be identified.

Taste buds are located on the tongue, palate, pharynx and epiglottis. The receptors for taste are specialized cells surrounded by nerve endings. The cells contain receptor molecules called gustiducins which convert taste stimuli into nerve impulses. The impulses from them are transmitted via three nerves: nervus intermedius, part of the facial nerve (VII) (chorda tympani) for the anterior two-thirds of the tongue; the glossopharyngeal (IX) for the posterior one-third and part of the pharynx; the vagus nerve (X) for the remaining taste buds in the pharynx and epiglottis.

When the impulses reach the ganglion associated with their nerve, they then pass to the rostral third of the nucleus solitarius. The pathway continues through the brainstem in the secondary ascending gustatory tract in the medial lemniscus to the contralateral ventral posteromedial nucleus in the thalamus. Some impulses may also travel to the hypothalamus. Connections to other cranial nerve nuclei link the taste pathway to reflexes involved in eating, such as swallowing. From the thalamus, the pathway runs to the lowermost part of the postcentral gyrus and limen insulae of the insula (Brodmann's area 43). In the postcentral gyrus, taste is processed in the same area as general sensations from the face and oral cavity.

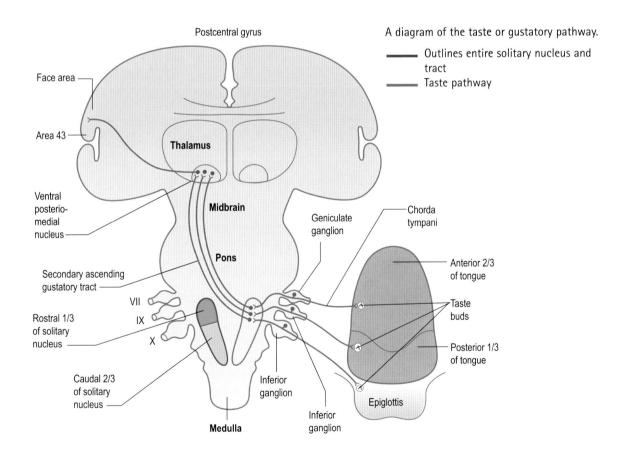

A diagram of the taste or gustatory pathway.

━━━ Outlines entire solitary nucleus and tract
━━━ Taste pathway

- *The caudal two-thirds of the nucleus solitarius (solitary nucleus) is a general visceral afferent nucleus receiving sensory information mainly from viscera supplied by the vagus (X) but also from the glossopharyngeal (IX) and facial (VII) nerves, in the digestive and respiratory tracts.*

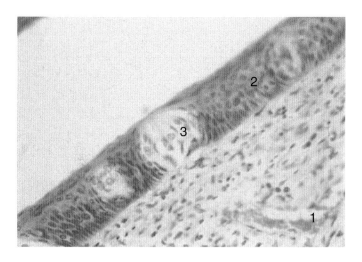

Fig. 23.1
Taste bud from the posterior part of the tongue. Hematoxylin and eosin stain. ×83

1 Blood vessel
2 Epithelium of tongue
3 Taste bud

● *The number of taste buds varies (2000–5000) from one individual to another. It has been estimated that each of the 10–12 circumvallate papillae bears about 250 taste buds.*

● *Taste buds are more numerous in infants than adults, and decrease with age, at a rate of about 1% per year.*

Fig. 23.2
Transverse section of the medulla oblongata illustrating the solitary tract (tractus solitarius). Solochrome cyanin stain. ×2.9

1 Cerebellum
2 Fourth ventricle
3 Hypoglossal nucleus
4 Inferior cerebellar peduncle
5 Inferior olivary nucleus
6 Medial lemniscus
7 Pyramidal tract
8 Reticular formation
9 Solitary nucleus (gray matter surrounding the tract)
10 Solitary tract

Dr. A. Fletcher LRI

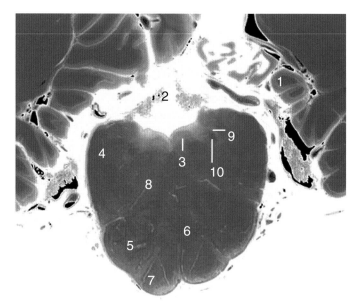

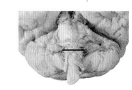

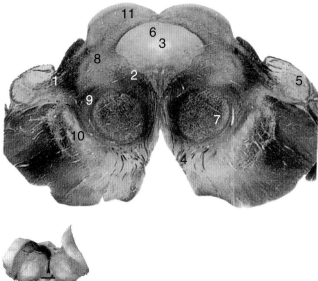

Fig. 23.3
Transverse section of the midbrain passing through the superior colliculi to demonstrate the secondary ascending gustatory tract. Weigert stain. ×2.3

1 Brachium of the inferior colliculus
2 Central tegmental tract
3 Cerebral aqueduct
4 Fibers of oculomotor nerve (III)
5 Medial geniculate body of the thalamus
6 Periaqueductal gray substance
7 Red nucleus
8 Reticular formation
9 Secondary ascending gustatory tract
10 Substantia nigra
11 Superior colliculus

- *Stimulation of the tongue by heating or cooling evokes sensations of taste. This "thermal taste" may be due either to taste bud cells themselves possessing dual sensitivity to both taste and temperature or to their being innervated by both taste and somatic sensory nerves.*

- *Monosodium glutamate is used in many foods as a "flavor enhancer". Some taste buds have specialized glutamate receptors, and strongly glutamate-responsive neurons have been demonstrated in gustatory pathways.*

- *In experiments to investigate the function of taste receptors, extracts of the plant Gymnema sylvestre were found to selectively abolish the ability to detect sweet tastes.*

- *Spicy foods stimulate pain receptors in the mucosa of the tongue. These are naked nerve endings, outside the taste buds, supplied by the trigeminal nerve.*

- *Phenylthiocarbamide is a substance that has a bitter taste to approximately two-thirds of the population. To the remaining third, it is tasteless due to a genetic variation in their taste sensitivity.*

Summary

1. Taste is a chemical sense triggered by substances dissolved in saliva.
2. There are four basic tastes: salt, sweet, sour and bitter. "Flavor" combines taste with smell, temperature and texture.
3. The sensory receptors are taste buds, mainly located on the dorsum of the tongue.
4. The taste or gustatory pathway resembles a somatic sensory pathway, with first-, second- and third-order neurons.
5. The first-order neurons lie in the ganglia of cranial nerves VII, IX and X. The second-order neurons lie in the solitary nucleus. The third-order neurons lie in the thalamus. The gustatory pathway terminates in the parietal lobe.

24 Motor Pathways (Descending Tracts)

In its widest sense, the term "motor" embraces all forms of active response by the body, whether actual movement as a result of muscle contraction or secretomotor activity of a gland. Movements generated by skeletal muscle are termed somatic motor activity. Visceral motor activity involves smooth or cardiac muscle, and glandular secretion. This section is concerned with the neural pathways controlling somatic motor activity, both voluntary movement itself and the systems in the brain that ensure it is smoothly coordinated. The brain also possesses systems by which movements are planned before being actually performed. There are also motor memory mechanisms so that movements can be learned. Planning of movements involves the premotor or supplementary motor cortex of the frontal lobe (Brodmann's areas 6, 8, 9), and possibly also the cingulate gyrus. The anatomical localization of memory for motor skills is uncertain. The cerebellum, corpus striatum and motor cortex all appear to be needed.

Cells in a variety of structures in the brain are motor in function. They are connected by motor pathways or descending tracts to the cells that directly innervate muscles and cause them to contract. Cells in the first category are called upper motor neurons and those in the second are lower motor neurons.

Upper motor neurons that directly give rise to descending (motor) tracts are those in the precentral gyrus of the frontal lobe (Brodmann's area 4, the primary motor cortex), and those of the red nucleus, colliculi, vestibular nuclei, reticular formation and inferior olivary nucleus. Those that are indirectly connected to descending tracts are the cerebellum, the basal ganglia and the ventral nuclei of the thalamus.

Lower motor neurons comprise the anterior (ventral) horn cells of the spinal cord and the cells of motor cranial nerve nuclei supplying striated muscles. These are the oculomotor (III), trochlear (IV), trigeminal (V) (motor nucleus), abducens (VI), facial (VII) (motor nucleus), hypoglossal (XII) and the nucleus ambiguus, supplying glossopharyngeal (IX), vagus (X) and accessory (XI).

The corticospinal (pyramidal) and corticobulbar tracts

These tracts are the principal tracts responsible for voluntary movement. About one-third of their fibers arise from the motor cortex of the precentral gyrus (Brodmann's area 4), the remainder from premotor and precentral areas. There the cells are arranged in a very specific pattern. If you imagine a very small person (homunculus) hanging upside down with the feet positioned in the longitudinal fissure and the head at the edge of the lateral fissure, you have a general description of the pattern of distribution of the cell bodies for each part of the body (see p. 288). The area supplying the hand is disproportionately large in order to control the fine movements required of the hand. Similarly, the area supplying the face is increased and axons from this area descend in the internal capsule to the motor cranial nerve nuclei listed above. This tract is the corticobulbar pathway. The corticospinal tract, which supplies the trunk and limbs, descends via the internal capsule and the basis pedunculi of the midbrain. It then continues into the brainstem. In the medulla oblongata 80–90% of the axons decussate to the contralateral side to form the lateral corticospinal tract. The remaining 10–20% of the axons descend on their own side as the anterior (ventral) corticospinal tract.

On entering the spinal cord the lateral corticospinal tract lies in the lateral white column and the anterior corticospinal tract lies in the anterior (ventral) white column. The fibers of the anterior corticospinal tract decussate in the spinal cord at or close to the segmental level at which they terminate.

At each level of the spinal cord axons from the lateral and anterior corticospinal tracts enter the gray matter. Those from cells controlling the fine movements of the digits synapse directly on the lower motor neurons but the majority of corticospinal tract axons interact indirectly with the cells of the anterior horn via one or more internuncial neurons. Some axons in the corticospinal tract synapse on cells in the posterior (dorsal) horn of the spinal cord and the dorsal column nuclei that give rise to ascending sensory tracts. These may modulate transmission of sensory information.

- *A cerebrovascular accident (CVA) above the decussation will result in paralysis associated with an upper motor neuron lesion, the muscles on the opposite side of the body being affected. This is because both lateral and anterior corticospinal tracts decussate before reaching the lower motor neurons.*

- *If the axon of the upper motor neuron is damaged below the decussation, the muscles on the same side of the body will be affected, causing paralysis. In addition, the suppressor neurons are no longer effective so that the lower motor neurons fire spontaneously or overdischarge to stimuli, resulting in spasticity.*

- *The effects of disrupting the blood supply to the motor cortex often indicate which artery is affected in a CVA. The "lower limb" portion of the motor homunculus, on the medial side of the cerebral hemisphere, is supplied by the anterior cerebral artery. Loss of blood flow will disable the leg and/or foot. The middle cerebral artery supplies the "upper limb and face" areas on the lateral side. Arm, hand or facial movements are damaged by loss of this supply.*

- *During recovery from a CVA affecting the corticospinal pathways, proximal limb muscles recover first followed by distal muscles. Fine finger movements are the last to reappear and are also the most likely to be permanently impaired or lost.*

Suppression of corticospinal activity

Though the majority of the axons in the tract arise from neurons in the precentral gyrus, there are some that originate from neurons anterior to the precentral gyrus (areas 4s and 6). These neurons inhibit the activity of the lower motor neurons, especially when responding reflexly to sensory stimuli.

- *When a complex movement is made, primary and supplementary motor cortex are active. Imagined movements activate only the "motor planning" area in the supplementary cortex.*

- *A positive Babinski sign can be elicited with upper motor neuron lesions. If the outside of the sole of the foot is stroked from heel to toe, the toes fan out and the big toe extends. A normal adult would respond by curling the toes in plantar flexion.*

- *The arm and hand area of the primary motor cortex, Brodmann's area 4, can be subdivided into anterior (4a) and posterior (4p) zones. Movements requiring specific conscious attention to the action are controlled by 4p, learned movements not needing conscious attention by 4a.*

- *Lower motor neuron paralysis is flaccid. This can occur, for example, in poliomyelitis when the ventral horn cells are selectively attacked. There is also atrophy or wasting of affected muscles, deprived of substances known as "trophic factors" normally released into them by the motor nerves.*

A diagram of the corticospinal and corticobulbar tracts. For clarity each tract is drawn on one side only and not all corticobulbar pathways are included.

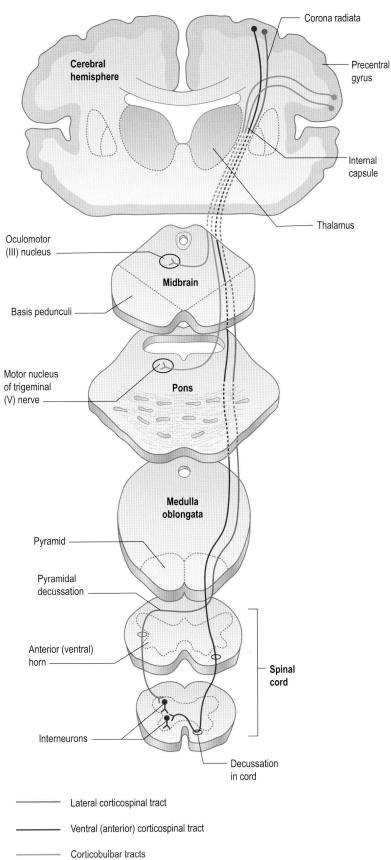

Corona radiata

Precentral gyrus

Cerebral hemisphere

Internal capsule

Thalamus

Oculomotor (III) nucleus

Midbrain

Basis pedunculi

Motor nucleus of trigeminal (V) nerve

Pons

Medulla oblongata

Pyramid

Pyramidal decussation

Anterior (ventral) horn

Spinal cord

Interneurons

Decussation in cord

——— Lateral corticospinal tract

——— Ventral (anterior) corticospinal tract

——— Corticobulbar tracts

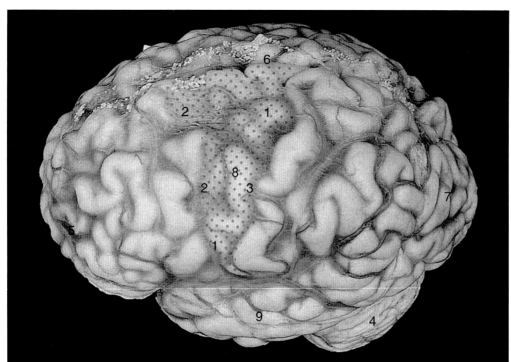

Fig. 24.1
A lateral view of the brain with a colored overlay illustrating the corticospinal (pyramidal tract) region. ×0.82

1 Area 4
2 Area 6 and 4s
3 Central sulcus
4 Cerebellum
5 Frontal lobe
6 Longitudinal fissure
7 Occipital lobe
8 Precentral gyrus
9 Temporal lobe

Fig. 24.2
A coronal section of area 4 with a superimposed homunculus. ×0.97

1 Area 4   3 Homunculus
2 Corpus callosum 4 Lateral sulcus

- *A "sensory homunculus" similar to the motor homunculus relates the sensory innervation of the body to appropriate areas of the primary sensory cortex.*

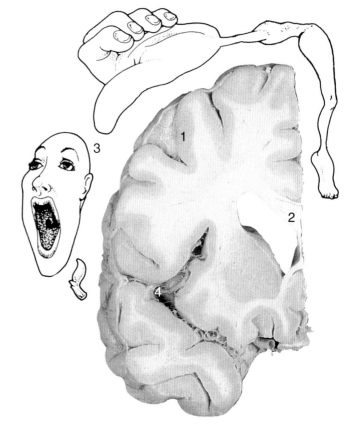

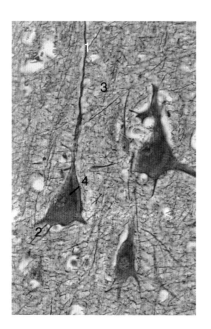

Fig. 24.3
An histological section illustrating the pyramidal shape of the Betz cell bodies of the upper motor neurons. Silver stain. ×334

1 Apical dendrite
2 Basal cell processes
3 Gray matter of the motor cortex
4 Upper motor neuron cell body

CAM

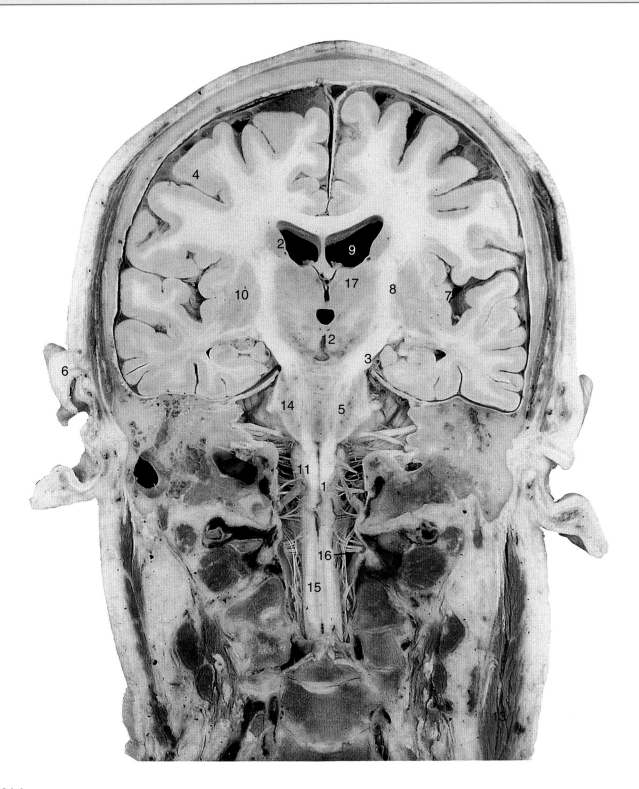

Fig. 24.4
A coronal section through the cerebral cortex, internal capsule and brainstem illustrating the continuity of the corticospinal tract ×0.9. Words in bold type denote structures labeled for orientation.

1 Brainstem	**7** Insula	**13 Neck muscles**
2 Caudate nucleus	**8** Internal capsule	**14** Pons
3 Cerebral peduncle	**9** Lateral ventricle	**15 Spinal cord**
4 Cerebral cortex (parietal lobe)	**10** Lentiform nucleus	**16** Spinal nerves
5 Corticospinal tract	**11** Medulla oblongata	**17** Thalamus
6 Ear	**12 Midbrain**	UN

Fig. 24.5
A coronal section of the midbrain showing the positions of the corticospinal tract. Van Gieson stain. ×3.4

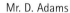

1 Blood vessel
2 Cerebral aqueduct
3 Corticospinal tract
4 Cortico-ponto-cerebellar fibers, intermingled with some corticospinal fibers
5 Crus cerebri
6 Frontopontine tract
7 Medial longitudinal fasciculus
8 Periaqueductal gray substance
9 Reticular formation
10 Substantia nigra
11 Temporo-parieto-occipito-pontine tract   Mr. D. Adams

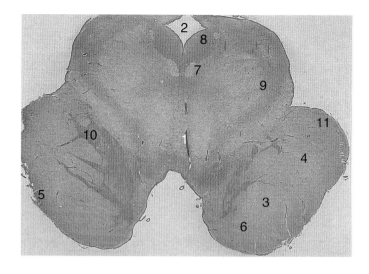

Fig. 24.6
The pons and cerebellum viewed from the anterior aspect to illustrate the corticospinal tract coursing through the pons. The anterior surface has been dissected to demonstrate the tracts. ×1

1 Cerebellar hemispheres
2 Corticospinal tract
3 Medulla oblongata
4 Pons

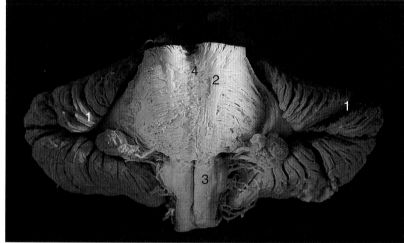

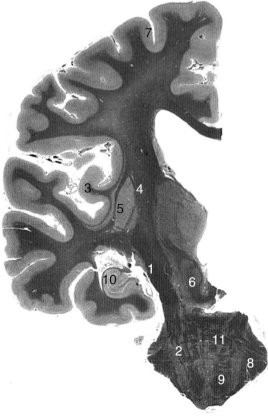

Fig. 24.7
A coronal section showing the course of the corticospinal tract through the internal capsule and into the brainstem. Note how the tract splits into fiber bundles as it passes through the pons, and regroups as it leaves the pons to enter the medulla. Solochrome cyanin and nuclear fast red stain. ×0.58

1 Cerebral peduncle
2 Corticospinal fiber bundles
3 Insula
4 Internal capsule
5 Lentiform nucleus
6 Midbrain
7 Motor cortex
8 Pons
9 Regrouping corticospinal fibers
10 Temporal lobe
11 Transverse pontine fibers

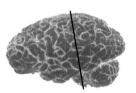

Dr. A. Fletcher LRI

Fig. 24.8

A coronal section of pons showing the position of the corticospinal tract fiber bundles. Weigert stain. ×2.9

1 Basilar portion of pons
2 Corticospinal tract fibers
3 Fourth ventricle
4 Medial longitudinal fasciculus
5 Superior cerebellar peduncle
6 Superior medullary velum
7 Transverse pontine fibers

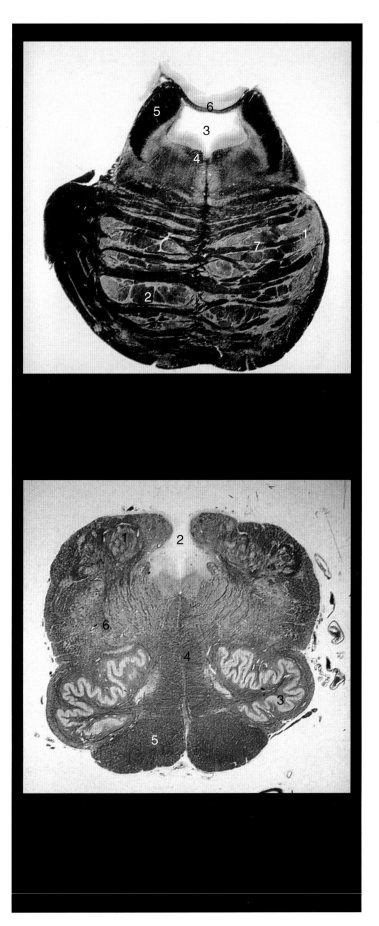

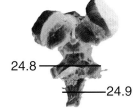

Fig. 24.9

A coronal section of medulla oblongata showing the pyramids. Myelin stain. ×4.4

1 Fasciculus and nucleus cuneatus
2 Fourth ventricle
3 Inferior olivary nucleus
4 Medial lemniscus
5 Pyramid of medulla oblongata
6 Reticular formation

MHMS

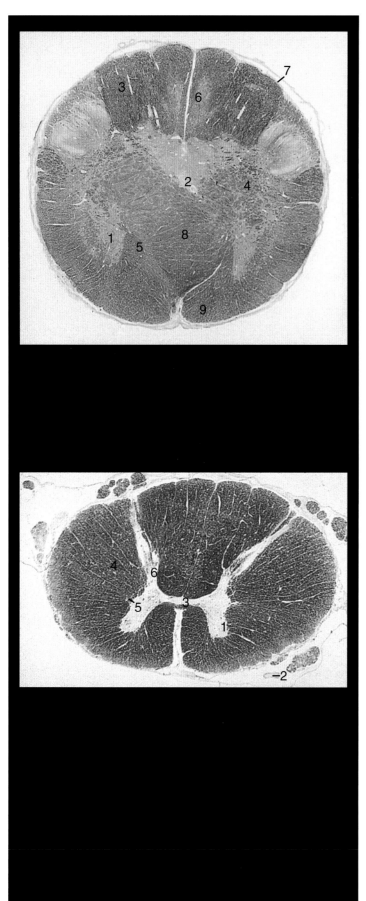

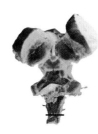

Fig. 24.10
A coronal section of medulla oblongata showing the motor decussation and the lateral and ventral corticospinal tracts. Weigert-Pal stain. ×6.6

1 Anterior horn of the spinal cord
2 Central canal
3 Fasciculus cuneatus
4 Lateral corticospinal tract
5 Medial longitudinal fasciculus
6 Nucleus gracilis
7 Pia mater
8 Pyramidal (motor) decussation
9 Ventral corticospinal tract

Fig. 24.11
A thoracic spinal cord cut transversely to illustrate the position of the corticospinal tract above thoracic spinal level T6. Weigert stain. ×6.7

1 Anterior horn
2 Blood vessels
3 Central canal
4 Lateral corticospinal tract
5 Lateral horn
6 Posterior horn

OXF

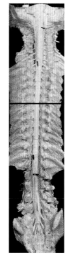

Extrapyramidal motor pathways

A number of subcortical structures in the brain give rise to descending tracts that connect to lower motor neurons and are mainly concerned with automatic movements, such as walking, with posture, and with movements of muscle groups. These tracts do not pass through the pyramid of the medulla oblongata as they descend through the brainstem into the spinal cord; hence they are termed extrapyramidal pathways. They are the rubrospinal, tectospinal, vestibulospinal, reticulospinal and olivospinal tracts.

The rubrospinal and tectospinal tracts arise in the midbrain. The rubrospinal tract is a small tract that originates from the red nucleus, decussates almost immediately and terminates above the mid-thoracic level of the spinal cord. It predominantly controls the tone of the flexor muscles. The medial and lateral tectospinal tracts arise in the colliculi, decussate almost immediately and terminate in the cervical and upper thoracic regions of the spinal cord. The tectospinal tracts control reflex turning of the head and neck to auditory or visual stimuli. The vestibulospinal tract arises from the lateral vestibular nucleus (Dieter's nucleus) in the rostral part of the medulla oblongata and descends without decussating. It controls the muscles that maintain normal posture and balance. The reticulospinal tracts arise from the pontine and medullary reticular formation. They are partly crossed and concerned with regulating automatic movements in locomotion. The small olivospinal tract, originating in the inferior olivary nucleus, descends after decussating to cervical levels of the spinal cord and coordinates movements of the head and neck and upper limbs, contralateral to its origin.

The thalamus, red nucleus, vestibular nuclei, inferior olivary nucleus and reticular formation all receive substantial connections from the cerebellum. It is by means of these connections that the cerebellum influences lower motor neurons; the cerebellum has no descending tracts connecting to the spinal cord.

Diagrams of the extrapyramidal motor pathways. Each tract is shown on one side only for clarity.

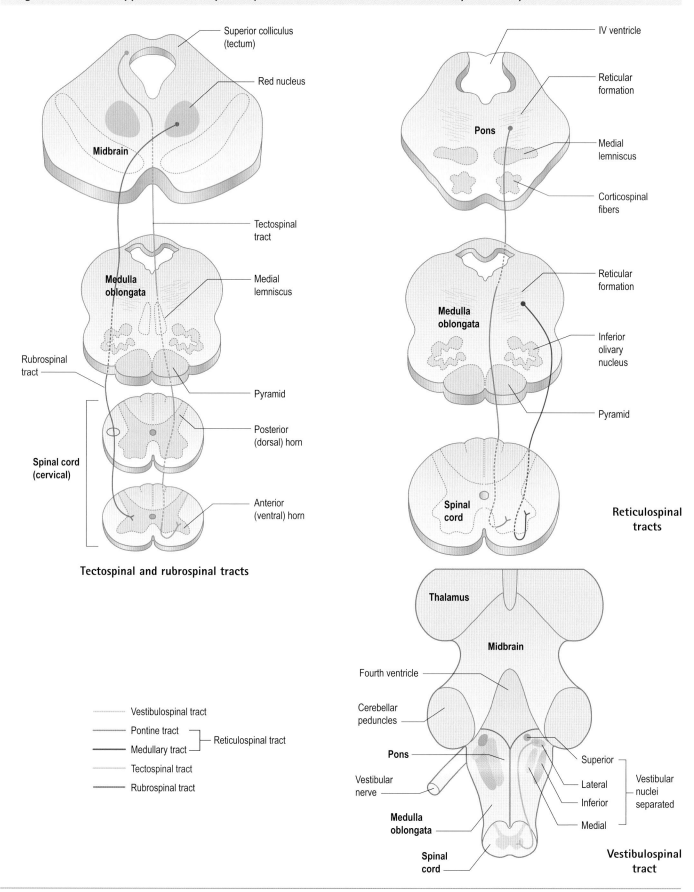

Superior colliculus (tectum)

Red nucleus

Midbrain

Tectospinal tract

Medulla oblongata

Medial lemniscus

Rubrospinal tract

Pyramid

Posterior (dorsal) horn

Spinal cord (cervical)

Anterior (ventral) horn

Tectospinal and rubrospinal tracts

IV ventricle

Reticular formation

Pons

Medial lemniscus

Corticospinal fibers

Reticular formation

Medulla oblongata

Inferior olivary nucleus

Spinal cord

Pyramid

Reticulospinal tracts

Vestibulospinal tract
Pontine tract ⎤
Medullary tract ⎦ Reticulospinal tract
Tectospinal tract
Rubrospinal tract

Thalamus

Midbrain

Fourth ventricle

Cerebellar peduncles

Pons

Vestibular nerve

Medulla oblongata

Spinal cord

Superior
Lateral
Inferior
Medial

Vestibular nuclei separated

Vestibulospinal tract

Figures 24.12–24.14 Sections illustrating the origin and course of all the extrapyramidal motor pathways in the brainstem and spinal cord.

Fig. 24.12
A section of midbrain showing the red nucleus and the rubrospinal tract. Myelin stain. ×2.6

1 Cerebellorubrothalamic fibers
2 Cerebral aqueduct
3 Interpeduncular fossa
4 Medial lemniscus
5 Oculomotor nerve fibers
6 Periaqueductal gray matter
7 Red nucleus
8 Rubrospinal tract
9 Substantia nigra
10 Superior colliculus

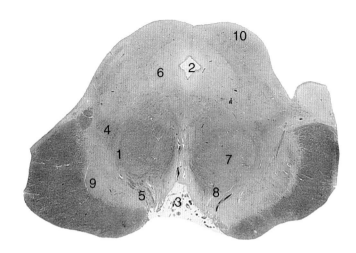

Fig. 24.13
A section of midbrain showing the tectospinal and rubrospinal tracts, at the level of the inferior colliculus. Weigert stain. ×2.9

1 Cerebral aqueduct
2 Cerebral peduncle
3 Decussation of superior cerebellar peduncle
4 Inferior colliculus
5 Interpeduncular fossa
6 Medial lemniscus
7 Medial longitudinal fasciculus
8 Periaqueductal gray matter
9 Rubrospinal tract
10 Tectospinal tract

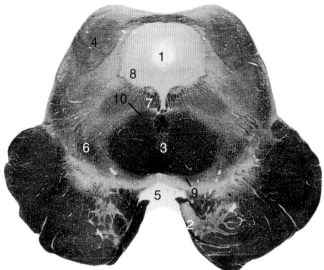

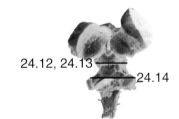

24.12, 24.13
24.14

Fig. 24.14
A transverse section through the rostral part of the pons to demonstrate the position of the rubrospinal and tectospinal tracts as they descend through the brainstem. Weigert stain. ×3.2

1 Basilar portion of pons
2 Fourth ventricle
3 Lateral lemniscus
4 Medial lemniscus
5 Reticular formation
6 Rubrospinal tract
7 Superior cerebellar peduncle
8 Superior medullary velum
9 Tectospinal tract
10 Transverse pontine fibers

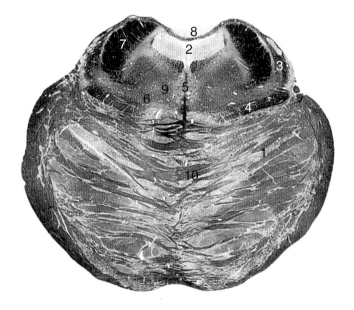

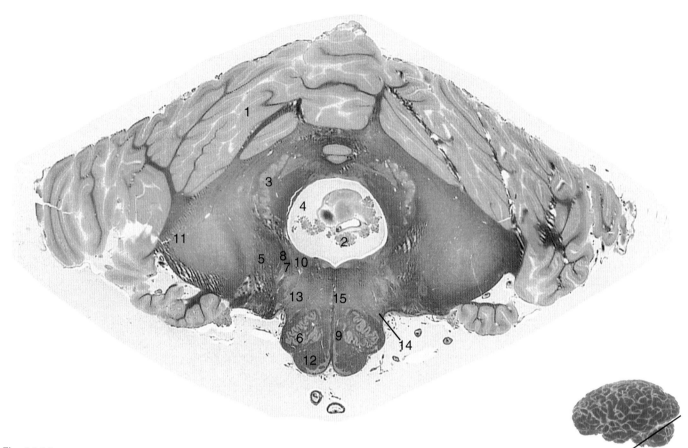

Fig. 24.15
A coronal section through the medulla oblongata and cerebellum showing the vestibular nuclei, inferior olivary nucleus and reticular formation. There are the origins of the vestibulospinal, olivospinal and reticulospinal tracts. Weigert-Pal stain. ×1.8

  1 Cerebellum
  2 Choroid plexus
  3 Dentate nucleus
  4 Fourth ventricle
  5 Inferior cerebellar peduncle
  6 Inferior olivary nucleus
  7 Inferior vestibular nucleus
  8 Lateral vestibular nucleus
  9 Medial lemniscus
10 Medial vestibular nucleus
11 Middle cerebellar peduncle
12 Pyramid
13 Reticular formation
14 Rubrospinal tract
15 Tectospinal tract

MHMS

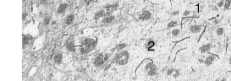

Fig. 24.16
Detail of the medial vestibular nucleus showing vestibulospinal tract fibers passing through the substance of the nucleus. Palmgren stain. ×63

1 Medial vestibular nucleus
2 Vestibulospinal tract, fiber bundles

● *The rubrospinal tract, and the spinocerebellar tracts and spinothalamic tracts are crowded together in the area shown and cannot be demarcated clearly.*

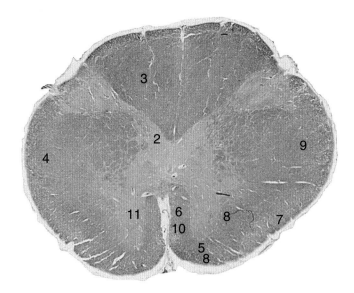

Figures 24.17–24.19 Transverse sections of the spinal cord demonstrating the position of extrapyramidal motor pathways and the different levels to which they descend in the cord. They share the following labels:

1 Cauda equina
2 Dorsal (posterior) horn
3 Dorsal (posterior) white column
4 Lateral white column
5 Lateral vestibulospinal tract
6 Medial longitudinal fasciculus and medial vestibulospinal tract
7 Olivospinal tract
8 Reticulospinal tract
9 Rubrospinal tract
10 Tectospinal tract
11 Ventral (anterior) horn

Fig. 24.17
A histological section through the first cervical (CI) segment of the spinal cord. Weigert stain. ×8.9

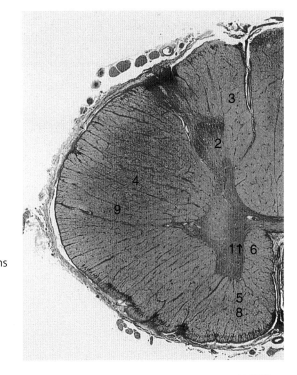

Fig. 24.18
A hemisection through an upper thoracic segment. Van Gieson stain. ×8.5

Mr. D. Adams

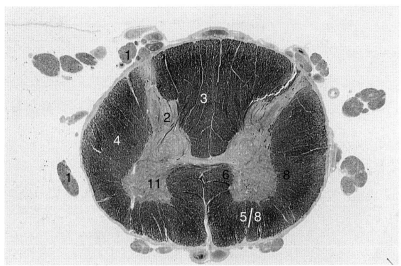

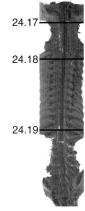

Fig. 24.19
A histological section through a lower lumbar segment. Weigert stain. ×8.4

Summary

1. The lowest involuntary level of movement control is by lower motor neurons which lie in the spinal cord and brainstem and directly innervate muscles.
2. Voluntary movements require an additional level of control by upper motor neurons in the brain.
3. The highest level of voluntary movement control is in the motor and premotor cortex of the frontal lobe. Other motor control centers lie in the brainstem.
4. Upper motor neurons influence lower motor neurons via descending tracts.
5. The most important descending tracts are the corticospinal and corticobulbar tracts, also known as the pyramidal tracts.
6. There are also extrapyramidal pathways: the rubrospinal, tectospinal, reticulospinal, vestibulospinal and olivospinal tracts.
7. Most descending tracts decussate, so that lesions of the motor cortex or descending tracts impair movement contralaterally.
8. Lower motor neuron disorders cause flaccid paralysis, muscle wasting and loss of reflexes.
9. Upper motor neuron lesions cause spasticity and hyper-reflexia. There is no muscle wasting.

25 Systems for Movement Control

Fig. 25.1
Horizontal section of the brain illustrating the level of
the plane of section in Figures 25.2 and 25.3. ×0.5

1 Cerebellum
2 Frontal lobe
3 Insula
4 Lateral ventricle
5 Longitudinal fissure
6 Occipital lobe
7 Parietal lobe
8 Temporal lobe

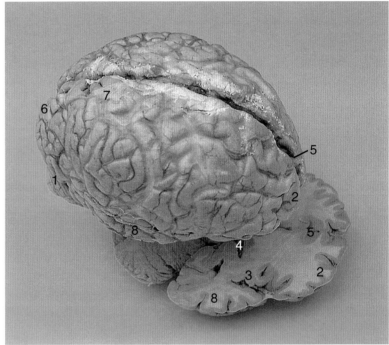

Fig. 25.2
A nuclear magnetic resonance (NMR) image of a horizontal section through
the head to show the thalamus and basal ganglia.

 1 Caudate nucleus
 2 Corpus callosum
 3 Frontal bone
 4 Frontal lobe
 5 Globus pallidus ⎫
               ⎬ Lentiform nucleus
 6 Putamen ⎭
 7 Insula
 8 Internal capsule
 9 Lateral ventricle
10 Lentiform nucleus
11 Meninges
12 Occipital bone
13 Occipital lobe
14 Temporal lobe
15 Thalamus
16 Third ventricle

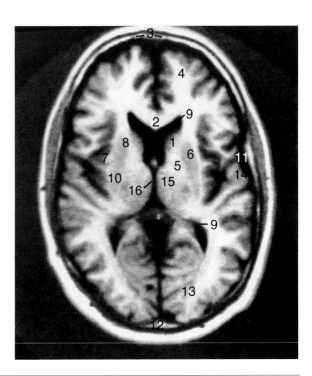

Dr G. Bydder

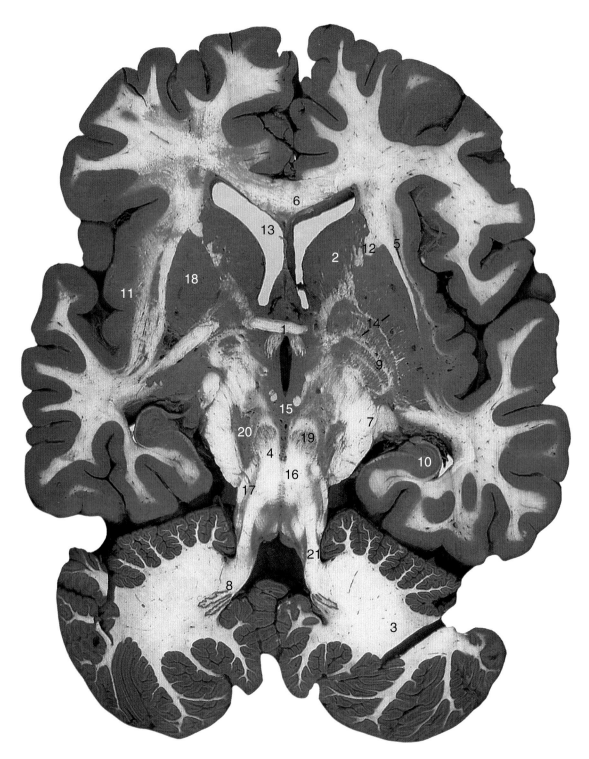

Fig. 25.3
Horizontal thick section of brain showing details of the cerebellum and the basal ganglia, both important in the control of movement.
Mulligan stain. ×1.2

1 Anterior commissure	**8** Dentate nucleus	**15** Mamillary body
2 Caudate nucleus	**9** Globus pallidus	**16** Midbrain
3 Cerebellum	**10** Hippocampus	**17** Pons
4 Cerebellorubrothalamic fibers	**11** Insula	**18** Putamen
5 Claustrum	**12** Internal capsule	**19** Red nucleus
6 Corpus callosum	**13** Lateral ventricle	**20** Substantia nigra
7 Crus cerebri	**14** Lentiform nucleus	**21** Superior cerebellar peduncle

The Cerebellum in Movement Control

The cerebellum is one region where sensory and motor integration can take place. It may be likened to a reference library to which the motor cortex can "refer". As already explained, it has no direct link to lower motor neurons. There are two ways in which it influences movement indirectly. Firstly, it has connections to motor areas of the cerebral cortex via relay in the thalamus. Secondly, it also connects to the red nucleus, olivary complex, reticular formation and vestibular nuclei, then through these to extrapyramidal motor pathways.

The nature of the interaction between the cerebellum and the motor cortex in movement coordination is poorly understood. One theory is that the cerebellum participates in the planning stage, before the movement is made. Patterns of neural activity are generated in the cerebellum and transmitted to the motor cortex. There they are used in programming the muscles that will be needed to perform the movement. Sensory feedback to the cerebellum during the movement can be compared to the original cerebellar "plan" and adjustments made to ensure that the movement is smooth and of the appropriate speed, strength and direction.

The cerebellum may be divided into three functional units: the archicerebellum, paleocerebellum and neocerebellum. The archicerebellum is composed of the flocculonodular lobe and fastigial nucleus which are linked to the vestibular nuclei. The paleocerebellum receives general sensory information, especially proprioception. Its extent is a little uncertain but it includes the anterior lobe, pyramid, uvula and the globose and emboliform nuclei. The neocerebellum is the largest part and comprises the remaining cortex which receives olivary afferents and a large input from the cerebral cortex via the pontine nuclei. Its major efferent deep nucleus is the dentate nucleus.

This functional subdivision parallels the order in which parts of the cerebellum have appeared in the course of evolution as movement control became more complex.

The inferior cerebellar peduncle connects cerebellum and medulla oblongata. It conveys the dorsal (posterior) spinocerebellar tract, olivocerebellar fibers from the contralateral inferior olivary complex, vestibulocerebellar fibers, trigeminocerebellar fibers, cuneocerebellar fibers from the accessory cuneate nucleus, and afferents from the reticular formation and arcuate nuclei (anterior external arcuate fibers and the striae medullares). Efferent fibers in the inferior peduncle pass to the vestibular nuclei and possibly to the reticular formation and olivary nuclei.

The middle peduncle is exclusively afferent. Its fibers originate from the contralateral cerebral cortex. Afferents from wide areas of the cortex synapse in the pontine nuclei. These in turn are connected to the cerebellum. This is the main route for sensory information to reach the cerebellum from cortical sensory areas, and also connects the motor cortex to the cerebellum. The pontine nuclei relay information to the cerebellar cortex.

The superior cerebellar peduncle contains only two afferent tracts, the anterior (ventral) spinocerebellar tract and tectocerebellar fibers from the midbrain colliculi. Efferent fibers run from the dentate nucleus to the contralateral red nucleus and ventrolateral nucleus of the thalamus, thence to the motor cortex of the cerebrum. Efferent fibers also link the fastigial nuclei to the lateral vestibular nucleus, and the globose and emboliform nuclei to the red nucleus and thalamus. The superior peduncle decussates in the midbrain.

The inferior olivary complex also receives afferent fibers from cerebral motor cortex, and the central tegmental tract from the corpus striatum and red nucleus.

The red nucleus projects to lower motor neurons via the rubrospinal tract. In addition to its connections from the cerebellum, it receives afferent fibers from motor cortex and corpus striatum, sends efferents to the thalamus and is reciprocally linked to the substantia nigra.

No cells are lost from the inferior olivary nucleus in old age. Its cells accumulate lipofuscin (age pigment) in greater amounts and earlier in life than those in any other brain nucleus. Damage to the inferior olivary nucleus produces similar tremors and uncoordinated movements to those produced by lesions in the cerebellum itself. Experimental evidence from animal brains shows that during habitual movements, groups of cells in the inferior olivary nucleus discharge impulses synchronously. This is followed by synchronized activity in the Purkinje cells to which they are connected. These observations may indicate that the function of the olivocerebellar connections is to create patterns of neural activity in the cerebellum that underlie the performance of unconsciously controlled learned movements.

● *There may also be afferent adrenergic connections to the cerebellum from the locus ceruleus (see p. 166). The functions of the locus ceruleus are not well understood. It has been shown to have a role in maintaining diurnal rhythms of activity and behavior.*

● *Animal studies suggest cerebellar connections with the autonomic system, possibly via the reticular formation.*

● *The flocculonodular lobe is phylogenetically the oldest part of the cerebellum, the archicerebellum, which is present in all vertebrates.*

● *Lesions in the midline of the cerebellum mainly affect its postural and balance functions. The patient cannot sit or stand upright without overbalancing.*

- *Because many cerebellar connections do not decussate, unilateral lesions of the cerebellar hemispheres affect the same side of the body as the brain damage. The gait becomes unsteady because one arm and leg are uncoordinated. There is also a tremor in the limbs as a movement is started (intention tremor).*

- *Bilateral cerebellar lesions can occur in general neurological diseases such as multiple sclerosis. The limbs are uncoordinated on both sides of the body, producing an abnormal gait known as cerebellar ataxia. The patient walks with the legs wide apart in an attempt to maintain balance. Speech becomes slow and slurred (dysarthria) due to the uncoordination of speech muscles. Rapid side-to-side eye movements called nystagmus are also characteristic of cerebellar disease.*

- *For further consideration of vestibular nuclei see pp. 191–192.*

- *For further consideration of ventral lateral thalamic nuclei see pp. 310–311.*

Diagram summarizing the connections between the cerebellum, extrapyramidal motor pathways and lower motor neurons, through which the cerebellum can influence movement control at brainstem or spinal level.

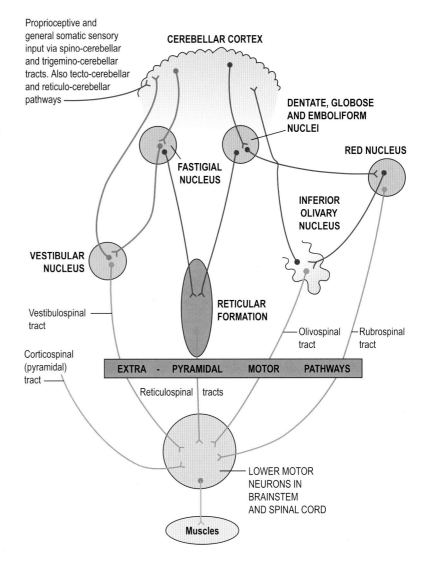

Proprioceptive and general somatic sensory input via spino-cerebellar and trigemino-cerebellar tracts. Also tecto-cerebellar and reticulo-cerebellar pathways

CEREBELLAR CORTEX

DENTATE, GLOBOSE AND EMBOLIFORM NUCLEI

RED NUCLEUS

FASTIGIAL NUCLEUS

INFERIOR OLIVARY NUCLEUS

VESTIBULAR NUCLEUS

RETICULAR FORMATION

Vestibulospinal tract

Olivospinal tract

Rubrospinal tract

Corticospinal (pyramidal) tract

EXTRA - PYRAMIDAL MOTOR PATHWAYS

Reticulospinal tracts

LOWER MOTOR NEURONS IN BRAINSTEM AND SPINAL CORD

Muscles

Diagram summarizing the connections through which the cerebellum can influence movement via an effect on the cerebral cortex.

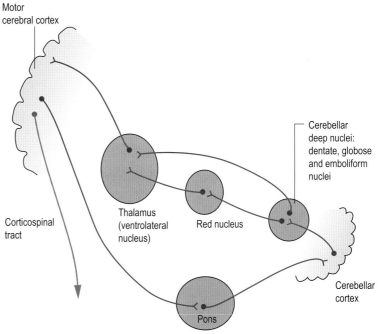

Motor cerebral cortex

Cerebellar deep nuclei: dentate, globose and emboliform nuclei

Corticospinal tract

Thalamus (ventrolateral nucleus)

Red nucleus

Cerebellar cortex

Pons

Figures 25.4 and 25.5 The relationship between brainstem and cerebellum.

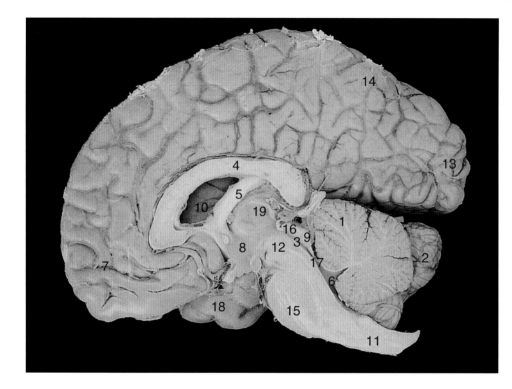

Fig. 25.4
A sagittal section of the brain to show the position and relationships of the cerebellum. ×0.75

1 Arbor vitae
2 Cerebellum
3 Cerebral aqueduct
4 Corpus callosum
5 Fornix
6 Fourth ventricle
7 Frontal lobe
8 Hypothalamus
9 Inferior colliculus
10 Lateral ventricle
11 Medulla oblongata
12 Midbrain
13 Occipital lobe
14 Parietal lobe
15 Pons
16 Superior colliculus
17 Superior medullary velum
18 Temporal lobe
19 Thalamus

Fig. 25.5
Sagittal section of brainstem showing some structures with cerebellar connections. Myelin stain. ×2.5

1 Cerebellum
2 Choroid plexus
3 Corticospinal tract
4 Fourth ventricle
5 Inferior colliculus
6 Inferior olivary nucleus
7 Medulla oblongata
8 Midbrain
9 Pons
10 Superior cerebellar peduncle
11 Superior colliculus
12 Thalamus

CAM

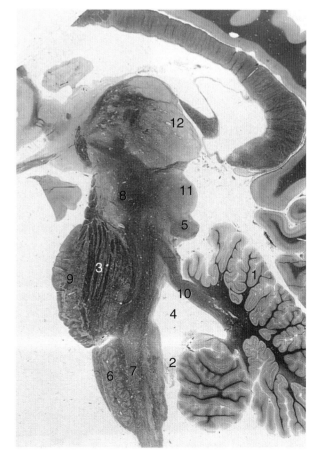

Figures 25.6–25.9 The inferior and middle cerebellar peduncles and their connections.

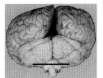

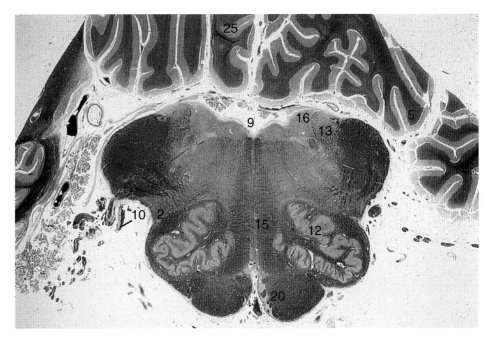

Fig. 25.6
Transverse section of medulla and cerebellum showing vestibular nuclei and inferior cerebellar peduncle. Myelin stain and counterstain. ×3 See p. 306 for key.

MHMS

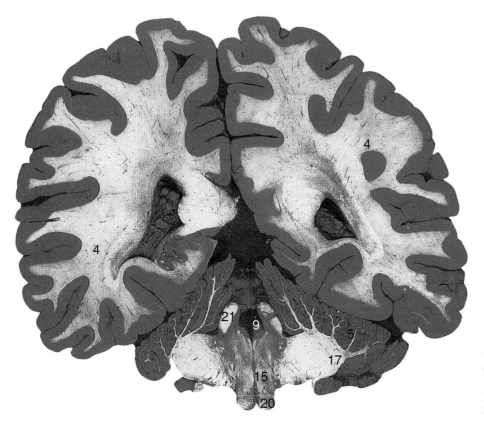

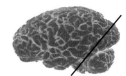

Fig. 25.7
A coronal thick slice of the cerebral hemispheres and brainstem to show the three cerebellar peduncles. Mulligan stain. ×0.88 See p. 306 for key.

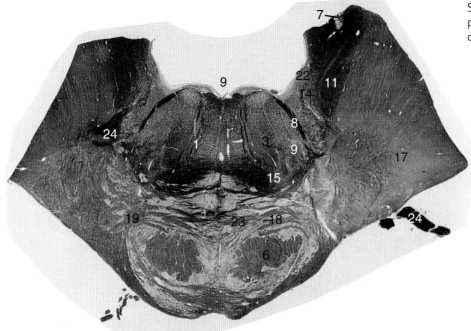
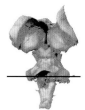

Fig. 25.8
Section of lower pons showing pontocerebellar fibers entering the middle cerebellar peduncle. Weigert stain. ×3

1 Abducens nerve (VI)
2 Anterior (ventral) spinocerebellar tract
3 Central tegmental tract
4 Cerebral hemispheres
5 Cerebellar hemisphere
6 Corticospinal tract
7 Dentate nucleus
8 Facial nerve (VII)
9 Fourth ventricle
10 Glossopharyngeal nerve (IX)
11 Inferior cerebellar peduncle
12 Inferior olivary nucleus
13 Inferior vestibular nucleus
14 Lateral vestibular nucleus
15 Medial lemniscus
16 Medial vestibular nucleus
17 Middle cerebellar peduncle
18 Pontine nuclei (circled)
19 Pontocerebellar fibers
20 Pyramid (of medulla oblongata)
21 Superior cerebellar peduncle
22 Superior vestibular nucleus
23 Transverse pontine fibers
24 Trigeminal nerve (V)
25 Vermis

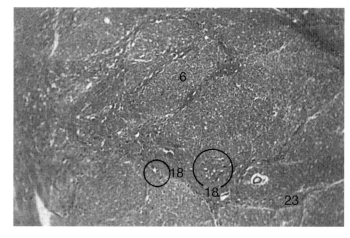

Fig. 25.9
A histological section of the pontine nuclei and transverse pontine (pontocerebellar) fibers. Luxol fast blue and cresyl violet stain. ×63
CXWMS

Figures 25.10–25.13 Sections to show the inferior olivary nucleus and some connecting structures.

Fig. 25.10
A coronal section through the brain, cutting the medulla oblongata through the middle of the inferior olivary nucleus. Mulligan stain. ×0.9

1 Central tegmental tract
2 Cerebellum
3 Dentate nucleus
4 Fourth ventricle
5 Hilum of inferior olivary nucleus
6 Inferior cerebellar peduncle
7 Inferior olivary nucleus
8 Medial accessory olivary nucleus
9 Medial lemniscus
10 Medulla oblongata
11 Occipital lobe
12 Olive
13 Pyramid

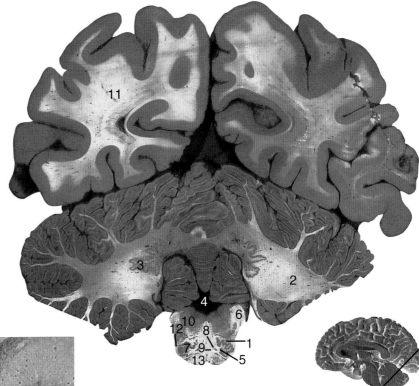

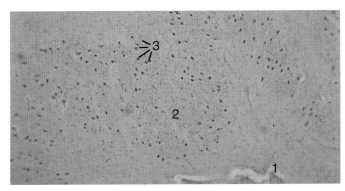

Fig. 25.11
An histological section to show the afferent and efferent fibers of the inferior olivary nucleus. Luxol fast blue stain. ×65

1 Afferent fibers
2 Efferent fibers
3 Inferior olivary nucleus

CXWMS

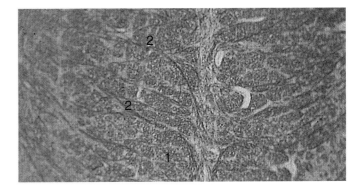

Fig. 25.12
An histological section to show the cellular organization of part of the inferior olivary nucleus. Cresyl violet stain. ×80

1 Blood vessel
2 Inferior olivary nucleus
3 Neuronal cell bodies

Fig. 25.13
A paraffin wax section to show olivocerebellar efferent fibers intersecting with the medial lemniscus. Luxol fast blue stain. ×100

1 Medial lemniscus
2 Olivocerebellar fibers

Figures 25.14–25.17 The pathway from the cerebellum through the superior cerebellar peduncle to the red nucleus.

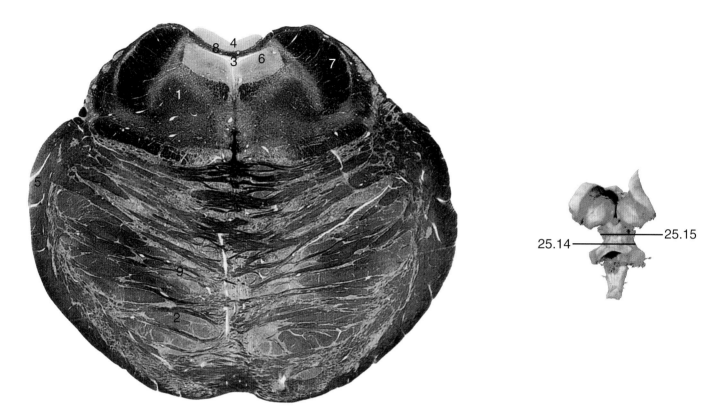

Fig. 25.14
A transverse section of pons passing through the superior and middle cerebellar peduncles. Weigert stain. ×4.2

1 Central tegmental tract
2 Corticospinal fibers
3 Fourth ventricle
4 Lingula of cerebellum
5 Middle cerebellar peduncle
6 Periaqueductal gray matter
7 Superior cerebellar peduncle
8 Superior medullary velum
9 Transverse pontine fiber

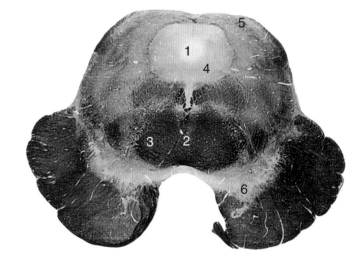

Fig. 25.15
A transverse section of the midbrain showing the decussation of the superior cerebellar peduncle. Weigert stain. ×2.7

1 Cerebral aqueduct
2 Decussating fibers
3 Decussation of the superior cerebellar peduncle
4 Periaqueductal gray matter
5 Inferior colliculus
6 Substantia nigra

Fig. 25.16
A high magnification photomicrograph of decussating fibers from the decussation of the superior cerebellar peduncle. Luxol fast blue and cresyl violet stain. ×120

1 Decussating fibers
2 Neuroglial cells

CXWMS

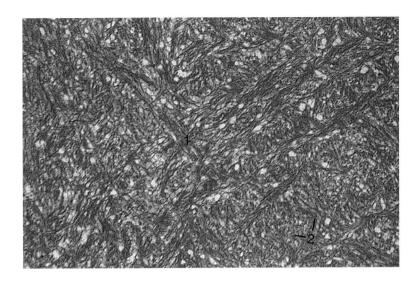

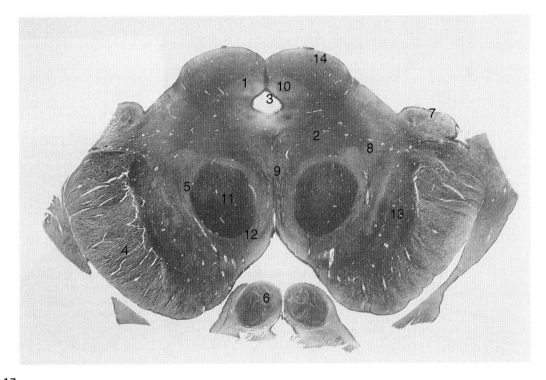

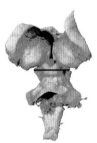

Fig. 25.17
A transverse section through the midbrain to show the red nucleus, dentatorubrothalamic fibers (from superior cerebellar peduncle) and the rubrospinal and central tegmental tracts. Luxol fast blue and acid fuchsin stain. ×2.85

1 Central gray matter	**6** Mamillary body	**11** Red nucleus
2 Central tegmental tract	**7** Medial geniculate body	**12** Rubrospinal tract
3 Cerebral aqueduct	**8** Medial lemniscus	**13** Substantia nigra
4 Crus cerebri	**9** Oculomotor nucleus	**14** Superior colliculus
5 Dentatorubrothalamic tract	**10** Periaqueductal gray matter	

Summary

1. The cerebellum exerts unconscious control over complex movements.
2. The cerebellum is connected to sensory pathways, to the brainstem and to the motor cortex.
3. The cerebellum has no direct connections to lower motor neurons.
4. The cerebellum coordinates movement by interacting with the motor cortex and with motor control centers in the brainstem.
5. Most cerebellar pathways are uncrossed, so that cerebellar disease usually impairs movements on the same side of the body as the lesion.

The Thalamus in Movement Control

The ventral lateral and ventral anterior nuclei of the thalamus are known as the motor thalamic nuclei because they are components of several motor pathways. The ventral lateral nucleus receives afferent tracts from the cerebellum, either directly or via the red nucleus, from the substantia nigra, the globus pallidus and the corpus striatum. It projects efferent fibers to motor and premotor areas of the frontal lobe cortex. The ventral anterior nucleus is an intermediary between the basal ganglia and the motor cortex. It receives pathways from the globus pallidus and substantia nigra and has afferent and

efferent connections with the premotor and supplementary motor cortex of the frontal lobe. Thus, the motor thalamic nuclei link subcortical structures having motor functions to the motor cortex. Through these links the subcortical structures can affect movement by influencing cortical function.

Dentatothalamic and rubrothalamic fibers adjacent to the red nucleus form field H of Forel or the prerubral area. They join with fibers from the globus pallidus to the thalamus to form the thalamic fasciculus, or field H1 of Forel.

Figures 25.18–25.24 Preparations to demonstrate structures in the basal ganglia and diencephalon, which are involved in movement control.

Figures 25.18 and 25.19 Histological sections to illustrate the parts of the thalamus involved in movement control.

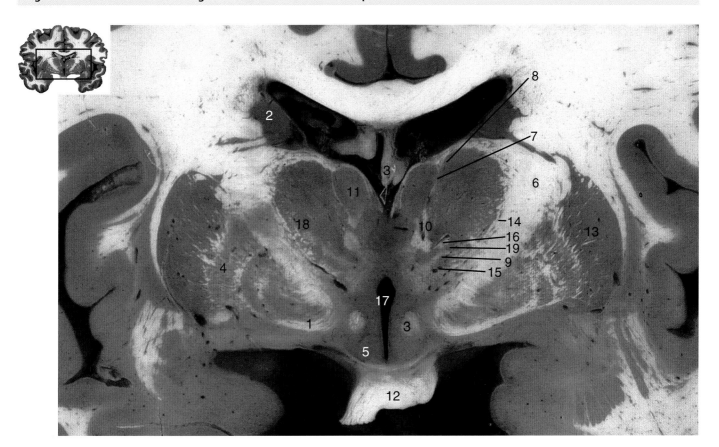

Fig. 25.18
A coronal thick slice through the thalamus and adjacent forebrain structures to show the subthalamus and the ventral lateral nucleus of the thalamus. Mulligan stain. ×2.3

1 Ansa lenticularis	9 Lenticular fasciculus or field H2 of Forel	17 Third ventricle
2 Caudate nucleus	10 Mamillothalamic tract	18 Ventral lateral thalamic nucleus
3 Fornix	11 Medial thalamic nuclei	19 Zona incerta
4 Globus pallidus	12 Optic chiasma	
5 Hypothalamus	13 Putamen	● *Auguste H. Forel (1848–1931) was a*
6 Internal capsule	14 Reticular nuclei of thalamus	*Swiss neurophysiologist who*
7 Internal medullary lamina	15 Subthalamic nucleus	*described the areas in the subthalamus*
8 Lateral dorsal thalamic nucleus	16 Thalamic fasciculus (field H1 of Forel)	*that bear his name.*

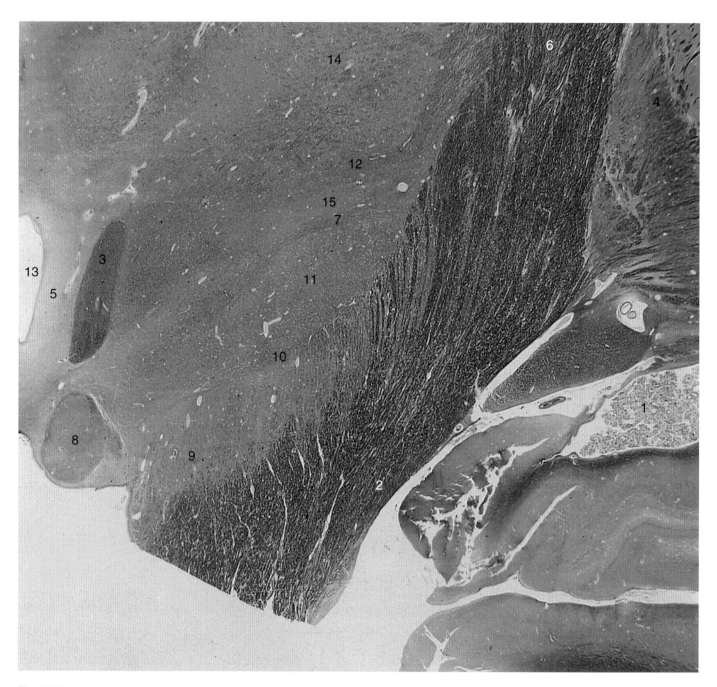

Fig. 25.19
Part of a coronal section through the diencephalon to illustrate the detailed anatomy of the subthalamic area.
Light green and solochrome cyanin stain. ×7.8

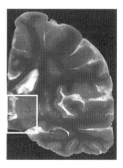

1	Choroid plexus	**9**	Substantia nigra
2	Crus cerebri	**10**	Subthalamic fasciculus
3	Fornix	**11**	Subthalamic nucleus
4	Globus pallidus	**12**	Thalamic fasciculus
5	Hypothalamus	**13**	Third ventricle
6	Internal capsule	**14**	Ventral lateral thalamic nucleus
7	Lenticular fasciculus	**15**	Zona incerta
8	Mamillary body		

The Basal Ganglia in Movement Control

These are a group of nuclei that interact with each other and with the ventral thalamic nuclei and with motor and premotor areas of the frontal lobe cortex to facilitate smooth, controlled, voluntary movement by acting at cortical level.

The basal ganglia comprise the caudate nucleus, lentiform nucleus, subthalamic nucleus and substantia nigra. The lentiform nucleus has two parts, the putamen and the globus pallidus. Connecting fibers crossing the internal capsule link the caudate nucleus and putamen together as the corpus striatum. Connections from the globus pallidus to the thalamus run via the pallidothalamic tracts (ansa lenticularis, lenticular fasciculus). Connecting pathways through the basal ganglia and thalamus form a looplike circuit. This loop acts as a feedback system through which the basal ganglia can facilitate movements in progress and eliminate unwanted movements, specially in habitual and postural movements, by interacting with the motor and premotor cortex of the frontal lobe. The structural components of the basal ganglia and their major functional connections (though not their complex three-dimensional arrangements) are illustrated in the diagrams below. There are two important additional circuits through which the corpus striatum is linked to the substantia nigra. They are known as the direct and indirect pathways. The direct pathway is a simple loop of afferent and efferent connections between the substantia nigra and the caudate nucleus and putamen. In the indirect pathway, efferent connections from the caudate nucleus and putamen pass through the external segment of the globus pallidus and subthalamic nucleus en route to the substantia nigra. Connections between the globus pallidus and the subthalamic nucleus form the subthalamic fasciculus, which contains both afferent and efferent fibers.

Electrophysiological evidence has shown that the direct pathway to the substantia nigra supports existing movement in progress while the indirect pathway suppresses unwanted movements. Lesions affecting these pathways, therefore, have different clinical consequences.

Diseases of the basal ganglia mainly affect the motor function on the contralateral side of the body. Abnormal inhibition of movement may be described as akinesia, such as in Parkinson's disease. Abnormal movements are known as dyskinesia. Such movements, when excessive, are described as hyperkinetic, as in Huntington's disease. The unwanted movements may be repetitive (tremor), writhing (athetoid) or jerky (chorea).

Lesions in the "direct pathway" reduce muscle tone and may lead to akinesia, while lesions in the "indirect pathway" are associated with dyskinesia.

A variety of transmitter substances have been identified and localized in the basal ganglia. In some cases, their functions are well understood. As in other parts of the central nervous system, glutamate is the major excitatory transmitter and GABA the main inhibitory transmitter. Dopamine is important as the main efferent transmitter from the substantia nigra and can be both excitatory and inhibitory. Acetylcholine, nitric oxide, substance P, enkephalins, dynorphine and neuropeptide Y have also been identified but their functions are unclear. Specific staining techniques have shown that they often colocalize in the same cells as the major transmitters.

- *The substantia nigra is unpigmented at birth.*

- *In Huntington's disease, there is degeneration of cells in the striatum projecting to the external segment of the globus pallidus. The GABA-ergic cells are particularly affected. It is a fatal hereditary disease caused by an autosomal dominant gene, causing involuntary movements and dementia.*

- *Parkinson's disease affects both direct and indirect pathways so that patients may show both akinesia and dyskinesia. It is a disease of the elderly in which cell degeneration in the substantia nigra leads to loss of dopaminergic pathways to the corpus striatum.*

- *L-DOPA is one of the drugs effective in the treatment of Parkinson's disease. It can be converted to dopamine and so replace that lost from the substantia nigra.*

A diagram to show the caudate nucleus, lentiform nucleus, subthalamic nucleus and substantia nigra, and some of their anatomical relationships.

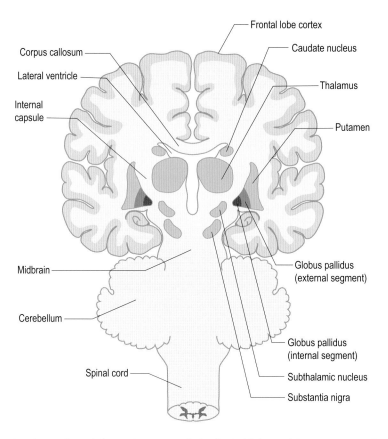

The "feedback loop" between the basal ganglia and the motor cortex of the frontal lobe, and its neurotransmitters.

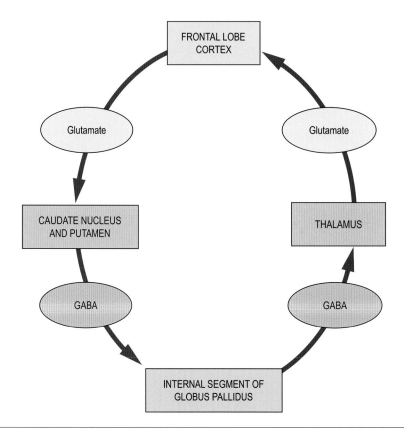

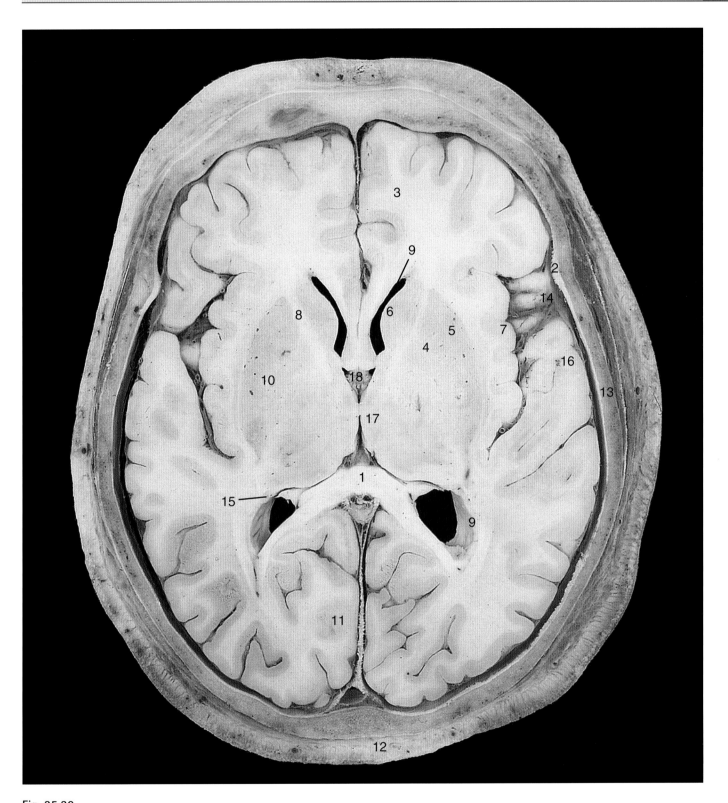

Fig. 25.20
A horizontal section through the head passing through the caudate and lentiform nuclei. ×1.2

1 Corpus callosum	**7** Insula	**13** Skull (parietal bone)
2 Dura mater	**8** Internal capsule	**14** Subarachnoid space
3 Frontal lobe	**9** Lateral ventricle	**15** Tail of caudate nucleus
4 Globus pallidus ⎱ Lentiform nucleus	**10** Lentiform nucleus	**16** Temporal lobe
5 Putamen ⎰	**11** Occipital lobe	**17** Thalamus
6 Head of caudate nucleus	**12** Scalp	**18** Third ventricle

UN

Fig. 25.21

A coronal section of the base of the forebrain to demonstrate connections between the caudate nucleus, putamen and globus pallidus. Phosphotungstic acid and hematoxylin stain. ×3.2

1	Amygdaloid nucleus	8	Extreme capsule
2	Anterior thalamic nuclei	9	Fornix
3	Claustrum	10	Globus pallidus
4	Connections between caudate nucleus and putamen	11	Hypothalamus
		12	Internal capsule
5	Connections between putamen and globus pallidus	13	Lateral ventricle
		14	Optic tract
6	Corpus callosum	15	Putamen
7	External capsule		

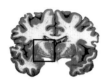

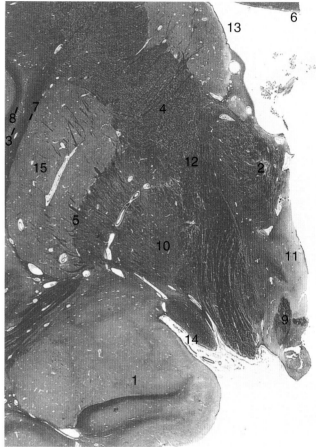

Figures 25.22 and 25.23 Sections to illustrate the structure of the substantia nigra.

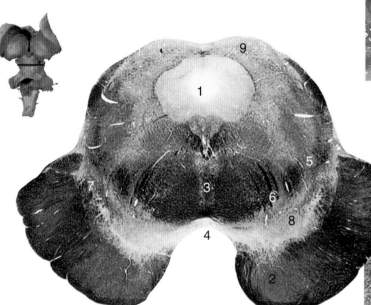

Fig. 25.22

A transverse section of midbrain showing the position of the substantia nigra and the pallidonigral and nigrostriatal connecting fibers. Weigert stain. ×2.4

1 Cerebral aqueduct
2 Crus cerebri
3 Decussation of superior cerebellar peduncle
4 Interpeduncular fossa
5 Medial lemniscus
6 Oculomotor nerve fibers
7 Pallidonigral and nigrostriatal fibers
8 Substantia nigra
9 Superior colliculus

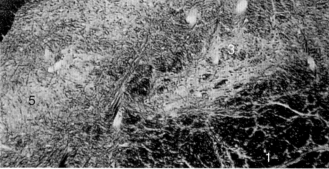

Fig. 25.23

Detail of the substantia nigra and the pallidonigral and nigrostriatal fibers. Weigert stain. ×39

1 Crus cerebri
2 Medial lemniscus
3 Pallidonigral and nigrostriatal fibers
4 Pigmented neurons of substantia nigra
5 Substantia nigra

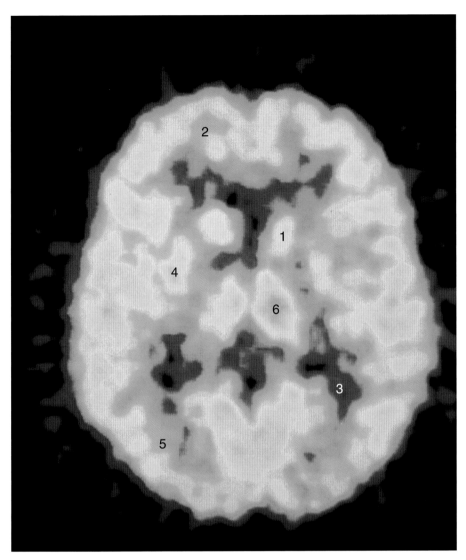

Fig. 25.24
Positron emission tomography (PET) scan showing the thalamus and corpus striatum in a horizontal section. Areas of high neural activity, mainly gray matter, are shown in yellow, and less active areas, mainly white matter, in green. Non-neural tissues and cerebrospinal fluid appear blue.

1 Caudate nucleus
2 Frontal lobe
3 Lateral ventricle
4 Lentiform nucleus
5 Occipital lobe
6 Thalamus

Wellcome Library, London

Summary

1. The thalamus links subcortical movement control centers in the cerebellum and basal ganglia to the motor cortex.
2. The motor nuclei of the thalamus are the ventral lateral nucleus and the ventral anterior nucleus.
3. The motor connections of the thalamus are part of the feedback mechanisms by which the cerebellum and basal ganglia can influence movement at the upper motor neuron level.
4. The corpus striatum, substantia nigra and subthalamic nucleus coordinate movement by interacting with the motor cortex.
5. Their function is to reinforce wanted movements and suppress unwanted movements.
6. Their most important neurotransmitters are glutamate, GABA and dopamine.
7. Anatomical lesions or abnormal transmitter levels in the basal ganglia can cause movement disorders.

26 Limbic System

The limbic system comprises a number of forebrain structures that are connected anatomically and have a common functional role in emotional aspects of behavior. It is concerned both with subjective emotional experience and with changes in bodily functions associated with emotional states. Particularly, it is involved in aggressive, submissive and sexual behavior, in pleasure, memory and learning, and in generating emotional responses, both subjective and physical, to external sensory stimuli.

These functions are based on the anatomy and connections of components of the limbic system. The limbic system contains both cortical and subcortical structures, and is connected to non-limbic, mainly sensory, parts of the cerebral cortex and to autonomic centers in the hypothalamus and brainstem.

1. Cortical Components of the Limbic System

The major cortical components of the limbic system comprise the cingulate gyrus, parahippocampal gyrus, and the hippocampus or hippocampal formation. These areas form a rim (limbus) on the medial side of the cerebral hemisphere, almost encircling the corpus callosum and diencephalon. The temporal pole, the prefrontal and orbital gyri of the frontal lobe, and the insula are also considered part of the limbic system because they are functionally related to the main limbic areas.

The cingulate gyrus is connected to the sensory association cortex and to the thalamic anterior nuclei. The parahippocampal gyrus has two-way connections with the olfactory system, blending with olfactory cortex at the uncus. It is connected to the hippocampus and to the sensory association cortex of all the sensory systems by afferent and efferent pathways. The hippocampus is the inrolled medial border of the temporal lobe. It has a specialized three-layered allocortex. It also has extensive afferent and efferent connections to the hypothalamus, especially the mamillary body, via its major tract, the fornix. The hippocampus contains large amounts of acetylcholine, dopamine, serotonin and norepinephrine (noradrenaline).

The temporal pole of the frontal lobe overlies the amygdaloid nucleus (see below). It is connected to the amygdaloid nucleus, and to the dorsomedial nuclei of the thalamus. The connections of the prefrontal cortex are

similar. The orbital gyri of the frontal lobe are part of the olfactory system (see p. 275), and have connections with the hippocampus. The insula is connected to olfactory, gustatory, auditory and somatic sensory areas of the cerebral hemisphere. These connections are both afferent and efferent, and the somatic sensory connections are bilateral.

2. Subcortical Limbic Nuclei

Subcortical components of the limbic system include the amygdaloid nucleus, the septal nuclei including the nucleus accumbens, the hypothalamus (particularly the mamillary body), the thalamus (especially the anterior and dorsomedial nuclei) and the habenular nuclei.

The amygdaloid nucleus and nucleus accumbens are anatomically part of the basal ganglia (see p. 130), though functionally they are not directly involved in movement control. However, there is a close link between movement and emotion, for example in hand gestures and facial expression. In basal ganglia disorders such as Parkinson's disease, there are both changes in mood and loss of expressive facial movements. Experimental evidence suggests that the basal ganglia may also be involved in the control of motivation and reward, and in the perception of time.

The amygdaloid nucleus lies in the temporal lobe and is anatomically continuous with the tail of the caudate nucleus. It is widely connected to the temporal lobe and frontal lobe cortex, and with the thalamus and hypothalamus. It contains many opiate receptors.

The nucleus accumbens underlies the paraterminal gyri of the frontal lobe and merges with the head of the caudate nucleus. A pathway extends from limbic areas of the cerebral cortex, via the nucleus accumbens to the substantia nigra. A dopaminergic connection also exists from the midbrain tegmentum to the nucleus accumbens. Above the nucleus accumbens lies the septum pellucidum, containing small septal nuclei. All are linked to the olfactory system and to the hippocampus. The septal nuclei are also connected to the thalamus and habenular nuclei.

The hypothalamus provides a link between the limbic system and the autonomic nervous system, through which physiological changes, such as an altered heartbeat, accompany emotional states. A further link between the limbic system and autonomic pathways is via the habenular nuclei, which link the limbic system to the reticular formation of the brainstem (see p. 326).

3. Connecting Tracts of the Limbic System

One important connecting pathway forms a circuit known as the Papez circuit.

The majority of the connections between components of the limbic system carry both efferent and afferent fibers, so there is no obligatory starting point for neural activity in the limbic system. There are many opportunities for interaction between cortical and subcortical parts. Clinical and imaging studies reveal complex interconnections between the cortical and subcortical parts of the limbic system. Detailed anatomical pathways are incompletely understood, but some major tracts are well defined.

The important limbic tracts are the fornix, between the hippocampus and the hypothalamus; the mamillothalamic tract, between the mamillary body and anterior thalamus; the cingulum, underlying the cingulate gyrus; and the stria terminalis, carrying amygdaloid efferent fibers and joining the medial forebrain bundle, which is the main longitudinal pathway of the hypothalamus.

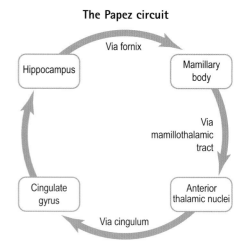

The Papez circuit

- *The name "Ammon's horn" sometimes given to the hippocampal formation in a coronal section refers to its resemblance to a ram's horn. Ammon was a ram-headed ancient Egyptian god. When viewed from above, the hippocampal formation is also named because of an imagined resemblance to a seahorse (hippocampus).*

- *In Alzheimer's disease, there is extensive cellular degeneration, especially in the hippocampus. Loss of the hippocampal formation by disease or injury causes severe anterograde amnesia.*

- *Caffeine stimulates neurons in the hippocampus to develop additional cellular processes.*

- *Stimulation of the septal area in conscious patients produces euphoria.*

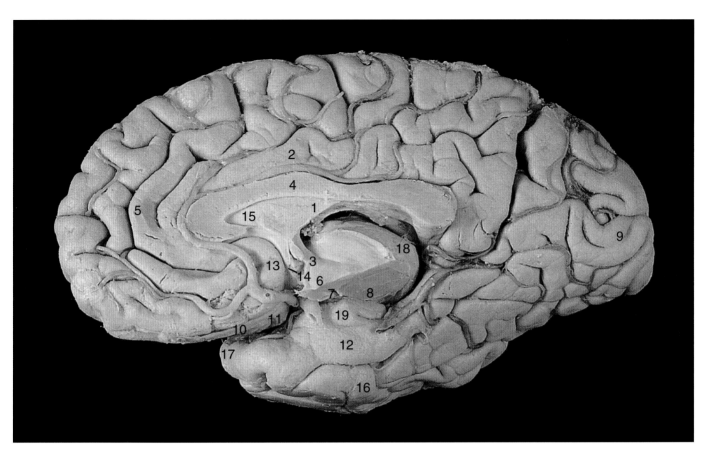

Fig. 26.1
The medial side of the brain with the brainstem sectioned through the midbrain to illustrate the components of the limbic system. ×0.9

1 Body of fornix	**8** Midbrain	**14** Paraterminal gyrus
2 Cingulate gyrus	**9** Occipital lobe	**15** Septum pellucidum
3 Column of fornix	**10** Olfactory tract	**16** Temporal lobe
4 Corpus callosum	**11** Orbital gyri	**17** Temporal pole
5 Frontal lobe	**12** Parahippocampal gyrus	**18** Thalamus
6 Hypothalamus	**13** Paraolfactory gyrus	**19** Uncus
7 Mamillary body		

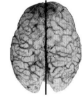

● *Both physical pain and emotional distress, such as social rejection, stimulate activity in the prefrontal cortex and the anterior part of the cingulate gyrus.*

● *The hippocampus has a very complex structure of fibrous and cellular layers. The different regions have different names. At its rostral end the hippocampus widens into the pes hippocampi.*

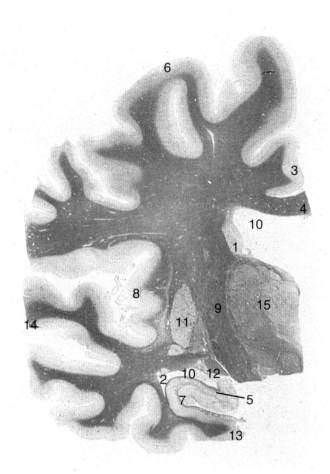

Fig. 26.2
A coronal section of a cerebral hemisphere and diencephalon showing the parahippocampal gyrus and the hippocampus. Solochrome cyanin and nuclear fast red stain. ×1.1

1 Caudate nucleus (head)
2 Caudate nucleus (tail)
3 Cingulate gyrus
4 Corpus callosum
5 Fimbria of fornix
6 Frontal lobe
7 Hippocampus
8 Insula
9 Internal capsule
10 Lateral ventricle
11 Lentiform nucleus
12 Optic tract
13 Parahippocampal gyrus
14 Temporal lobe
15 Thalamus

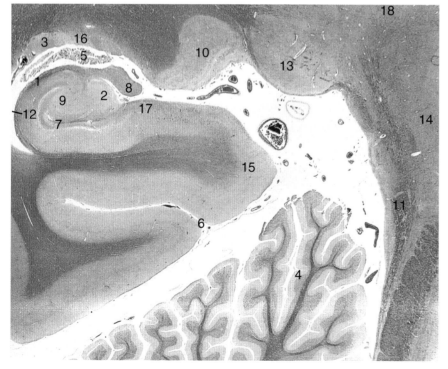

Fig. 26.3
A longitudinal section through the rostral end of the brainstem and the medial border of the temporal lobe showing the parts and relationships of the hippocampus (hippocampal formation). Solochrome cyanin and nuclear fast red stain. ×5.5

1 Alveus of hippocampus
2 Ammon's horn of hippocampus
3 Caudate nucleus
4 Cerebellum
5 Choroid plexus of the lateral ventricle
6 Collateral sulcus
7 Dentate gyrus of hippocampus
8 Fimbria of fornix
9 Hippocampus (hippocampal formation)
10 Lateral geniculate body
11 Lateral lemniscus
12 Lateral ventricle
13 Medial geniculate body
14 Midbrain
15 Parahippocampal gyrus
16 Stria terminalis
17 Subiculum of hippocampus
18 Thalamus

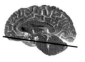

Figures 26.4–26.6 Histological sections illustrating the structure of the dentate gyrus and Ammon's horn.

Fig. 26.4
A section through the pes hippocampi showing the dentate gyrus and Ammon's horn. Cresyl violet stain. ×7.5

1 Alveus (nerve fiber layer)
2 Ammon's horn (pyramidal cells)
3 Choroid plexus of the lateral ventricle
4 Dentate gyrus (granular cells)
5 Lateral ventricle
6 Subiculum

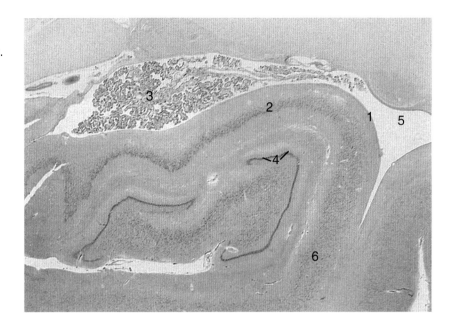

Fig. 26.5
A section showing the granular cells of the dentate gyrus. Cresyl violet stain. ×102

1 Granular layer
2 Molecular layer
3 Polymorphic cell layer   CAM

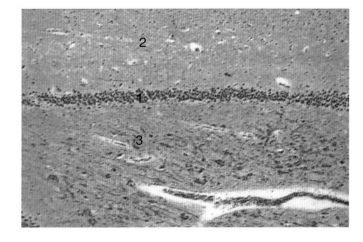

Fig. 26.6
A section showing the pyramidal cells of Ammon's horn. Cresyl violet stain. ×257

1 Nerve fibers of alveus
2 Pyramidal neurons   CAM

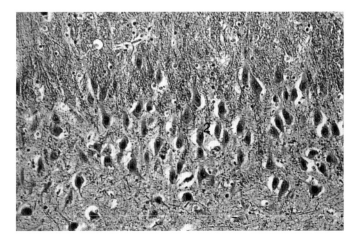

● *The indusium griseum is a thin layer of gray matter on the superior surface of the corpus callosum that is continuous with the dentate gyrus of the hippocampus.*

Figures 26.7 and 26.8 Histological sections showing the amygdaloid nucleus.

Fig. 26.7
A coronal section through one cerebral hemisphere showing the position and relationships of the amygdaloid nucleus. Carmine stain. ×.98

1 Amygdaloid nucleus	8 Frontal operculum
2 Arachnoid mater	9 Hypothalamus
3 Caudate nucleus	10 Insula
4 Cingulate gyrus	11 Internal capsule
5 Cingulum	12 Lentiform nucleus
6 Corpus callosum	13 Temporal lobe
7 Frontal lobe	14 Temporal operculum

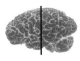

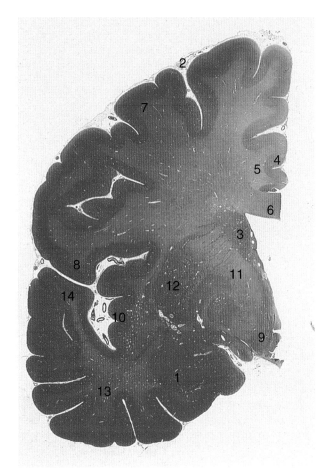

The amygdaloid nucleus is not a single nucleus but a complex consisting of several nuclei with different connections. The medial or corticomedial nuclei have olfactory connections. The lateral basal or basolateral nuclei have links to the hippocampus and indirectly to the cingulate gyrus and the orbital cortex of the frontal lobe. Left and right amygdaloid nuclei connect via the anterior commissure.

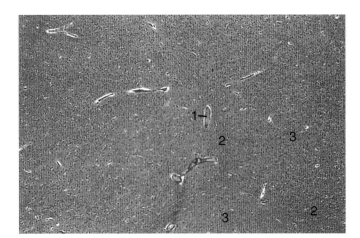

Fig. 26.8
A medium-power photomicrograph of the amygdaloid nucleus showing the separation of individual nuclei within it by nerve fiber bundles. Phosphotungstic acid and hematoxylin stain. ×25

1 Blood vessel	3 Nucleus
2 Fiber bundle	

Fig. 26.9
Coronal fMRI scan showing bilateral amygdala responses (left stronger than right) to the presentation of fearful faces and voices.

1 Insula
2 Lateral ventricle
3 Left amygdala
4 Lentiform nucleus
5 Right amygdala
6 Temporal lobe

Dr. J. S. Morris IN

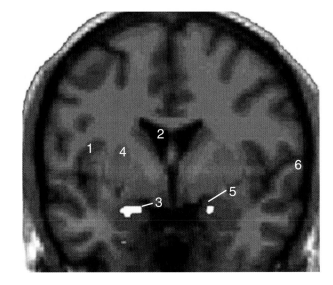

● *Porpoises have an extremely reduced or absent sense of smell and the corticomedial portion of their amygdaloid nucleus is small.*

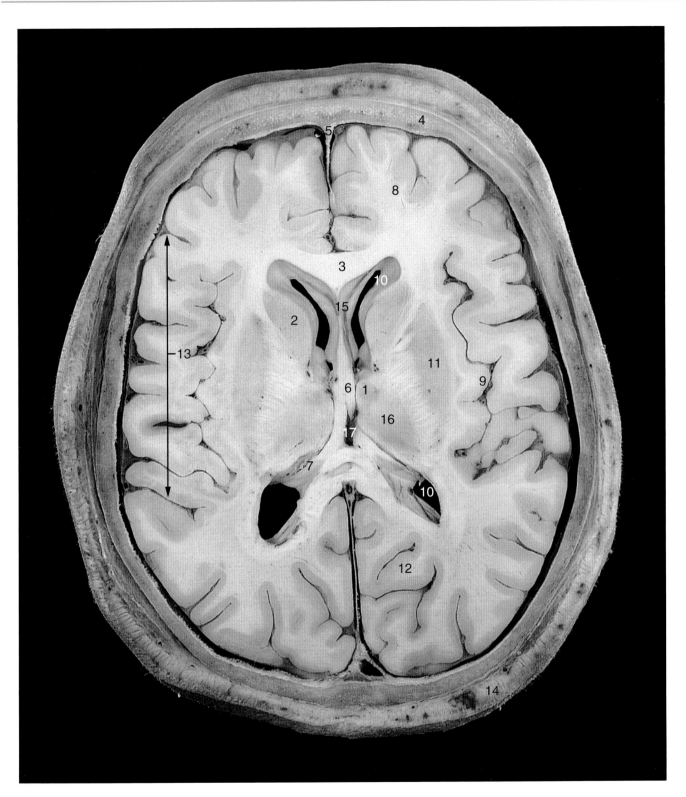

Fig. 26.10
Horizontal section of the brain *in situ* showing the anterior thalamus and the fornix. ×1

1 Anterior thalamus (thalamic nuclei)
2 Caudate nucleus
3 Corpus callosum
4 Cranium
5 Falx cerebri
6 Fornix (body)

7 Fornix (crus)
8 Frontal lobe
9 Insula
10 Lateral ventricle
11 Lentiform nucleus
12 Occipital lobe

13 Parietal operculum
14 Scalp
15 Septum pellucidum
16 Thalamus
17 Third ventricle

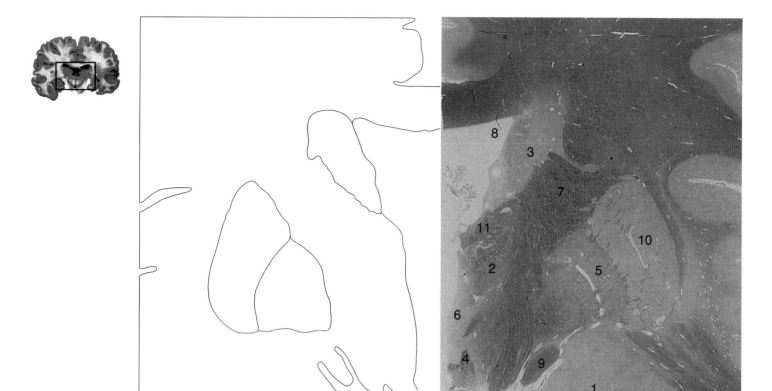

Fig. 26.11

Part of a coronal section through the forebrain at the level of the interventricular foramen to show the anterior thalamic nucleus, amygdaloid nucleus, stria terminalis and the fornix passing through the hypothalamus. Weil stain. ×1.8

1 Amygdaloid nucleus	**5** Globus pallidus	**9** Optic tract
2 Anterior thalamic nucleus	**6** Hypothalamus	**10** Putamen
3 Caudate nucleus (head)	**7** Internal capsule	**11** Stria terminalis
4 Column of fornix	**8** Lateral ventricle	

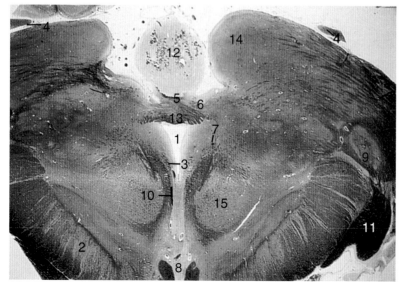

Fig. 26.12

A coronal section of the caudal end of the diencephalon showing the habenular nucleus and associated tracts. ×2.1

1 Cerebral aqueduct becoming third ventricle
2 Crus cerebri
3 Dorsal longitudinal fasciculus
4 Fornix
5 Habenular commissure
6 Habenular nucleus
7 Habenulopeduncular tract or
 fasciculus retroflexus
8 Hypothalamus
9 Lateral geniculate body
10 Mamillotegmental tract
11 Optic tract
12 Pineal organ
13 Posterior commissure
14 Pulvinar of thalamus
15 Red nucleus

MHMS

Figures 26.13 and 26.14 Histological preparations illustrating the anatomy of the septal nuclei and nucleus accumbens.

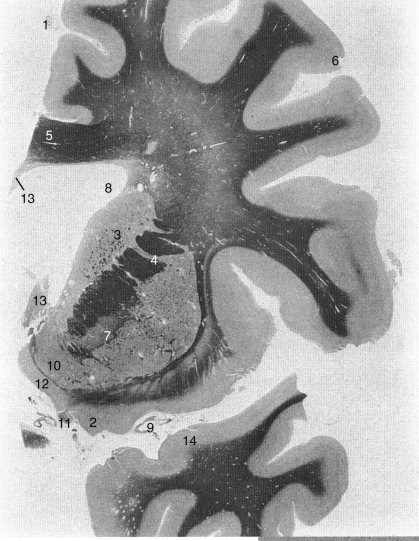

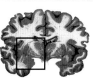

Fig. 26.13
A histological section through one cerebral hemisphere passing through the paraterminal gyrus showing the underlying nucleus accumbens (septi). Solochrome cyanin and nuclear fast red stain. ×2.5

1 Anterior cerebral artery
2 Anterior perforated substance
3 Caudate nucleus
4 Continuity of caudate nucleus with putamen
5 Corpus callosum
6 Frontal lobe
7 Globus pallidus
8 Lateral ventricle
9 Middle cerebral artery
10 Nucleus accumbens (septi)
11 Olfactory tract
12 Paraterminal gyrus
13 Septum pellucidum
14 Temporal lobe

Fig. 26.14
A vertical histological section through the septum pellucidum showing how it is formed by fusion of the septa pellucida of the two cerebral hemispheres. Cresyl violet stain. ×50

1 Blood vessel
2 Ependyma
3 Fusion of left and right septa pellucida
4 Septum pellucidum

Figures 26.15–26.18 Dissections and histological preparations showing the fornix, mamillary body, mamillothalamic tract, stria terminalis and medial forebrain bundle.

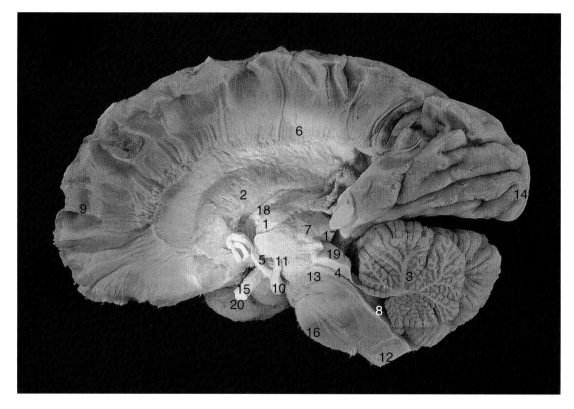

Fig. 26.15

Brain dissected from the medial side to show the fornix, mamillothalamic tract and stria terminalis. The mamillothalamic tract and the columns of the fornix are embedded in the hypothalamus. ×0.84

1 Anterior thalamic nuclei	**8** Fourth ventricle	**15** Optic nerve
2 Caudate nucleus	**9** Frontal lobe	**16** Pons
3 Cerebellum	**10** Mamillary body	**17** Pulvinar of thalamus
4 Cerebral aqueduct	**11** Mamillothalamic tract	**18** Stria terminalis
5 Column of fornix	**12** Medulla oblongata	**19** Tectum
6 Corona radiata	**13** Midbrain	**20** Temporal lobe
7 Dorsomedial thalamic nucleus	**14** Occipital lobe	

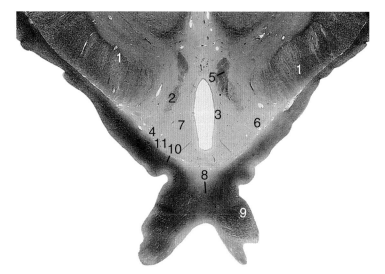

Fig. 26.16

A coronal section of the hypothalamus showing the columns of the fornix, mamillothalamic tract and medial forebrain bundle. Weigert stain ×2.75

1 Cerebral peduncle
2 Column of fornix
3 Hypothalamus
4 Lateral hypothalamic area
5 Mamillothalamic tract
6 Medial forebrain bundle
7 Medial hypothalamic area
8 Optic chiasma
9 Optic nerve
10 Optic tract
11 Supraoptic nucleus of hypothalamus

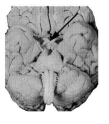

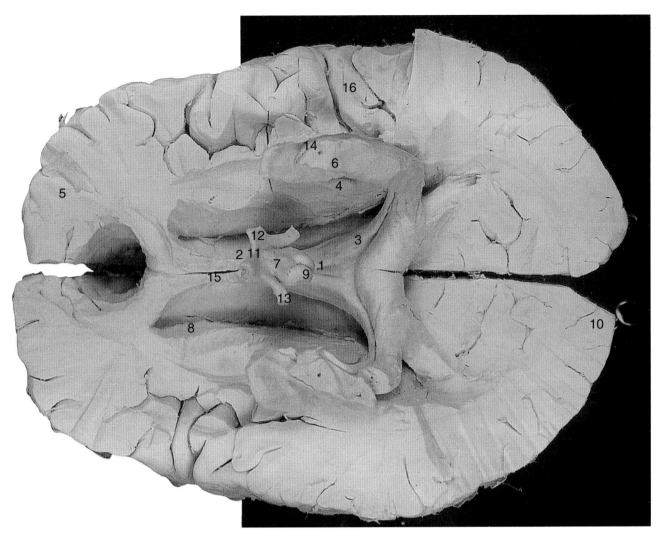

Fig. 26.17
The brain viewed from below and dissected to show the hippocampus and the fimbria, crura and body of the fornix. ×1.1

1 Body of fornix
2 Corpus callosum
3 Crus of fornix
4 Fimbria of fornix
5 Frontal lobe
6 Hippocampus
7 Hypothalamus
8 Lateral ventricle
9 Mamillary body
10 Occipital lobe
11 Optic chiasma
12 Optic nerve
13 Optic tract
14 Parahippocampal gyrus
15 Septum pellucidum
16 Temporal lobe

OXF

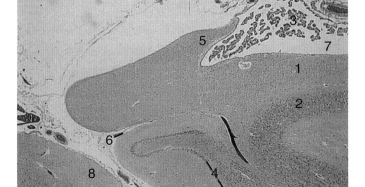

Fig. 26.18
Histological section of the hippocampus showing the alveus, a superficial layer of nerve fibers and the fimbria of the fornix, into which these fibers aggregate. Cresyl violet stain. ×25

1 Alveus
2 Ammon's horn
3 Choroid plexus of lateral ventricle
4 Dentate gyrus
5 Fimbria
6 Hippocampal sulcus
7 Lateral ventricle
8 Subiculum

CAM

● *The fornix contains approximately one million fibers.*

● *The medial forebrain bundle is poorly myelinated and hence is difficult to see in histological sections.*

Summary

1. The limbic system is largely located in the forebrain, and is involved in complex behavior such as emotion and memory.
2. It comprises specialized areas of cerebral cortex, subcortical nuclei and the tracts connecting them.
3. Some brain regions that are parts of the limbic system are also functionally or anatomically parts of other systems, e.g. the basal ganglia or the autonomic nervous system and the endocrine system.
4. Limbic structures are widely connected to sensory and motor cortex. These connections involve the limbic system in both subjective (feeling) and objective (action or physiological change) aspects of emotional expression.

27 Guide for Student Examination of the Brain

The student can perform a simple examination of the formalin and alcohol-fixed brain by following the sequence given in Figures 27.1–27.9. Protective gloves and clothing should be worn during this study.

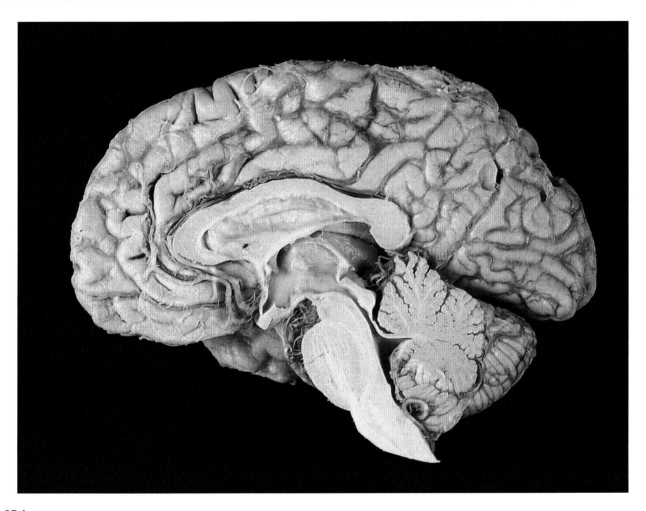

Fig. 27.1
Make a sagittal cut through the brain and identify the following structures. ×0.9

1 Cerebellum
2 Corpus callosum
3 Gyrus
4 Fourth ventricle
5 Frontal lobe
6 Hypothalamus
7 Inferior colliculus
8 Infundibulum
9 Interventricular foramen

10 Mamillary body
11 Medulla oblongata
12 Midbrain
13 Occipital lobe
14 Olfactory bulb and tract
15 Optic chiasma
16 Parietal lobe
17 Pia-arachnoid membranes

18 Pineal stalk
19 Pons
20 Posterior commissure
21 Septum pellucidum
22 Sulcus
23 Superior colliculus
24 Thalamus
25 Third ventricle

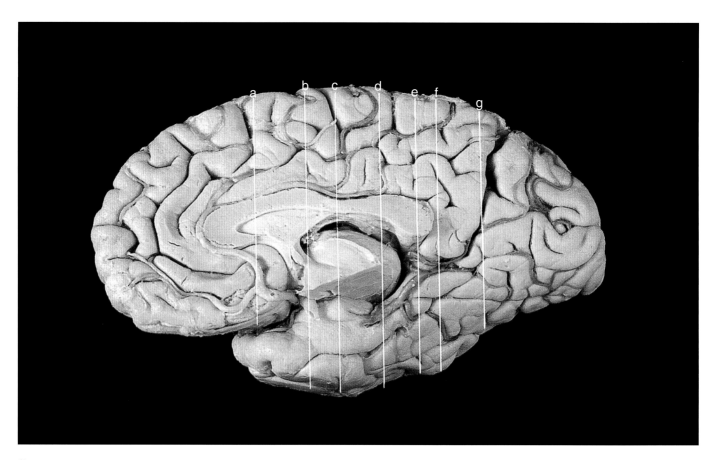

Fig. 27.2
Cut through the midbrain and remove the cerebellum and brainstem. This photograph illustrates the right hemisphere following removal of the cerebellum and brainstem. Make the incision shown at **a**. ×0.88

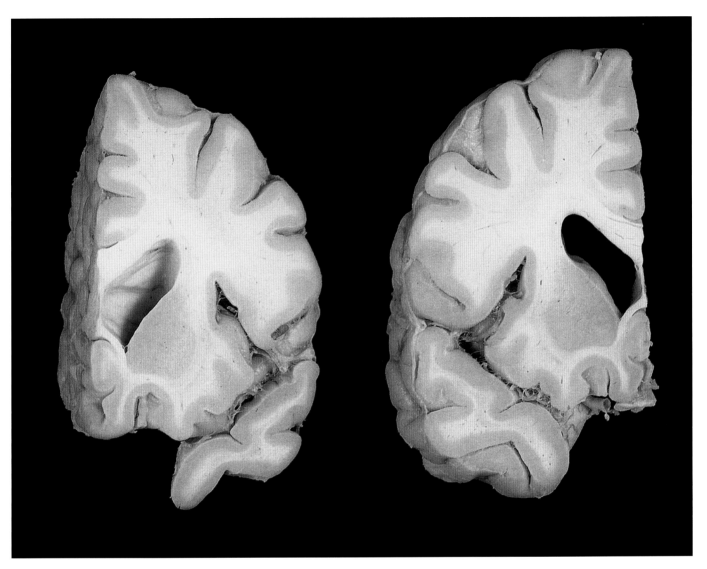

Fig. 27.3
Identify the following landmarks in the section at **a**. The frontal pole of the cerebral hemisphere is on the left. ×1.1

 1 Anterior cerebral artery
 2 Caudate nucleus
 3 Cerebral cortex
 4 Claustrum
 5 Corpus callosum
 6 External capsule
 7 Insula
 8 Lateral sulcus (with middle cerebral vessels)
 9 Lateral ventricle (anterior horn)
10 Lentiform nucleus
11 Temporal lobe
12 White matter

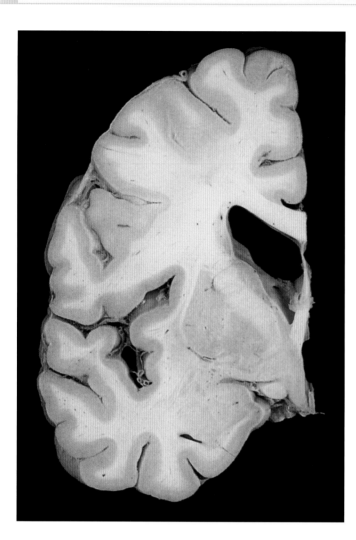

Fig. 27.4
The section cut at **b**. Identify the following structures. ×1.3

1 Amygdaloid nucleus
2 Caudate nucleus
3 Choroid plexus of lateral ventricle
4 Corpus callosum
5 External capsule
6 Insula
7 Internal capsule
8 Lateral sulcus
9 Lateral ventricle (body)
10 Lentiform nucleus
11 Optic nerve
12 Septum pellucidum
13 Temporal lobe

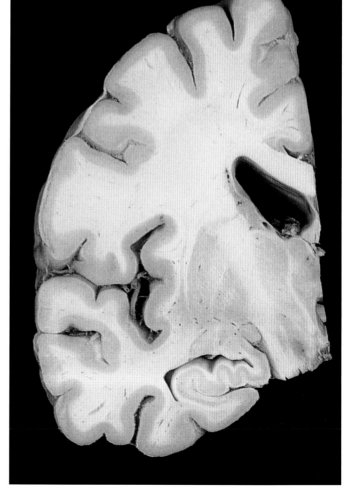

Fig. 27.5
The section cut at **c**. Identify the following landmarks. ×1.2

1 Claustrum
2 Corpus callosum
3 External capsule
4 Hippocampus
5 Hypothalamus
6 Insula
7 Internal capsule
8 Lateral ventricle (body and inferior horn)
9 Third ventricle

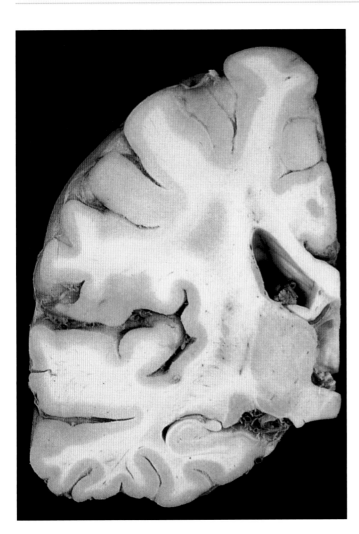

Fig. 27.6
The section cut at position **d**. The following landmarks should be identified. ×1.2

1 Corpus callosum
2 Hippocampus
3 Insula
4 Internal capsule
5 Lateral geniculate body
6 Lateral ventricle (with choroid plexus)
7 Lentiform nucleus
8 Parahippocampal gyrus
9 Thalamus

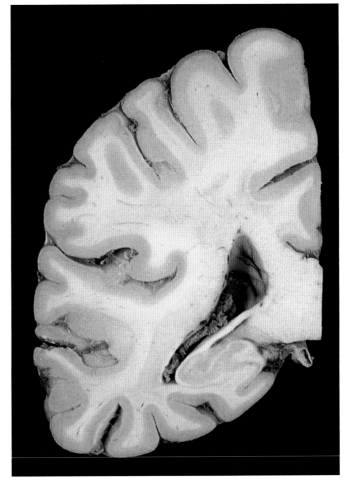

Fig. 27.7
The section cut at position **e**. The following structures should be identified. ×1.1

1 Corpus callosum (splenium)
2 Lateral ventricle (inferior and posterior horns)
3 Posterior cerebral artery
4 Temporal lobe

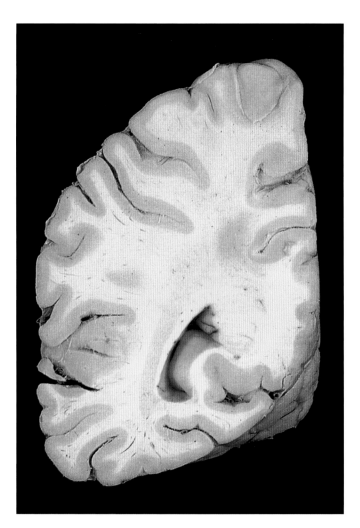

Fig. 27.8
The section cut at **f**. Identify these landmarks. ×1.2

1 Lateral ventricle (posterior horn)
2 Occipital lobe
3 Parietal lobe

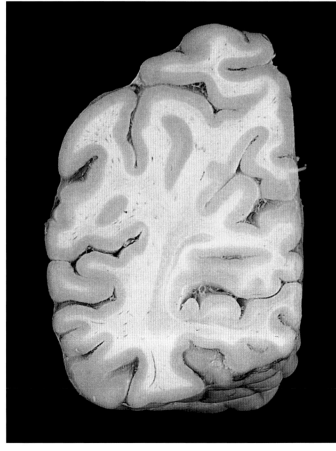

Fig. 27.9
The final section has been cut. Examine the section at **g** and identify these landmarks. ×1.4

1 Calcarine sulcus
2 Gray matter
3 Occipital lobe
4 Primary visual cortex
5 White matter

28 Student Guide to Imaging

Fig. 28.1
Examine this image and identify the following:

1 The imaging technique
2 The direction of view

Then identify:

3 Anterior cerebral artery
4 Internal carotid artery
5 Middle cerebral artery
6 Nasal cavity
7 Occipital bone
8 Petrous temporal bone

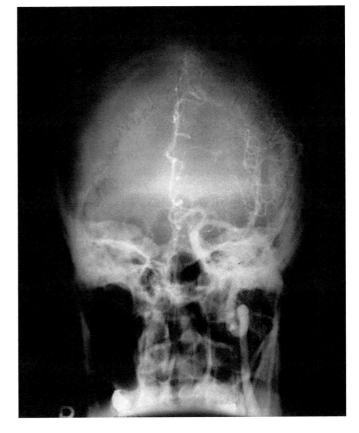

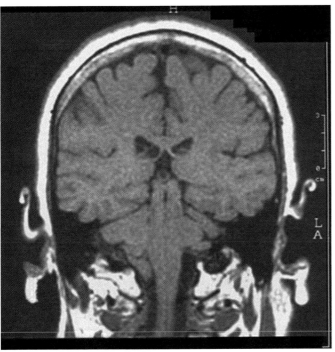

Fig. 28.2
Examine this image and identify the following:

1 The imaging technique
2 The plane of section

Then identify:

3 Cerebellum
4 Lateral ventricle
5 Medulla oblongata
6 Middle cerebellar peduncle
7 Parietal lobe
8 Spinal cord
9 Subarachnoid space
10 Superior sagittal sinus

Fig. 28.3
Examine this image and identify the following:

1 The imaging technique
2 The plane of section

Then identify:

3 Corpus striatum
4 Falx cerebri
5 Frontal lobe
6 Insula
7 Lateral ventricle
8 Midbrain
9 Temporal lobe
10 Third ventricle

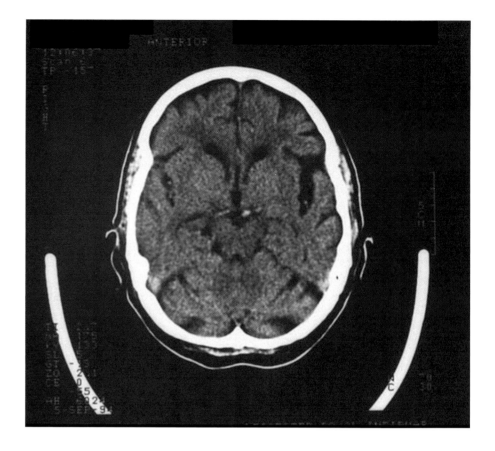

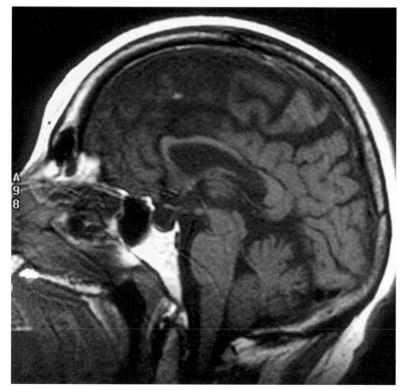

Fig. 28.4
Examine this image and identify the following:

1 The imaging technique
2 The plane of section

Then identify:

3 Body of sphenoid bone
4 Cerebellum
5 Corpus callosum
6 Frontal sinus
7 Medulla oblongata
8 Midbrain
9 Pituitary gland
10 Pons

Figs 28.1–28.4 from Dr. R. Abbott LRI

Glossary

Abducens nerve   6th cranial nerve (VI)

Accessory nerve   11th cranial nerve (XI)

Afferent   Towards (sensory if towards the central nervous system)

Agnosia   Sensory unawareness

Akinesia   Abnormal impairment of movement

Angiogram   Display of blood vessels *in vivo* for diagnostic purposes, by using contrast medium and X-rays

Apoptosis   Cell death (e.g. as part of a normal developmental process)

Arachnoid (mater)   Middle layer of meninges

Ascending tract   Central sensory pathway, usually from spinal cord to brain

Association fibers   Fibers connecting parts of the same cerebral hemisphere

Autonomic nervous system   Visceral innervation; sympathetic and parasympathetic divisions

Axon   Process of a nerve cell, usually long and generally conducts impulses away from the cell body

Basal ganglia (nuclei)   Nuclei involved in modification of motor control, the caudate and lentiform nuclei, subthalamus and the substantia nigra

Basilar artery   One of the arteries supplying the brain

"Blue slice"   Thick brain section stained with Mulligan stain; gray matter appears blue

Brainstem   Medulla, pons and midbrain (some authors include the diencephalon)

CAT or CT scan   Computed (axial) tomography: a diagnostic imaging technique

Cauda equina   "Horse's tail": the lower lumbar, sacral and coccygeal spinal nerves as they lie in the vertebral canal

Caudal   Towards the tail, or hindmost part of neuraxis

Caudate nucleus   One of the basal ganglia forming part of the corpus striatum

Cell body   Part of neuron containing nucleus

Central nervous system   Brain and spinal cord

Cerebellar hemisphere   One of two lateral components of the cerebellum

Cerebellar peduncle   Inferior, middle and superior, fiber tracts linking cerebellum and brainstem

Cerebellum   "Little brain", a dorsal outgrowth from the embryonic hindbrain

Cerebral aqueduct (of Sylvius)   Passage through midbrain, part of ventricular system

Cerebral hemisphere   One half of the cerebrum

Cerebral peduncle   One crus cerebri plus one half of the midbrain tegmentum

Cerebrospinal fluid (CSF)   Fluid in ventricles and in subarachnoid space

Cerebrum   Largest part of the brain, consists of two hemispheres

Cervical   Referring to the neck region

Chorda tympani   Part of the 7th cranial nerve (VII) (see facial nerve)

Choroid plexus   Vascular structure secreting CSF into ventricles

Circle of Willis   Anastomosis between internal carotid and basilar arteries around hypophysis

Cisterna   Expanded portion of subarachnoid space

Claustrum   Gray matter superficial to external capsule

CNS   Abbreviation for "central nervous system"

Colliculi   Parts of tectum, sensory/motor integration centers: auditory (inferior colliculi) and visual (superior colliculi)

Commissure   Connection of fibers between similar points on left and right sides of the brain

Contralateral   On the opposite side

Contrast medium   Substance introduced into the body to enhance contrast in diagnostic images

Corpus callosum   The largest commissure, connects the two cerebral hemispheres

Corpus striatum   Caudate, putamen and globus pallidus, nuclei inside cerebral hemisphere

Cortex   Superficial layer of gray matter covering the cerebrum, midbrain (colliculi) and cerebellum

Corticobulbar tract   Descending tract connecting motor cortex with motor cranial nerve nuclei

Corticospinal tract   Descending tract, from motor cortex to anterior (ventral) horn cells of the spinal cord

Cranial nerve nuclei   Collections of cells in brainstem giving rise to or receiving fibers from cranial nerves; may be sensory or motor

Cranial nerves   12 pairs of nerves arising from the brain

Crus cerebri (basis pedunculi)   Basal part of cerebral peduncle of midbrain, containing corticospinal and corticobulbar tracts

CSF   Cerebrospinal fluid

Decussation   Crossing over of fibers

Demyelination   Loss or destruction of myelin

Dendrite   Receptive process of a neuron, normally conducts impulses towards cell body

Descending tract   Central motor pathway from brain to spinal cord

Diencephalon   The posterior part of the embryonic forebrain; made up of the thalamus, hypothalamus and epithalamus of adult

Dorsal columns   Fasciculus gracilis and fasciculus cuneatus, pathways for fine touch and conscious proprioception

Dorsal root   Afferent sensory component of spinal nerve

Dura (mater)   Outermost layer of meninges

Dural venous sinuses   Large venous channels for draining blood from the brain; run in dura mater

Dyskinesia   Abnormal, unwanted movements

Effector   A neuron functioning in producing a response to a stimulus, innervating a muscle or gland

Efferent   Away from (motor if away from the central nervous system)

External capsule   White matter superficial to lentiform nucleus

Extrapyramidal motor pathways   Descending tracts (motor pathways) other than the corticospinal tract

Facial nerve   7th cranial nerve (VII) (see chorda tympani)

Falx cerebelli   Fold of dura mater between cerebellar hemispheres

Falx cerebri   Fold of dura mater between cerebral hemispheres

Fasciculus   A tract or bundle of nerve fibers

Fasciculus cuneatus   Ascending tract for conscious proprioception and discriminating touch above T6 segment of the spinal cord

Fasciculus gracilis   Ascending tract for conscious proprioception and discriminating touch below T6 segment of the spinal cord

Flocculus   Part of cerebellum

fMRI (functional MRI)   A diagnostic imaging method displaying brain function and general structure

Folium   A flat leaflike fold on the surface of the cerebellum

Foramen   An opening, aperture

Foramen of Luschka   Lateral foramen (of fourth ventricle)

Foramen of Magendie   Median foramen (of fourth ventricle)

Forebrain   Anterior division (vesicle) of embryonic brain; cerebrum and diencephalon of adult

Fornix   Archlike tract below corpus callosum

Fourth ventricle   Cavity in hindbrain, containing CSF

Frontal lobe   Part of cerebral hemisphere

Funiculus   A large aggregation of white matter in the spinal cord; may contain several tracts

Ganglion   Swelling on nerve or nerve root, contains cell bodies, e.g. dorsal root or sympathetic ganglion

Geniculate bodies   Lateral and medial parts of thalamus, relay centers on visual (lateral) and auditory (medial) pathway, respectively

Germinal matrix   Site of new cell formation in the developing cerebral hemisphere

Glial cell (neuroglial cell)   Supporting cell in central nervous system

Globus pallidus   Part of lentiform nucleus

Glossopharyngeal nerve   9th cranial nerve (IX)

Gray matter   Nervous tissue, mainly nerve cell bodies

Gyrus   A convoluted fold on a cerebral hemisphere

Hindbrain   Posterior division of the embryonic brain; pons and medulla oblongata and cerebellum of adult

Hippocampus or hippocampal formation   Specialized area of phylogenetically old cortex in floor of inferior horn of lateral ventricle, in temporal lobe; part of limbic system

Hypoglossal nerve   12th cranial nerve (XII)

Immunocytochemistry   Staining technique using specific antibodies to localize substances in cells

Innervation   Nerve supply, sensory or motor

Insula   Buried portion of cerebral hemisphere below lateral sulcus

Internal capsule   White matter between lentiform nucleus and thalamus and head of caudate nucleus

Interventricular foramen   Opening from lateral into third ventricle

Ipsilateral   On the same side

Lacunae   Irregularly shaped venous "lakes" or channels draining into the superior sagittal sinus

Lateral foramen   Foramen of Luschka, opening in roof of fourth ventricle for escape of CSF into subarachnoid space surrounding the brain

Lateral ventricle   Cavity in cerebral hemisphere

Lemniscus   A bandlike bundle of nerve fibers, e.g. medial lemniscus

Lentiform nucleus   Part of corpus striatum, composed of putamen and globus pallidus

Leptomeninges   Arachnoid and pia mater

Limbic system   Part of brain associated with emotional behavior

Lower motor neurons   Anterior horn cells and their axons of spinal cord, or cell in motor cranial nerve nucleus

Lumbar   Referring to the lower back region

Medial lemniscus   Brainstem portion of sensory pathway for fine touch and conscious proprioception, after synapse in nucleus gracilis and nucleus cuneatus

Median foramen   Foramen of Magendie, opening from fourth ventricle into cisterna magna of subarachnoid space for escape of CSF surrounding the brain

Medulla oblongata   Narrow caudal part of the hindbrain

Meninges   Covering layers of the central nervous system

Midbrain   The middle division of the embryonic brain; also part of the adult brainstem

Monosynaptic reflex arc   A reflex arc containing only one synapse

Motor   To do with movement or response

Myelin sheath   Covering of nerve fiber, part of Schwann cell or oligodendrocyte

Nerve fiber   Neuronal cell process, plus sheathing cells, plus myelin if present; if in peripheral nervous system enclosed in basal lamina

Neuraxis   The straight longitudinal axis of the embryonic or primitive neural tube, bent in later evolution and development

Neuron   Nerve cell

Neuropil   A complex meshwork of axon terminals, dendrites and neuroglial processes

NMR   Nuclear magnetic resonance, also known as magnetic resonance imaging (MRI); a diagnostic imaging method

Node of Ranvier   Gap in myelin sheath between two successive Schwann cells or oligodendrocytes

Nucleus   An aggregation of nerve cells within the CNS

Nucleus cuneatus   Nucleus at upper end of fasciculus cuneatus

Nucleus gracilis   Nucleus at upper end of fasciculus gracilis

Occipital lobe   Part of cerebral hemisphere

Oculomotor nerve   3rd cranial nerve (III)

Olfactory nerve   1st cranial nerve (I)

Operculum   Frontal, parietal and temporal folds of cerebral hemisphere, covering and so concealing the insula

Optic chiasma   X-shaped union between optic nerves, with fiber decussation

Optic nerve   2nd cranial nerve (II)

Pachymeninx   The dura mater

Papilledema   Bulging of the optic disk; sign of raised intracranial pressure

Parietal lobe   Part of cerebral hemisphere

Pathway   A chain of functionally interconnected neurons making a connection between one region of the CNS and another, a tract or tracts and nuclei connected, e.g. visual pathway

Peduncle   A thick stalk or stem, bundle of nerve fibers

Peripheral nervous system   Nerve roots, nerves and ganglia outside the CNS

PET (positron emission tomography)   A diagnostic imaging method for brain function and blood flow

Pia (mater)   Innermost layer of meninges

Polysynaptic reflex arc   A reflex arc containing more than one synapse

Pons   Enlarged middle portion of the brainstem, part of hindbrain

Proprioception   The sense of body position (conscious or unconscious)

Putamen   Part of lentiform nucleus

Pyramidal tract   Corticospinal tract; pyramidal system is the corticospinal and corticobulbar tracts

Receptor   Sense organ

Red nucleus   Structure in the midbrain, red in fresh material

Reticular formation   Diffuse nervous tissue in brainstem

Rostral   Towards the nose, or the most anterior end of the neuraxis

Rubrospinal tract   Descending tract from red nucleus of midbrain to spinal cord

Sacral   Referring to the pelvic region

Schwann cell   Sheathing cell of peripheral nerve fibers

Secretor   Motor nerve supply to a gland

Sensory   To do with receiving information from the environment

Septum pellucidum   Two layers of thin membranes separating the anterior horns of the lateral ventricles

Somatic senses   Touch, pain, temperature, pressure, proprioception, vibration

Special senses   Sight, hearing, balance, taste (gustatory) and smell (olfactory)

Spinocerebellar tracts   Ascending tracts for unconscious proprioception

Spinothalamic tracts   Ascending tracts for pain, temperature, non-discriminative touch, pressure

Subarachnoid space   Space between arachnoid and pia mater

Subcortical   Not in the cerebral cortex, i.e. at a functionally or evolutionarily "lower" level in the central nervous system

Substantia nigra   Area in midbrain, appears dark in fresh material

Sulcus   Groove between adjacent gyri

Synapse   Area of structural and functional specialization between neurons where transmission occurs

Tectum   Roof of midbrain

Tegmentum   The dorsal portion of the medulla oblongata and pons, and the part of the midbrain between the tectum and crus cerebri; contains nuclei, tracts and reticular formation

Telencephalon   Rostral part of embryonic forebrain; primarily cerebral hemisphere of adult

Temporal lobe   Part of cerebral hemisphere

Tendon reflex   Reflex contraction of a muscle when its tendon is stretched

Tentorium cerebelli   Fold of dura mater overlying cerebellum

Third ventricle   Cavity in diencephalon, containing CSF

Thoracic   Referring to the chest region

Tract   A bundle of nerve fibers within the CNS, with a common origin and destination, e.g optic tract

Trigeminal nerve   5th cranial nerve (V)

Trigeminothalamic tracts   Ascending tracts for sensations from the face

Trochlear nerve   4th cranial nerve (IV)

Ultrasonography   Diagnostic imaging method utilizing high-frequency sound waves

Upper motor neuron   Cell in motor cortex or other motor area in the brain, connected by descending tract to lower motor neurons

Vagus   10th cranial nerve (X)

Ventral root   Efferent motor component of mixed spinal nerve

Ventricles   Cerebrospinal fluid-filled cavities inside the brain

Vermis   Unpaired midline portion of cerebellum between hemispheres

Vertebral artery   An artery supplying spinal cord and brainstem

Vestibulocochlear or acoustic nerve   8th cranial nerve (VIII)

Vestibulospinal tract   Descending tract from vestibular nuclei of medulla to spinal cord

Visceral   Referring to internal organs

White matter   Nervous tissue made up mainly of nerve fibers

Suggestions for Further Reading and Further Reference

Suggestions for Further Reading (First Edition)

Barr, M.L. and Kiernan, J.A. (1988) *The Human Nervous System – An Anatomical Viewpoint*, Philadelphia, J.B. Lippincott Company.

Carpenter, M.B. (1985) *Core Text of Neuroanatomy*, 3rd edn, London, Williams and Wilkins Company.

Fitzgerald, M.J.T. (1985) *Neuroanatomy Basic and Applied*, London, Baillière Tindall.

Kahle, W., Leonhardt, H. and Platzer, W. (1986) *Color Atlas and Textbook of Human Anatomy*, Vol. 3 Nervous System and Sensory Organs, New York, Georg Thieme Verlag Thieme Inc.

Liebman, M. (1987) *Neuroanatomy Made Easy and Understandable*, 3rd edn, Aspen Publishers U.S.A.

Snell, R.S. (1980) *Clinical Neuroanatomy for Medical Students*, 2nd revised edn, Boston, Little, Brown and Company.

Suggestions for Further Reference (First Edition)

Gluhbegovic, N. and Williams, T.H. (1980) *The Human Brain: A Photographic Guide*, Philadelphia, Harper and Row.

Young, J.Z. (1978) *Programs of the Brain Based on the Gifford Lectures, 1975-1977*, Oxford, Oxford University Press.

Suggestions for Further Reading (Second Edition)

Barker, R.A. and Barasi, S. (2003) *Neuroscience at a Glance with Pharmacology by M.J. Neal*, 2nd edn, Oxford, Blackwell Publishing Ltd.

Briar, C., Lasserson, D., Gabriel, C. and Sharrack, B. (2003) *Crash Course Nervous System*, 2nd edn, London, Mosby.

Crossman, A.R. and Neary, D. (2000) *Neuroanatomy: An Illustrated Colour Text*, Edinburgh, Churchill Livingstone.

FitzGerald, M.J.T. and Folan-Curran, J. (2002) *Clinical Neuroanatomy and Related Neuroscience*, 4th edn, London, W.B. Saunders (Imprint of Elsevier Science Ltd).

Gertz, S.D. (1999) *Liebman's Neuroanatomy Made Easy and Understandable*, 6th edn, Gaithersburg, Aspen Publishers Ltd.

Greenfield, S. (1998) *The Human Brain: A Guided Tour*, London, ScienceMasters.

Haines, D.E. (2000) *Neuroanatomy: An Atlas of Structures, Sections, and Systems*, 5th edn, Baltimore, Lippincott Williams & Wilkins.

Hirsch, M.C and Kramer, T. (1999) *Neuroanatomy 3D – Stereoscopic Atlas of the Human Brain, Berlin*, Springer-Verlag.

Suggestions for Further Reference (Second Edition)

Duvernoy, H.M. (1992) *The Human Brain*, 2nd edn, Paris, Springer.

Nolte, J. and Angevine, Jr., J.B. (2000) *The Human Brain in Photographs and Diagrams*, 2nd edn, St Louis, Mosby.

Woolsey, T.A., Hanaway, J. and Gado, M.H. (2003) *The Brain Atlas, A Visual Guide to the Human Central Nervous System*, 2nd edn, Hoboken, John Wiley & Sons, Inc.

Index